INDIGENOUS ANCESTORS AND HEALING LANDSCAPES

Sidestone Press

INDIGENOUS ANCESTORS AND HEALING LANDSCAPES

CULTURAL MEMORY AND INTERCULTURAL COMMUNICATION IN THE DOMINICAN REPUBLIC AND CUBA

JANA PESOUTOVA

Published by Sidestone Press, Leiden
www.sidestone.com

Lay-out & cover design: Lino Valcárel & Sidestone Press
Photograph cover: Lino Valcárcel

ISBN978-90-8890-764-7 (softcover)
ISBN 978-90-8890-762-3 (hardcover)
ISBN 978-90-8890-763-0 (PDF e-book)

The research leading to this dissertation received funding from the European Research Council (ERC) under the European Union´s Seventh Framework Programme (FP7/2007'2013)/ ERC-Synergy project NEXUS 1492, grant agreement nr. 319209.

Contents

1. Rhizomes of Healing Landscapes **9**

Colonial discourse and the question of cultural continuity 11

Forgetting Indigenous Peoples of the Greater Antilles 16

Approaching Healing Landscapes 19

Data collection and fieldwork methodology 21

Ethics 23

Outline of the dissertation 26

PART 1: THEORETICAL AND HISTORICAL DIMENSIONS OF CARIBBEAN LANDSCAPES **27**

2. Healing Landscapes from a theoretical perspective **29**

Introduction to landscape studies 30

Memory landscapes 33

Healing Landscapes 40

3. Natural Man in the Caribbean Paradise: the origins of colonial discourse **53**

The noble savage idea in Lesser Antilles 61

Indigenous past as the beginning of the Dominican nation 62

Indigenous ancestors during the formation of the Cuban nation 63

The indigenous past in Dominican and Cuban History textbooks 64

The Alienation from Natural Man in the collective memory 65

4. Empty Pages in the Biography of Healing Landscapes **67**

Indigenous ancestors transforming Caribbean Landscapes 69

West African ancestors shaping Caribbean landscapes 73

European ancestors reshaping Caribbean landscapes 76

The multidirectional circulation of the medicinal knowledge in the Greater Antilles 82

Concluding remarks 88

5. Crossroads of Cultural landscapes: the indigenous base of demographic changes **91**

Brief account of indigenous ancestors in colonial Hispaniola 94

African ancestors in Dominican demographic history 102

The interactions among the colonized strata 105

The subsequent historical development of Dominican society 106

A brief overview of demographic background of selected Dominican sites 108

Major tendencies in Cuban ethnogenesis 119

Colonial history of Indigenous Cuban ancestors 119

The heterogeneity of the Cuban ancestors of African origin 127

A brief overview of demographic background of selected Cuban sites 130

Revising the indigenous component in demographic histories 135

PART 2: CONTEMPORARY TRADITIONS **137**

6. Qualities of the landscape in daily life **139**

Flora as a source of alimentation 140

Concluding remarks 157

7. Healing in sacred and animated landscapes **159**

Other spiritual beings in Cuban and Dominican landscapes 163

Illness and cure 164

Healing specialists 166

Healing Plants 171

Ancestral roots and rhizomes 185

Concluding remarks 192

8. The subaquatic realm of ancestors and other beings **195**

Dominican Ancestral Subaquatic Dwellings 196

Caribbean waterbodies as reservoirs of indigenous past 219

Concluding remarks 223

9. Re-membering Ancestors in Caves **225**
Mana Landscape 226
Cave of La Mancha: Healing with Indigenous Lwas 228
The Cave of Saint Francis as a Healing and Memory Place of Bánica 236
Healing among Spiritists, Managuaco cavern, Holguín, Cuba 247
Cueva De los Santos Gibara, Cuba 250
Cuban and Dominican caverns as memory places of indigenous past 253
Concluding remarks 259
10. Synthesis and Conclusions. At the Crossroads of Healing Landscapes **261**
Remembrance and Oblivion 261
Historical formation of Cuban and Dominican Medicinal Cultures 261
Constituents of healing landscapes 266
Memory of indigenous ancestors 269
Water sources and caves as ancestral places 270
Healing landscapes as expressions of cultural memories of indigenous past 274
Healing landscapes within landscape theories 291
Future directions of research 296
Bibliography **299**
Attachment **327**
Abstract **341**
Resumen **347**
Samenvatting **353**
Acknowledgments **359**
Curriculum vitae **363**

1

Rhizomes of Healing Landscapes

The research for this dissertation has been conducted within a broader project, 'Nexus 1492', which investigates the first interactions between the Old and the New World. Nexus 1492 focuses on the histories and legacies of the indigenous Caribbean across the historical divide introduced by European colonization and addresses the ensuing complex intercultural dynamics over the past five centuries (Hofman, Davies, Brandes & Willems 2012). This study has been funded by the European Research Council under the European Union's Seventh Framework Programme (FP7/2007-2013)/ERC Synergy grant agreement no. 319209 (NEXUS1492: New World Encounters In A Globalizing World). Within the framework of that project, this study focuses on current healing practices in relation to intercultural dynamics, paying special attention to the indigenous legacy. Concretely, this research examines current Dominican and Cuban healing landscapes as expressions of cultural memory.

By combining data from ethnographic fieldwork and critical historical analysis, this thesis explores the perceptions about connections between people's health and the surrounding natural environment. The main problem that informs this research is: how do healing landscapes encapsulate cultural memories of the indigenous past? In order to gather a better understanding of the contemporary healing landscapes this study offers first insights into how contemporary medicinal cultures have been historically constructed. Fieldwork was carried out in order to explore how community members relate some landscape features to the indigenous past and how these associations play a role in traditional healing practices. A further analysis of the historical and ethnographic data will help us to situate the concept of the healing landscape within current landscape theories.

This study builds on insights from previous studies, which have discussed the material and nonmaterial aspects of healing practices in order to sketch the contours of a rich environmental symbolism and the values displayed in healing rituals. Following studies that address healing practices from a holistic perspective, humans are seen as a part of landscapes together with different living and other-than-human beings, which are interconnected and relevant to people's health and worldmaking. Within the context of healing practices, of particular interest is the human interaction with divine and ancestral beings residing or manifested in places, plants and natural features, with the aim to promote physical, mental, and spiritual healing. This interaction defines 'healing landscapes', an etic term which use to summarize some of emic concepts.

This study highlights the importance of local epistemologies, which help us to further nuance some of the contradictions and ambiguities in local medicinal histories. In doing so, it hopes to contribute to the understanding of landscape transformations in the Caribbean after the European conquest and to the deconstruction of representations of present-day Caribbean societies in terms of uprooted hybridity or impurity, and as being too fragmented (*i.e.* by colonization) to have any spiritual relation with the local landscape.[1]

In contrast, current healing landscapes seem to be testimonies of how people recreated their relationships with the new environment according to their own worldviews and in relation to new socio-cultural contexts. One of the authors who have put forward interesting insights into how Caribbean communities constructed relations with newly inhabited landscapes was the Cuban ethnologist Lydia Cabrera. In her pioneering work *El Monte* (Cabrera 1954) she addressed some aspects of environmental symbolism within Cuban religions. Inspired by her approach, this study aims to further understand the importance of landscapes within healing rituals by integrating information about medicinal plant properties (Roig y Mesa 1974; Portorreal 2011, Germosén-Robineau 2005, Ososki 2004, Roersch 2016), their religious symbolisms (Bolívar Aróstegui et al. 1998; Quiroz-Moran 2009; Rodríguez Reyes 1998) and those of other landscapes features, within the context of Caribbean religions and healing practices (*e.g.* Deive 1988; Tejeda Ortíz 2013; Brendbekken 1998).

The concept of 'cultural memory' is applied here to investigate how people engage with the past through healing practices, and how these practices in turn are continuations and/or reinterpretations of past beliefs, knowledge and customs. One of the motives for approaching healing landscapes from a cultural memory perspective is that, current understanding of healing landscape is ultimately linked to the present-day conceptualization of the past, and its role in the present. According to local etiologies, illnesses may be caused and remediated by ancestors. Their role and identification of and with their heritage is enweaved in the broader socio-cultural transformations after the European invasion. The healing landscapes also convey historical and religious knowledge, which can be indicative of past landscape transformations.

Medicinal histories within the Caribbean are not to be separated from the construction of knowledge about the different Caribbean peoples and their past, a process that is based on archives formed through centuries of colonial power relations. Historically

1 Glissant (1997) counterpoises the relation and root identity the latter defined by a claim of legitimacy based on proclaimed entitlement to the possession of land, vision of distant past, and a myth of the creation of the world. In Glissant's view the claim for the legitimacy of the land possession becomes the Caribbean context problematic. The root identity based on the thought of self and territory related to the myth of creation and remote past has been invalidated in the Caribbean through *"the massacre of the Indians, uprooting the sacred"* (Glissant 1997, p. 146). The colonization and the massive import of new population implied construction of a new relation as a rhizome land defined through relation with others, not as *"absolute ontological possession regarded as sacred but the complicity of relation"* (Glissant 1997, p. 147). Does not, however, the root identity follow too much the Eurocentric vision of nationhood and its relation to the territory? Instead, here the relation identity is conceived as an opportunity to think about how the manifestation of numinous and sacred has been perceived by various ancestors in newly occupied natural environments and changing societies of the Caribbean.

there has been great interest in Caribbean natural resources, including botanical knowledge, starting with the first written accounts of the Caribbean (for overview see Deive 2002). After brief approximations to Cuban medicinal history (Górdon y Acosta 1894; López Sánchez 1997), the understanding of contemporary healing practices requires more information about the contribution of non-institutional medical experts including those that were historically marginalized.

The Spanish historical sources about indigenous peoples, enslaved peoples, and free peoples of color are marked by beliefs of the authors concerning their own cultural and religious superiority. This bias has generated many instances of silencing historically marginalized peoples and of replacing their voices with stereotypical descriptions in conformity with the interests of dominant groups. This process of silencing the colonized peoples in history was not only instigated by the colonial authorities but may also have occurred as a particular form of resistance through perpetual concealment (Glissant 1996). Consequently, histories of healing practices of different population strata have been power-saturated.

This historical bias then became integrated into scholarly theories about cultural change, which influence the interpretation of existing medicinal cultures until today. Before embarking on our research, it is therefore imperative to examine a set of theoretical and methodological issues that emerge from this situation.

Colonial discourse and the question of cultural continuity

As the Caribbean has become an emblematic case of colonial enterprise, neocolonialism and anticolonial resistance, there has been a lot of reflection about its legacy of colonialism in the last decades. The persistence of colonial biased attitudes was addressed within the campaign to dignify Afro-Caribbean heritage. Since Fernando Ortiz, one of the pioneers in advocating acknowledgment of the importance of enslaved peoples' heritage for the national identity, and his followers like Cabrera (1940, 1954) in Cuba, there have been many Caribbean scholars who have denounced the still persistent nexus of power and knowledge displayed in the studies of enslaved and indigenous peoples.[2]

Martinican author Aimé Césaire (1972 [1955]), one of the founders and most famous representatives of the *négritude* movement, denounced racism as one of the live legacies from the colonial period. Césaire condemned historians for refusing to acknowledge any merits of non-white races, and condemned psychologists and sociologists for their views on "primitivism", their insistence on the marginal, separate character of non-whites, and their ethnocentric applications of the term 'rational'. The recent French government policies emphasizing the country's former colonial enterprise in a more positive light make clear that Césaire's criticism is not just about the past, but also challenges present-day practices.[3] Similarly, the authorization of the French state to use pesticides in Guadeloupe and Martinique while the same were prohibited in France and while authorities were aware of their detrimental effects on

2 For a brief overview of how the Afro-Cuban ancestors have been discussed in Cuban historiography see (Barcia Zequeira 2004).

3 For a critique of Césaire read Glissant's *Caribbean Discourses* (1996).

human and environmental health has been interpreted as a continuation of colonial legacies (Ferdinand 2017).

Césaire's call for more attention to the language of "neutral" academic definitions, such as *e.g.* "colonial contact", for its trivialization of the detrimental impact of colonialism was also followed by his students, for example Fanon. Fanon denounced that a researcher's "objectivity" is often used as an excuse to not pay attention to the social realities of injustice, and so in fact hinders the understanding of the so-called "Black Problem" (2012 [1952]). This distancing of researchers from their "objects of study", "the poor traditional other", was also criticized by scholars like Fabian (1983). Fanon's analysis suggests that the bias in the academic literature has impact on constructing public knowledge through educational formation. More particularly, he argued that stereotyping representations of black Martinicans in popular culture and in children's textbooks as people without culture, history, and civilization has a strong alienating effect (Fanon 2006).

Various other authors have acknowledged the impact of ideologies in Dominican historiography that justified the conquest and enslavement of peoples from the island and of those kidnapped from West and Central Africa (Cassa 1999). Deive (2009) showed the dichotomies that marked the accounts of Dominican populations throughout the centuries in which the descriptions of peoples were politically manipulated: many of them exalted the kindness and warmth of Dominican people as inviting the foreign occupation, and others caricatured Hispaniola inhabitants in negative terms when resisting these occupations.

Although different historical trajectories have marked both countries of this study, their past and consequently their cultural memories are marked, among others, by domination and resistance. When addressing cultural memory in societies with a colonial past, one of its main defining traits is the influence of colonial discourse.[4] In short, a discourse is seen as a way of representing different material and immaterial aspects of the world (Fairclough 2003). Though this discourse is fluid and changing over time, it is rooted in human practices and institutions. In this sense, historians, as well as other individuals, are part of the discursive process. Whether based on observation or imagined, the colonial discourse was formed in direct connection with the process of colonization in order to rationalize and justify colonial conditions, and as such it had a real impact on human lives, bodies, and on human interaction with landscapes. The 16th century European raids of the Lesser Antilles capturing people accused of cannibalism are only one illustrative example of how a biased image of people from foreign lands can have real impact on the lives of those people.

The persistence of colonial discourse in current research has been a concern of many Caribbean scholars. Edward Said's conceptualization of the colonized being constructed as different and Other, as well as Foucault's reminder that every regime of

4 Caribbean criticism of colonial discourse has developed in conjunction with modern ideas about discourse as such. Several European scholars, such as Foucault (1970 in Loomba 1997), Saussure (1960 in Loomba 1997), and Lacan (1967 in Fanon 1967) have questioned the Enlightenment's assumption that individuals are the sole source of meaning; they rather consider language as a socially determined system. According to Foucault, all ideas are ordered by some medium that imposes a pattern that is called a discourse (Loomba 1997). This discourse is then modified by various rules that form a whole domain within which language is used.

representation is a regime of power/knowledge, was very influential. Jamaican cultural theorist Stuart Hall has drawn attention to the difficulty of decolonizing the discourse while accepting its total hegemony.[5] Hall (1992) addressed the problematic nature of decolonizing the mind. He shows that stereotyped notions from colonial times still persist in present-day sociological assumptions about the Third World through influential figures such as Marx or Weber. [6] In his view, the discourse about the West was formed in relation to the "Indigenous others" during the colonization of the Caribbean, and in diverse transformed manifestations this discourse continues to inflict its image of self and other on social practices and relations. In contrast to Césaire's view of racism as a direct legacy of colonialism, Hall sees present-day discourses not so much as direct continuities of previous ones but rather as framed by the human tendency to create in-and-out groups. In accordance with Foucault, Hall sees knowledge about the past as never neutral, because it is shaped and exercised by structures of hegemony but he also acknowledges the limits of this hegemony. Hall highlights the importance of the interpretative processes, the ambiguity of the message being transmitted, and the agency of those decoding the discourse.

Power is encoded in knowledge not just from the top down but also from the bottom up. As Haitian historian Trouillot (1995) has emphasized, the construction of historical knowledge relies not just on academic texts but also on public contribution. While there are multiple views about past events, not all people have the same opportunity to voice their views, and scholars should make more of an effort to record marginalized voices in the production of histories. As Trouillot suggests, it is not the case that the subaltern cannot speak, but rather that they are not heard. While it is clear that history can be silenced in different stages of the production of knowledge and manipulated to serve the interests of a particular group in power, there are some undervalued sources of historical information, which should be critically assessed (Trouillot 1995). Simply put, the past is constructed from the present, and there are multiple ways in which the past is interpreted and can be significant for the present. At the same time, the broader societal interpretations of the historian's studies should be taken into account (Trouillot 1995).

The formal construction and public production of knowledge have been discussed often in opposition, as history and memory, but both can also be seen as different modes of remembering (Erll 2008). The first hypothesis of this study is that a more inclusive view of Dominican and Cuban medicinal history can be achieved when looking at the intersection of official historiography with the formal construction of knowledge

5 Said (1978) also highlighted the dialectical relationship between texts and their social / historical context. Inspired by Gramsci's theory on the nexus between hegemony and knowledge, and by Foucault's concept of discourse, Said wrote one of the most influential books in colonial discourse studies: *Orientalism*. In this work, he shows how the colonial discourse was used to justify and maintain the exercise of power over *The Other*. One of his greatest contributions is to have revealed the strong bias in the representation of the colonized, as a consequence of colonial processes, and the influence of this bias and of the colonial process itself on the whole range of academic ideas about non-western cultures.

6 Posterior works such as that of Marxist author Amin (1989) have analyzed contemporary Eurocentrism as a distortion, a justification of capitalism. As some of the critics of this work argued, Marxism is one of social theories that did not escape from the rigid models of evolutionary thinking also evident in Amin's discussion of communal and tributary civilizations.

and public production of knowledge. Consequently, present-day healing practices are formed by formal and informal ways of knowledge production. Within this context, we may investigate how the current healing practices can inform us about the medicinal past of these societies.

Healing is performed in a particular time and space, in which the past is reenacted in a more or less conscious way. Thus, healing can be performed at historical places in which ancestors are actively commemorated and consulted concerning matters of health and wellbeing. Ancestral knowledge can also be transferred in a rather unconscious way, *e.g.* through bodily practices, or stored away in other forms of cultural memory formalized in collective origin narratives or communal celebrations. In practice, the distinction between collective and individual forms of remembering, and between formal and informal modes of knowledge transfer, is often difficult to make so that they merge into one common pool of knowledge.

As stated above, for centuries the production of historical knowledge has been part of a colonial power game, the legacy of which is still discernable in present-day processes of socialization. In accordance with this paradigm, the history textbooks of formal education transfer have selected pieces of information (top down) about the past, which may contrast with the contents of informal learning (bottom up, *e.g.* through oral traditions).[7] This may yield various counterpoints of different modes or facets of social memory, which sometimes lead to an erasure of local epistemologies under the influence of colonial perspectives, and in other cases allow those local epistemologies to continue to exist in spite of the hegemony, though possibly fragmented by or embedded in intercultural dynamics and power relations.

That formally produced knowledge is inseparable from broader ideologies becomes clear when one looks at current interpretations of legacies. Several authors have discussed how historical and ideological bias is reflected in theories that explain cultural change, and how this bias keeps influencing later academic interpretations of the contribution that particular population groups have made to national heritage.

A number of authors such as Gárcia Arevalo (2008), Sued Badillo (2003), Vega (1981), and Ulloa Hung and Valcárcel Rojas (2016), have criticized the exclusive focus on the Indigenous, Hispanic or African contribution to the national heritage and to particular cultural practices in Dominican and Cuban history. The overemphasis on such a particular influence was not just driven by ideologies but also caused by methodological issues due to the scarcity of historical and ethnographic literature. Deive addressed this issue in the study of Afro-Dominican heritage, which is complicated by fragmentary historical records and the general lack of studies on the forms of enslavement, consequently obscuring the nature of cultural change (Deive in Vega 1981).[8] Similarly, Ulloa Hung (2015) has addressed methodological issues in the study of material heritage of the African diaspora in the Dominican Republic. The scarcity of studies on material heritage, the focus on monumental heritage, the emphasis on

7 For more on problematics of teaching about the precolonial history in the Caribbean see Con Aguilar´s upcoming dissertation: Heritage Education Memories of the Past in the Present Caribbean Social Studies Curriculum: A View from Teacher Practice.

8 Some of the factors were the adaptation to the new environment, the degree of control imposing by official policies on assimilation (urban, plantation, household context, day laborers, and refugees) and the contact with other cultures.

acculturation instead of considering other models of cultural change such as transculturation or ethnogenesis seems to be driven by ideologies that deny the diversity and agency of enslaved peoples and further contribute to undervaluation of this heritage (Ulloa Hung 2015).

The ideological shifts have been related to methodological changes. Since the first pioneering works of Fernando Ortiz, the Cuban religions received a greater interest in and appreciation, and also their studies replaced earlier views that denigrated the practices of Regla de Ocha or Palo de Monte as mere "witchcraft" and "superstition". An emic perspective became important, while the position of the investigator shifted from that of a distant observer to that of a participant. Investigators of the institute Casa del Caribe developed a tradition of full immersion by initiation and actively sharing the system of beliefs that one studied (personal communication with Raul Ruiz Miyares 2015; James 1999).

The concerns of scholars who focus on African legacies have been shared by authors who study the indigenous heritage of the Dominican Republic, Cuba, and the Caribbean in general. The Caribbean criticism receives support from different anticolonial studies on and by indigenous peoples all over the world (Pérez Jimenez 2015; Artist 2016; Tuhiway Smith 1999; May Castillo & Stecker 2017; Jansen & Perez 2017). The relevance of Caribbean critique is still obvious, especially in contexts in which a formal process of decolonization was not yet completed, has not even begun or where violations of human rights, discrimination, and even killings of indigenous peoples continue. Among the many recent cases we might mention the murder of Bertha Cáceres in Honduras, or the forced disappearance of 43 students from Ayotzinapa, Mexico. Indigenous peoples' struggles against colonial legacies, climate change and neocolonial exploitation are connected to present-day social problems in Cuba, the Dominican Republic, Puerto Rico and other parts of the Caribbean.

The concerns voiced by Caribbean commentators about legacies of the colonial past in the present also resonate in other contexts marked by genocide, ethnic wars, injustice, institutional exploitation and discrimination. The decolonizing approach, as advocated by many Caribbean and indigenous scholars, is globally imperative in times of neocolonial forms of exploitation, in which the states are replaced as actors by multinationals, which create new dependencies in the so-called Third World.[9] In both study regions colonialism is not a closed chapter of history. The colonial discourse is preserved in school textbooks, colonial hierarchies of class/race are reproduced and especially in the Dominican Republic these are apparent in the persistent social marginalization.

Like the history of enslaved peoples and otherwise historically marginalized groups, the history of indigenous peoples is charged with methodological and ideological problems. The study of histories and legacies of indigenous peoples is obscured by a profound demographic decline, and possibly by the process of transculturation. The violent European invasion, accompanied by the no less violent spiritual conquest, has resulted in a profound transformation and loss of indigenous worldmaking in the Dominican Republic and Cuba. In combination with the introduction of diseases, the

9 See also Jansen and Pérez Jiménez' recent critique (2017) of studies about but without indigenous peoples.

conquest and enslavement have led to loss of lives, cultures, languages, and knowledge, including botanical science and medicinal skills.

Different studies have argued that current botanical knowledge and medicinal cultures in Cuba and the Dominican Republic originated from the worldviews and knowledge of indigenous peoples (Barreiro 2002; Estevez 2013; Beauvoir-Dominique 2008; Taíno Legacies Project; Ososki 2004; Portorreal 2011; Bisnauth 1989; Forte 2013).[10] Other authors, such as Deive (1988), while acknowledging certain indigenous influences, suggest on the contrary that current Dominican popular medicine is largely of Iberian heritage. In contrast, recent studies have emphasized the importance of the West African botanical legacy in healing practices and concepts in the Americas (Voeks & Rashford 2013; Carney 2003; Van Andel et al. 2015). In general, the transformations of the conceptual landscape after the European conquest and the role of the indigenous medicinal cultures or worldviews in these transformations are poorly understood. More studies are needed to understand the complex intercultural dynamics of the construction of present-day healing landscapes (Vega 1981).

Although it is clear that the biography of Dominican and Cuban landscapes begins long before the Europeans invaded in the Caribbean, the role of the indigenous peoples according to general historiography seems to have ended rather quickly after the introduction of the *encomiendas* in the early colonial period. The idea of the indigenous peoples' rapid disappearance has profoundly marked theories of cultural change used in explaining the societal makeup of Cuba and the Dominican Republic. In contrast, this idea leads to severe inconsistencies in the argument of different authors who present contemporary medicinal cultures as indigenous legacy. From a historical perspective it is then necessary to assess how the healing landscapes may have been conceptualized after the conquest.

Forgetting Indigenous Peoples of the Greater Antilles

More than seventy years ago, Felipe Pichardo Moya criticized the widely accepted notion that Cuban indigenous peoples were practically exterminated in the first decades after the conquest. First because of the bias of colonial historians who wished to justify

10 See also the website of the Taíno Legacies Project financed by Smithsonian Institute: https://global.si.edu/success-stories/caribbean-indigenous-legacies-project-celebrating-ta%C3%ADno-culture, see also Barreiro 2001, García Molina, Garrido Mazorra, Fariñas Gutierrez 2007). Different authors have argued that indigenous peoples have correlated their own belief systems with Catholicism (Mitchel 2006) and inserted their beliefs into the religion introduced by the colonizers. For example, Mitchel (2006) suggested that the Arawaks identified the Christian God the Father with their creator-god, Wamurreti-Kwonci, whom they otherwise knew as the benign Jocahuna. Jesus Christ could also be identified with Jocahuna, while the Virgin Mary was "confused" with Atabei [Atabex, Atabeira], a Goddess of Arawak belief (Bisnauth, 1989 in Mitchell, 2006: 12). Mitchell draws further parallels between the Holy Spirit and Hurakana, the role of *behiques* and Catholic priests, Kanaima and Santa, Heaven and Coyaba. However logical these parallels might seem, the author does not provide any further historical evidence to support his arguments. More studies have proposed that certain elements of contemporary beliefs have an indigenous origin. Beauvoir-Dominique (2008) identified *vévés*, *rara* feast, healing rituals such as the cleansing with chicken and bathing with tobacco smoke or the ritual use of corn, as indigenous spiritual heritage. Keegan and Carlson (2008) have searched some connection with the indigenous peoples in *opias* and *obeas* relating it to the current Jamaican belief in duppies living in ceibas and almond trees.

metropolitan control, and later due to the uncritical acceptance of the extinction of the indigenous population as part of a critique of the colonial regime in the context of constructing the national identity, many historical references to the presence of Cuban indigenous peoples after 1550s have been passed over in silence (Pichardo Moya 1945).

The rapid extinction of the indigenous peoples as portrayed in history books, was also later transferred into the theories of cultural change. The first models of the transformation of indigenous cultures in the region of study attributed a low degree of agency and cultural development to the original inhabitants. However, there is an increasing body of literature about (and evidence for) indigenous responses to the European conquest and colonization. The study of Valcárcel Rojas (2016) shows diverse modes in which indigenous peoples integrated into the new colonial context, which nuances the opposition of portraying the indigenous peoples as passive victims of genocide or exalting them as martyrs and rebels against the colonial regime. His results add to the complexity of the Cuban and Dominican ethnogenesis and are important in taking into account the models of cultural transformations after 1492.

Different concepts have been utilized to describe the transformations that occur when different cultures and peoples interact in colonial contexts: acculturation (Herskovits 1941, Malinowski 1963), assimilation, cultural crystallization (Foster 1960), bricolage (Levi-Strauss 1966), creolization (Brathwaite 1971), hybridity (Bhabba 1994), mestizaje (Freyre 1933), syncretism (Herskovits 1937) and transculturation (Ortiz 1994 [1947]). Here I will focus on the theory of transculturation of Fernando Ortiz, whose legacy is still influential in studies of history, society, culture and religion (Font et al. 2005). The concept of transculturation has been further developed in studies of cultural change (Restall 2005) and of transformation of indigenous cultures (Fariñas Gutiérrez 1995; Valcárcel Rojas 2012).

Ortiz proposed the term 'transculturation' in order to replace 'acculturation', as a way to describe the result of the extremely complex transformations of Cuban culture. In contrast to the concept of 'acculturation' that was popular in Ortiz's time, 'transculturation' was designed to describe mutual adaptations and influences going in different directions, not only from the dominant group to the subaltern. In this way, Ortiz reacted to a tendency in the research on acculturation, which assumed unidirectional cultural change, in which the dominant or "donor" culture (Europe) impacted indigenous cultures (a theory later also criticized by Foster 1960). Ortiz argued that the process of cultural transformations is more complex: it may include processes of acculturation but also involve deculturation (defined as the loss or uprooting of a previous culture), and the consequent creation of new cultural phenomena, called neoculturation (1994 [1947], p. 102). The latter term accentuates that a union of two cultures carries certain continuities from both these cultures but also leads to the creation of a new culture.

Even though Ortiz' initial work was considered to be heavily impacted by social Darwinism and a reductionist view of human development – and some of this discourse remained influential up to his last book (Ortiz 1975) – his *Cuban Counterpoint Tobacco and Sugar* has been read by cultural theorists as the first serious systematic attempt to grant more agency to non-Europeans in the process of cultural change and to understand Afro-Caribbean heritage (De Feo 2014). However, scarcity of studies on indigenous colonial history at the time when Ortiz wrote his Counterpoint has had a determining influence on how the theory of transculturation has been applied to Cuban indigenous peoples. For Ortiz, as far as the indigenous peoples are concerned, the transculturation failed in a biological and cultural sense. His idea of biological discontinuation was based on the lack of historical references for the period in question. The supposed biological discontinuity then became the point of departure for arguing cultural deculturation.

Ortiz' explanation of that "failure" seems to be guided, however, by his unilineal view of cultural development: "*First came the transculturation of the Paleolithic Indian to the Neolithic, and the disappearance of the latter because of his inability to adjust himself to the culture brought in by the Spaniards.*" The historical disappearance of Taíno was explained as the result of a clash of cultures in different stages of development, living in different historical times: *"Taínos in the stone age"* and *"Europeans in the Renaissance"* (Ortíz 1995, pp. 98-102).[11]

Some authors have taken Ortiz´s theory of transculturation to integrate the indigenous contributions (Morales Patiño & Pérez Acevedo 1945; García Castañeda 1949; Domínguez 1980). Following more up to date historical and archeological studies on the colonial history of the indigenous peoples of Cuba, Fariñas Gutiérrez (1995) showed that the indigenous presence in different locations was long-lasting, accompanied by integration into Catholic system (*e.g.* through baptism), or by resistance against this, as well as by material expressions of the transculturation. Fariñas Gutiérrez highlighted cases in which parallels could be drawn between different worldviews. To pinpoint the origin of these examples, like the appearances of the Virgin, in the Caribbean context remains challenging. As Mintz (1989) explained, to determine the origin of a particular cultural trait is problematic because there are at least three processes functioning at the same time: the internal forces within the particular culture (replacement, cultural loss, and invention), cultural change due to the contact between different cultures, and adaptations to the new natural and socio-cultural context.

In a culturally diverse region such as the Caribbean, there are many coincidences and directions that might influence the process of transculturation. This process is complicated by the presence of multiple ingredients, like in Cuban *ajiaco*, to follow Ortiz´s metaphor, and of diverse factors that influence the sometimes parallel processes, which gave foundations to present-day Caribbean societies. The origins of the cultural forms that result from such a process of transculturation are especially difficult to discern if there is a lack of historical sources or studies on their antecedents.

---

11 The discourse about fixed stages of development has been prominent for years in the disciplines of archaeology and anthropology during the period in which Ortiz developed his theory of transculturation. In fact, this idea was at the root of anthropology, marked by an expectation of the inevitable extinction of the indigenous peoples, which according to evolutionist logic had to make space for Western civilization in the near future. This led to efforts to map the knowledge about these «dying races» in order to capture the relevant data of human development towards civilization. With these objectives Schoolcraft and Gallatin founded the American Ethnological Society in 1844. Similar ideas were adopted by evolutionists such as Morgan, who considered indigenous peoples to be examples of a pre-stadium on the way to the real (western) civilization. He built a unilineal classificatory system around the idea that technology is the engine driving human moral and intellectual progress. Conceiving history in terms of universal progress, he identified *The Others* as savages and as survivals of ancient states of development.

The transfer of knowledge may be influenced by factors that can be culturally specific, one of which is our perception of time. Our perception of the nature of time motivates and determines how people interact with the past and how the past presents itself today. The current understanding of healing landscapes and their historical background is thus linked to cultural practice and memory. The reflection upon the past may be made more or less explicit during healing performances by, for example, ritual commemoration of ancestors in sacred places. The past might be stored away in individual bodily memory such as in the dispositions of *habitus* (Bourdieu 1990). People make and remake history and memory in their practices. Oral traditions, rituals, symbols and other representations are modes of handing down meanings from the past, which are reinterpreted according to the new sociocultural context. Healing practices conducted at ancestral places using ancestral botanical knowledge may inform us about historical continuity and change, but also about why it is considered important to remember, to engage with the history in this particular form.

The historical background of healing landscapes and their current character cannot be understood without the consideration of memory politics. Caribbean islands have been inhabited for thousands of years prior to European colonization. The indigenous voices may have been passed over in silence in the historical sources, but their imprints are still visible in the Caribbean landscapes. Enslaved people, freed people, and later Creoles when working the fields have encountered these imprints, materialized in artefacts and present in traditional notions of the spiritual importance of particular places.

Contemporary inhabitants are more or less consciously engaging with the past through dwelling in this landscape. Current healing practices may therefore be understood as an interaction with the surrounding material and immaterial world, as part of being-in-the-world, which is historically and spatially contingent. The study of healing landscapes in the region today holds crucial keys for understanding past landscape transformations (including material and conceptual change) after the European arrival, and vice versa: the study of the past contributes to an understanding (and appreciation) of heritage and identity in the present. Approaching the healing landscape as an expression of cultural memory permits us to learn from the engagement of present-day population with their history and with the heritage of peoples who were living in the Caribbean landscape before the European conquest.

Approaching Healing Landscapes

This research centers on the present-day character and historical background of healing landscapes in the Dominican Republic and Cuba. More specifically, the research questions interrogate the healing landscape from a memory perspective, in order to access their historical link with indigenous peoples. Specific questions are: How do healing landscapes encapsulate cultural memories of the indigenous past? How have contemporary medicinal cultures been historically constructed? Which landscape features are associated with the indigenous past, and how are these engaged during healing practices? How can interpretations of specific healing landscapes be situated within current landscape theories?

The first objective of this study is to identify contemporary healing landscapes in the Dominican Republic and Cuba, which until now have barely received scholarly attention. The concept of the healing landscape became immediately relevant during my first ethnographic encounter with the region. From the beginning of the fieldwork it became clear to me that the natural environment is not just a background or resource for herbal medicine, but often an agent and a constant referent in religious life, history and culture, which is consequently reflected in traditional healing practices. For devotees, healing is often a religious experience, embedded in a rich system of symbolism connected to their surrounding environment, which teaches them the knowledge and moral codes of the ancestors. The religious symbolism and multiple meanings of the landscape are directly related to its centrality in the lifeways and subsistence activities of the people.

The term 'landscape' enables us to go beyond an ethnobotanical focus on medicinal plants and their applications, and to consider more broadly the general role of the environment in the process of healing. Such an approach follows the school of human geography studies on healing places (Gesler 1993) and anthropological studies from the South American context, by focusing on the articulation of the connection between health and landscape, which have also been addressed in West Africa. The 'landscape' concept also makes it possible to situate the healing landscape within broader studies that address landscapes as mnemonic tools (Bollig & Bubenzer 2009; Santos-Granero 1998, 2004).

This reading of landscape as a healing agent was particularly motivated by discrepancy between the assumption of uprooted identities and Cabrera's insights about rich landscape symbolism within Cuban religions. As such it contrasts the widespread assumption that inhabitants of Caribbean islands were too fragmented and uprooted to have any spiritual relationship with the local landscape. However, investigation concerning sacred landscapes on Caribbean islands is rather scarce (Cabrera 1954; Dodson 2008). When compared to the copious literature on the same topic in other parts of the Americas, where a strong continuity of indigenous languages and cultural traditions is evident, Caribbean sacred landscapes remains rather undescribed. In fact, there is little understanding of how newcomers in the Caribbean interpreted the landscape they encountered and how (or from where and from whom) they obtained their botanical knowledge.

The second objective of this study is to provide some new insights into the ongoing process of the historical construction of healing landscapes. This includes the need to summarize some of the available data on plant histories, etiologies and worldviews of historically marginalized groups.

As Caribbean landscapes are in an ongoing process of cultural transformation, the significance of some historical, religious and other types of symbolic places is still being reinterpreted within healing rituals. The process of engagement with the past can be reflected in, for example, the selection of locations for healing practices. The selection might be motivated by the presence of physical remains of traditional *lieux de mémoires*, which are often monumental human built structures, but also by cosmologies and etiological narratives about the origins of disease, which guide the patients to certain plants, trees and natural healing shrines.

Memories emerge in social frameworks, which are influenced by hegemonic structures. Even those memories that are perceived as very inner and individual experiences are constructed within a social and cultural context. This context often includes institutional directives as to what ought to be remembered, especially in the form of a national top-down education system. There are also limits to the hegemonic influences on memory. This study has collected a considerable amount of data on cultural memory that relies fundamentally on informal education, received through oral traditions, rituals, and healing practices. A broader knowledge of the epistemic communities provides more nuances to the grand narratives of Caribbean history.

The focus on the "memory of the indigenous past" will help us to further understand the effect of alienation mentioned by Fanon (1952). Without doubt, the armed conflict, the forced labor, the introduced diseases, together with processes of (institutionally directed) cultural change and loss, profoundly marked the current status of what ought to be the Caribbean indigenous heritage and the way people identify with this heritage. How this identification is contextual and is the subject of official identity politics will become clear in the historical overview. This will later be contrasted with fieldwork data about how the valorization of this heritage is often displayed in current healing practices. Many people not only interact with ancestral places but also perceive indigenous ancestors as agents that influence human health and wellbeing.

Data collection and fieldwork methodology

This research started with an analysis of the colonial history of indigenous peoples, and their role in the medicinal histories of the region, consisting of a close reading, historical contextualization, and textual analysis of the main primary and secondary documents, which were used to better understand the medicinal cultures, as well as the cultural and religious transformation of the 16th century. Further research concerned documents relating to the history of the indigenous peoples in Hispaniola after the encomienda period. These texts were read "against the grain", assessing the author's motives, political agenda and intended meanings, and identifying agencies and internal contradictions in the texts. The sources on the Greater Antilles, in particular Cuba and the Dominican Republic, were complemented with historical and ethnographic accounts from the Lesser Antilles and from the Arawakan speaking communities on the South American mainland. The resulting insights were then incorporated into transculturation theory used to describe the cultural history of the region.

The main corpus of knowledge originates from ethnographic fieldwork, interactions with local experts and mentors in the field. The contributors to this study were approached by my guides, by the local authorities and by other contact persons, who introduced me as a student interested in the local customs and history. The settings of the interviews were the households of the contributors, patronal celebrations, certain sacred and ritual places or surroundings of their dwelling when *e.g.* collecting the plants. All information used in this dissertation was used with the contributors' explicit consent after having been informed about the purpose of the study and their rights. The majority of them are local experts and carriers of oral traditions, historical and cultural knowledge of various ages (predominantly above 50 years old). Nearly all agreed with the use of their names or nicknames in this dissertation. In the cases of those who did not consent, or when I believed that the information they provided might reflect negatively on them, their names were not included.

The selection of the locations was consistent with the goals of the Nexus 1492 project with respect to the transformations of indigenous cultures after the colonial powers invaded their territories. Therefore, more attention was paid to locations where archeological or historical indications of cultural contact between the different cultural groups were available. The overview of places that were visited is displayed in figure 7 and 10. In total, I have spent twenty weeks in the Dominican Republic in the periods of January-February, August-October 2014 and June-August 2015, and eight weeks in Cuba in May 2014 and May-June 2015. This time discrepancy was due to the fact that the region studied in Cuba was smaller and the work-permit and logistic restrictions were more complicated in rural areas.

The data set was collected during my participation in different rituals, informal conversations and semi-structured interviews with open-ended questions in different settings. The interviews were recorded, I kept a log with overviews on a daily basis and included photographical documentation.

Although no compensations were requested, a small present was offered and to those whom I visited repeatedly I brought some groceries. To my guides I paid a general salary since they spent the entire day with me, and I refunded their families for accommodations. In conformity with general customs, I often left "something for *misterios*" after the consultations with traditional healers.

After the fieldwork, all recordings were listened to again; the most important parts were transcribed, and coded with the program Atlast.ti. The interviews and recordingfrom which I later used direct quotes in this text are available through the Leiden University Depository and DANS.[12] The analysis of these interviews was based upon the constructivist version of grounded theory (Charmaz 2001) rooted in pragmatism and relativist epistemology, acknowledging that social realities are mutually constructed through interaction. The advantage of this method is that it draws upon the interviewee's concepts while acknowledging the investigator's influence. The data from these interviews were triangulated with my field notes. The final interpretation of the results was enriched by comments made by local researchers. Their insights were especially important for achieving a correct interpretation and representation of statements, given the aforementioned impact of colonial discourse in the social sciences and in society at large.

One of the influential factors in the collection and interpretation of the data is, as in other types of ethnographic studies, the researcher herself. Even though I tried to highlight the voices of the contributors as much as I could and to acknowledge their contribution by mentioning their names, some researcher bias will remain, reflecting my background as a 30 year old female, atheist, trained in linguistic and cultural studies, originating from the Czech Republic, living in the Netherlands with a partner of Mixtec-Dutch background, at the time of the migrant crises in Europe and rise of xenophobic and right wing sentiments. The different cultural background often helped in breaking the ice when initiating conversation, but without doubt it also led people to avoid discussion of certain customs because of some form of stigma, or to leave out aspects of the tradition that would be perceived as shared and well-known (*e.g.* the names and functions of Catholic Saints).

---

12 DANS stands for Data Archiving and Networked Services, available at https://dans.knaw.nl/.

Vansina (1987) already emphasized the importance of involving local scholars when recording oral histories and studying the meaning of such texts, as these often include metaphors so that their significance goes beyond the vocabulary. Some interviews – especially those made at the beginning of the fieldwork – were not without intercultural communication problems, which are also clear in the transcripts, where some question had to be repeated or reformulated. Although these communication differences were not considered a severe obstacle to the transfer of the message, my limited linguistic skills (confronted with a different vocabulary and accent), but also my unfamiliarity with certain concepts and other intercultural differences should – as in other ethnographic works – be taken into account. This experience was considered as valuable for a reflection upon colonial prejudices embedded in colonial inequality and upon intercultural misunderstanding still present today. Frequently, however, my interlocutors would surprisingly share very personal information with me. Obviously, some information was only communicated after prolonged contact, while other topics would just be omitted from the conversation with an outsider.

Caribbean scholars have pointed out the danger that a foreign investigator tends to impose Western epistemologies on the local frames of knowledge, and to pay most attention to unfamiliar habits, which may lead to "othering" in terms of time, culture and religion. Fabian (1983) reminds us that anthropology itself contributed to the intellectual justification of the colonial enterprise. The focus of earlier studies was usually on differences, which were situated on a fixed time line of human evolution, and as a consequence sometimes reinforced the distancing from the cultures and peoples described, making them into just an object of study, the other, which was portrayed as more savage, primitive, or traditional then the Self.

Being aware of these dangers, before going on the first fieldwork I focused on the analysis of the historical construction of the biased representation of the indigenous ancestors. During the various religious celebrations and rituals instead of just observing I actively participated. Part II contextualizes the ritual use of the landscape and approximate it to readers who might not share the same belief system by explaining their relevance in the daily and agricultural activities. By drawing examples from various Caribbean religions, including those of European origin, in general terms I aimed to show the universal value of the environment as a source of physical and mental health. This also shows the creativity and symbolic means through which Caribbean ancestors and contemporary communities established new relationships with their surrounding landscapes and overcame various obstacles including individual and communal ailments. These various examples should help to overcome an alienating language about *The Others.*

Ethics

In this study I have followed the Codes of Ethics of the AAA and of Leiden University.[13] The emphasis on the memory of the indigenous past should be considered as one of many possible approaches to healing landscapes. Here the focus on healing landscapes as cultural memory of the indigenous past highlights some problems that are still af-

13 Both codes coincide also to a large extent with the Nexus Code of Ethics.

fecting historically marginalized strata of the Caribbean population. This study by no means aims to prove that local medicinal cultures are solely the heritage of a particular group or an isolated ideology of a particular time.

The focus on the indigenous past within the healing landscapes is used here to enable me to show and discuss intercultural dynamics and politics of memory. Many previous reconstructions of the indigenous past, especially in the Dominican Republic, were proposed in opposition to African heritage, and more particular that of their Haitian neighbors. As this study took place when Law 169-14 was adopted, implying denial of basic human rights as access to higher education, formal employment or adequate health care to people of Haitian origin, the subsequent chapter and especially the third, fourth and fifth will show the undeniable importance of West African heritage in Dominican society. In no way does this text support the nationalistic use of the term "indigenous" or other practices of social exclusion.

It is worthwhile to emphasize that the definition of Indigenous Peoples as accepted in the international legislative framework was developed not on the basis of a particular ethnic origin but rather on the basis of a shared condition of experiencing the detrimental effects of colonial legacies. Indigenous peoples all over the world face the continued presence of colonial structures and mentalities, which results in discrimination, exploitation, marginalization, oppression and other forms of social injustice that primarily (though not exclusively) affects the communities which descend from the pre-colonial inhabitants of the territory. In the case of Cuba and the Dominican Republic there are few people who consciously identify as descendants of peoples that lived on these islands prior to the European conquest. Consequently, one might say, the majority of the population of these countries does not fit into the definition of indigenous peoples as descendants of the original people or occupants of lands before these lands were taken over or conquered by others. On the other hand, few contemporary Dominicans and Cubans, regardless of their race or ethnic origin, have ancestors who were not deprived of their original lands or who were not profoundly and negatively impacted by colonialism. The history of these ancestors, however, is often silenced and forgotten in favor of those who have been inscribed in the historical records preserved until today. When discussing the demographic hisotry and the process of the transculturation the term indigenous people (distinguished from the former by a lowercase letters) is used to refer to the ancestors who descend from peoples who populated Caribbean and Americas prior to the European conquest in order to avoid confusion with Indigenous Peoples which might originate in Africa or Caribbean.

The topic, as well as the approach, of this study also implies other ethical concerns. While I have obtained clear consent from local mentors to publish data, some of the information will not be included. The exact locations of the ritual places are not revealed because of concerns for vandalism and ongoing persecutions of the 21 Division in the Dominican Republic.[14] A small part of the collected data on the plants has been included to illustrate the richness of the local botanical knowledge and the potential of plants to narrate cultural history. Neither the project nor the author claim ownership of this intellectual property about the medicinal properties of the plants. All profits

14 21 Division is the term preferred by some contributors for Dominican Vudú. For more literature on this topic consult Deive (1988) or Tejeda Ortíz (2013).

based on the botanical knowledge facilitated by this study must therefore be directed to the local owners of this intellectual property.

The recent appeal of CARICOM (2014) for reparatory justice concerning crimes against humanity perpetrated during the colonial era and for more research providing an understanding of the imperial history from the local perspective reminds us of theoretical, methodological, ethical implications that still remain relevant in times of global imperialism, the war on terrorism, and the increasing privatization of cultural knowledge and communitarian resources.[15] This thesis supports the call for reflection upon this issue and hopes to stimulate more research in this sense and to construct more dialogue between different epistemological communities.

Studies generated by community experts and local investigators are an important contribution to the understanding of the relationship between health and environment, and at the same time an important step in the healing process after a long history of social injustice. One Puerto Rican historian, Morales (2001), suggested that revisionist approaches to history are potentially beneficial for healing from historical injustice. She proposes that the examination of imperial history should be grounded in a diagnosis of aspects that do the most harm in contemporary society. In her view, through a critical revision of the erasure of the historically marginalized groups, historical narratives can heal the traumas of oppression. Likewise, an emic understanding of colonial legacies and local responses is needed to develop tailored policies to address them.

As the studies by Cain (2015) and Phulgence (2015) show, memories and memorialization of slavery and its legacies should be important topics in both the Caribbean and Europe. The colonial history of slavery and its consequences in the Caribbean are often conveniently forgotten on the other part of the Atlantic. Is the recognition of suffering not an expression of fundamental norms of human dignity? Are the memorials of 18 million victims of the Transatlantic Trade and Slavery, as placed in New York or Amsterdam, the end or the precursors of efforts to establish the right means of restorative justice? The data collected on cultural memory about the indigenous past offer more points for the discussion about the current memory politics on this topic.

Caribbean healing landscapes are bridging generations by their materiality and memories encoding ancestral knowledge, conflicts and reconciliations. The current healing landscapes are deemed to be a legacy of histories of illness, displacement, disrupted communities, but they also demonstrate a people's capacity to resist, to survive, and to heal. As such these landscapes are testimonies of the human creativity with which communities responded to colonial oppression by integrating various religious and healing practices. The contemporary testimonies invite readers to think about the human capacity to heal not by forgetting but by remembering, a process in which memories are recalled in constant interaction with the outside world, impregnated with our common past.

15 There is renewed interest in cultural reparations of Caribbean cultural objects located in European museums. The legal status and history of these collections has been addressed by Françozo & Strecker (2017).

Outline of the dissertation

The main body of this dissertation consists of two parts, with consecutively numbered chapters. Part I, comprises chapters 2 to 5, and deals fundamentally with the historical dimension of the research question and its implications, but also relevant ethnographic data and contemporary reality are interwoven in the presentation and discussion.

Chapter 2 discusses the concepts of healing landscapes and cultural memory in more detail and situates them within the broader landscape and memory studies concerning various regions including African, American and European examples.

Chapter 3 reviews briefly the historical genesis of representation of the landscapes and indigenous peoples of the Dominican Republic and Cuba as an important node of collective memory.

Chapter 4 provides an overview of available historical data on the background of medicinal cultures of the 16th century. This highlights some aspects of broader landscape transformations, including intercultural encounters of heterogeneous worldviews underpinning the healing practices.

Chapter 5 includes the historical background of locations where the ethnographic fieldwork was conducted. It reveals the long-continued existence and social integration of the indigenous peoples during the colonial period. Together, these historical sources make it possible to assess the contested nature of the cultural memory of indigenous past.

Part II, which comprises chapter 6 to 9, describes different landscape features that are associated with the indigenous past and clarifies how these are engaged during traditional healing practices. Chapter 6 first shows the significance of natural resources in daily life, and then proceeds with discussing the landscape symbolism in agricultural, ritual time and the liminal life period of disease.

Chapter 7 provides a general overview of different landscape features as agents, and discusses related etiologies, the roles of healers, and their interaction with medicinal plants.

Chapters 8 and 9 deal in more detail with two types of natural sites that are often loci and settings of religious life and healing practices, associated with narratives concerning indigenous ancestors. The analysis of various examples of water sources and caverns will make it possible to draw connections between these elements and provide us with insights into the more and less conscious ways of remembering, which create links between present and previous generations.

Chapter 10, which entails the final discussion section of the dissertation, synthesizes the data from the previous chapters relative to the research questions and formulates the conclusions. It proposes a new interpretation of the historical background and contemporary character of the healing landscapes as well as of their relationship to the indigenous peoples of the Caribbean.

Part 1

THEORETICAL AND HISTORICAL DIMENSIONS OF CARIBBEAN LANDSCAPES

2

Healing Landscapes from a theoretical perspective

The interdependency between natural environment and health has been discussed for millennia (*e.g.* Hippocrates' *Airs Water Places*) and are at foundations of epidemiology.[16] In the past the reflections upon the link between human health and the environment were incorporated into ethnographic publications on magic, folklore, animism, and totemism, but most of the time these were examined in a rather traditional way as part of the traits and "survivals" of past cultures, which supposedly represented the "primitive thinking" of "the other" (see the next chapter). In contrast, the «Western" perceptions were discussed in terms of physical, medical, and therapeutic benefits of landscapes for the human body. The past two decades have experienced a general increase of environmental concerns in Western societies and academia, specifically regarding the relationships between the natural environment, health, and wellbeing, which has resulted in the development of research on this topic in human geography, environmental psychology, medicine, environmental anthropology, and anthropology of religion. The value of the natural environment in its relation to body is here addressed with the term *"healing landscapes"* (Russo 2008).

The first part of this chapter addresses the contribution of cultural memory theory to landscape studies, as a means that may help us to understand how healing landscapes are subject of historical changes, how landscape features facilitate knowledge transfer across generations, and how people, through healing rituals and medicinal cultures,

16 Hippocrates, the father of medicine, applying inductive reasoning, expressed in his work *Airs, Waters, and Places* (± 400 BC) his firm conviction that there was a relation between the geographical location and one's character and health. Hippocrates opposed the idea that illnesses were caused by divine intervention and could be cured through appealing to the deities. Instead, he argued that illness is a result of humoral imbalances. He distinguished four humors: blood, phlegm, black, and yellow bile, each of which had its own complexion (characteristics). An illness was to be diagnosed by determining the complexion of the illness, and its cause. The cure consisted of restoring the balance in the body by correcting the diet, the humoral imbalance of the body, or the relationship with the environment. Physicians following Hippocratic teaching believed in deterministic relations between seasons, waters, prevailing winds, physical geography, the soil of a place and the humoral balance, which all together influenced human health. Hippocrates and Galen's teaching were influential during the Renaissance at important Spanish medical centers such as Sevilla, Salamanca, and Alcalá de Henares. The humoral theory seems to have also been prominent in popular medicinal cultures in Spain. Spanish healers were said to heal with their breath, saliva or even touch, thanks to their natural complexion, because of a balance of the four humors (Castañega 1997 [1529]).

engage with the past. The second part reviews some of the literature on the value of the natural environment in its relation to the body, including its role in health and the quality of life. The concept of *"healing landscapes"* serves us to bring together some insights of studies that touch upon human relationships with the environment, focusing on improving individual and collective health and quality of life in the Caribbean, West Africa and South America.

Introduction to landscape studies

The concept of landscape has been variously used and debated within multiple disciplines ranging from geography and history to cultural anthropology, linguistics and archaeology. Until now, landscapes, as Bender (2002, p. 106) has said: *"refuse to be disciplined; they make a mockery of the oppositions that we create between time (history) and space (geography) or between nature (science) and culture (anthropology).*" Indeed, the differences in thinking about and perceptions of the landscape depend on the disciplinary perspective, on both the cultural and the personal background (gender, age, status, ethnicity) of the researcher and on the specific moment and context of the observation: as such they are rather to be understood as *"always in the making"* (Bender 2002). Given the historical particularity of western discourses, a critical reader might wonder whether and in what way the concept of "landscape" is accurate when speaking about the engagement with the past in the Caribbean or more specifically when assessing healing practices and knowledge. Before explaining the relevance of the concept we therefore will first have to reflect upon some of its meanings.

Many landscape studies start by tracing the etymological origin of the term "landscape" back to the term "landschap" from the Dutch language (Wiley 2007). First, in both current English and Dutch, landscape/landschap denotes a picture representing a natural inland scenery. Second, a prospect of natural inland scenery, such as what can be observed from a glance at one point of view towards a track of land with distinguishing characteristics and features – this is considered a product modified by geomorphological processes and changes introduced through human agency.[17] Finally, the English definition simply refers to a tract of land. While the most popular use of 'landscape' refers to a picture, probably because of the popularity of the Dutch landscape paintings in the 17th century, the word already occurred earlier, in the 13th century, when it denoted a *"landstreek,"* literally referring to a part of a country/area, or "*landelijke omgeving*", rural/pastoral surrounding. The latter definition denotes something that is physically out there, a physical material entity. This coincides also with one of the basic meanings in English. These different definitions are indicative of alternative disciplinary approaches, each of which emphasizes a particular concept of landscape. While sometimes described in dichotomies and oppositions, it is clear that also in present-day English this word has multiple meanings. The painterly view indicates the particularity of one's perception, which is embedded within a cultural historical context. For example, when Dutch landscape paintings gained popularity there was a shift from religiously oriented scenes to daily realities, and still life scenes, a change most likely motivated by religious changes during the period of reformation.

17 See the Oxford English Dictionary for these general definitions.

The Dutch landscape painting seems to be framed by a specific religious view, different from that of the Spanish Roman Catholic Church of early modern encounters in the Caribbean or from popular beliefs of the Spanish countryside.[18]

These meanings of the word landscape have guided landscape studies to address landscapes as cultural representations as well as material measurable landscapes (Wiley 2007). The interrelation of nature and culture returns repeatedly to the theoretical discussions, most recently because of the "ontological turn" in South American anthropology in the form of Viveiros Castro's perspectivism and its critiques (*e.g.* Halbmayer 2012, Rival 2012). The definition of the link between nature and culture has been discussed and refined for a much longer time than that of landscape (see also Descola & Pálsson 1996). One of the hallmarks of the nature/culture dichotomy is precisely its academic history, which has placed it at the foundation of geography studies, from where the concept of landscape has been transferred to other academic disciplines.

The current buzz word 'landscape' has gained popularity in Europe due to the work of German geographer Schlüter who used it in order to set the boundaries of geography, or in German *Landschaftkunde* (literally Landscape science) as a discipline (Martin 2005). A major task of this discipline was to trace changes in two types of landscapes: *Urlandschaft* (primeval landscape) and *Kulturlandschaft* (cultural landscape, *i.e.* landscapes modified by humans). In a reaction to the environmental determinism of his period, Sauer (1925) developed the concept 'cultural landscape' as an entity fashioned from natural landscape by cultural groups. Over the past two decades, however, there has been a dramatic increase in attention paid to the complex relations between culture and landscape. This new cultural geography went beyond landscapes as material expressions of culture to emphasize its cultural character, loaded with symbolic meanings. This approach was adopted, for example, by Cosgrove (1998 in Wylie 2007), who addressed how landscapes are portrayed, defined, and viewed as a reflection of processes of social formation at the time of its creation, so that they cannot be understood in purely aesthetic ways free of this context. More attention has also been paid to the question how the culturally constructed landscapes are products of social relations, including power, and economic circumstances (Wylie 2007). Post-structuralist´s currents in geography have further emphasized that this relational character of meaning is always present in the process of 'becoming' according to a particular context.

Within the Caribbean context the term 'landscape' has been implemented by UNESCO for a combination of works of humans and nature, which expresses a long intimate relationship between humankind and their natural environment.[19] UNESCO declared the cultural landscapes of Viñales Valley, the First Coffee Plantations in the Southeast Cuba, and the mixed site of Jamaican Blue and John Crow Mountains as heritage of universal value for humanity. The recognition of sites such as Blue and

18 See for more on the historical development of the landscape studies Hirsch & O'Hanlon (1997), Wiley (2007), or Hermans et al. (2013).

19 UNESCO distinguishes various subcategories under the heading 'landscape'. The world list includes the intangible aspect of landscapes, the first nominated sites being Tongariro National Park in New Zealand and the Uluru-Kata Tjuta National Park in Australia. Surprisingly few sites from the Americas have been recognized as cultural associative landscapes and most of them include monumental architecture. Among these are, for example, the Maya archaeological sites Calakmul and Tikal, the Inca site Machu Picchu, and Rio de Janeiro.

John Crow Mountains called also for more recognition of important non-monumental archaeological sites in the Caribbean and worldwide. Simultaneously, this highlights the importance of heritage for peoples without written history because it shows how Maroon memory of some historical events has been kept alive through ritual practices and narratives.[20]

Within this context, it is also clear that cultural landscapes or mixed sites are generic umbrella terms. The cultural landscapes and mixed sites maintain implicitly the constructivist view of humans being outside of their environment. This would speak to an audience that rarely experiences a daily engagement with landscapes that leave traces behind and evoke memories of past activities, persons and social relations. Similarly, such a spectator's view seems to undervalue the mutual agency of all living organism and the interdependency of humans and environments for their health and wellbeing.

Some tensions between the multiple meanings of the term 'landscape' have marked the anthropological research on this topic. Hirsch and O'Hanlon (1995) argue that at first landscapes were deployed as a framing background, which informs the way an anthropologist brings his or her study into view. In this approach, anthropologists were distancing themselves from emic views because they deemed their own perspective to be more 'objective'. Later, this approach moved towards capturing the emic meanings attributed to physical surroundings, to the extent that these could be made object of ethnographic description and interpretation. In general, such descriptions emphasized the cultural associations that were different from the researcher's own cultural background, which led to an overemphasis on the differences between cultures and on the 'exotic' character of the studied culture. In contrast, reacting to this distancing and alienating perspective, phenomenological approaches have sought to understand cultural landscapes in terms of embodiment, inhabitation, and dwelling.

Ingold (2007) has fundamentally criticized the human exceptionalism (separation of the human from nature) by observing that it is problematic to describe nature as a-human and a-cultural, yet knowable to the landscape scientist who supposedly can translate its value-free data into reliable theoretical constructions. To illustrate this point, Ingold argued that: "*If all meaning is thus culturally constructed then the environment on which it is imposed must originally be empty of significance. But if we hold that the culture is man's means of adaptation to the environment and if environment prior to its ordering through cultural categories is mere flux, devoid of form and meaning, it follows that culture is an adaptation to nothing at all*" (Ingold 2002, p. 39).

The awareness of the interdependence of culture and environment seems to be generated to a certain extent by intrinsic values that the environment affords to humans (Ingold 2002). Those who are dependent on the landscape for their living are also more likely to be aware of its vulnerability and threats such as climate change. Ingold (2002) understood this mutually constitutive relation between persons and environment as effectivities and affordances between the actions of capabilities of subjects and possibilities for action offered by objects. In these lines, environmental affordances should

20 The cultural heritage is materialized in form of the Nanny town heritage route and associated remains such as trails, settlements, archaeological remains and hiding places, which bear witness to Maroon history. The forests and their rich natural resources provided everything the Maroons needed to survive, to fight for their freedom, and to nurture their culture. Descendants of Maroons hold strong spiritual associations with these mountains.

be searched for not just in the visible, physical, or practical use, but also in terms of affordances for the process of construction of cultural meanings, which go beyond (but likely relate to) material satisfactions.

From a religious viewpoint, the landscapes are symbol and/or manifestation of a divine creative force, a locale of interaction between people as well as between humans and other beings, whose invisible superhuman powers can intervene in human well-being and health by causing sickness or curing it. Aspects of the environment can also become signs, which communicate information given by invisible and non-human agents. In material terms, natural environments can be beneficial to human physical health by affording green medicine and a healthy environment to dwell in. For their mental health landscape may give humans a sense of belonging and place by providing them a context of being-in-the world that transcends the human lifespan. This may help us to position ourselves in space and time (which, according to religious teachings, may go back all the way to creation itself). Such a positioning not necessarily refers to a linear sequence of historical events but may also involve culturally bounded notions of time and place. And as Bender has argued, "*people relate to place and time through memory, but the memories may be of other places and other times*" (Bender 2002, p. 107). As Halbwachs (1992 [1941]) suggested, even individual memories are of a social nature. In conclusion, even the most intimate memories and interaction are constructed on the basis of individual experiences of dwelling in familiar or foreign landscapes, which are negotiated in the framework of collective and cultural memory.

Memory landscapes

All different definitions of landscapes in western discourse entail the notion of the passage of time, be it geomorphological modification of land mass, or historical trajectories embodied in experience of the landscape at specific moments (Bender 2002). Ingold (1993) proposed to move beyond definitions of the landscape as a neutral, external backdrop to human activities, towards a particular cognitive or symbolic ordering of space by a 'dwelling perspective', "*according to which the landscape is constituted as an enduring record of – and testimony to – the lives and works of past generations who have dwelt within it, and in so doing, have left there something of themselves*" (Ingold 1993, p. 152). Following this understanding it is proposed here to use the concept of "*landscape*" as an opportunity to understand time and space as integral to each other.

In that connection heterogeneous human perception of time should be examined in order to understand its relation to or engagement with the landscape. Therefore, this study focuses rather on ways how present-day populations engage with these landscapes full of ancestral material imprints. It is not just that landscape narrates a story. We follow Ingold's observation that to perceive landscape is "*to carry out an act of remembrance, and remembering is not so much a matter of calling up an internal image, stored in the mind, as of engaging perceptually with an environment that is itself pregnant with the past*" (Ingold 2000, p. 189). As Kolen and Renes (2015) argued, landscapes contain also traces of those predecessors whose life and dwelling at occasions felt into oblivion in the collective memory or were never intended to be remembered. This capacity to narrate about the past was also recalled by Glissant, who suggested for Martinique: "*Our landscape is its own monument: its meaning can only be traced on the underside. It is all history*" (1996, p. 11). In a similar vein the project 'Nexus 1492' investigates the material traces of life and dwelling of the pre-colonial inhabitants of the Caribbean and the impact that the European conquest had on them.

The understanding of healing landscape also involves the consideration of its temporality. Distinct time dimensions may be found in the explanation of the origin of a specific disease or in the interference of the ancestors or deities in the health and well-being of the patients. The ancestors have been present already for a long time, deities have been living since the time of creation.[21] The engagement with the past can also be materialized in individual healing traditions, for example through particular healing locations associated with sacred narratives that explain the function of particular herbs, or interpret the environment in a symbolic manner as a communication of the invisible beings. In this way different perceptions of time are expressed in culturally diverse medicinal cultures.

The motives for recalling the past within healing practices might be guided by origin narratives which might be evoked to call attention to specific features of the landscape, in order to show and maintain their cultural importance (Ingold 2000), create a sense of belonging (Santos Granero 1998) or locate and perceive other worlds in this world (Halbmayer 2012). Herein also the past of the before time intervenes with a spacialization of memories into natural features or built sites (Pierre Nora 1997) that transcend at least one generation (Santos Granero 1998; Hill & Santos-Granero 2002). Until now built memory places have received more recognition as monumental heritage places. More attention should be given to alternative places or spacializations of history (incl. religious ones) or natural environmental features, which are not calling our visual attention but nonetheless might be of great importance for local history. This ought to be of particular importance when we try to understand the character of the healing landscapes in the Caribbean region today. The temporality of the landscape might be of particular importance during the healing ceremonies as many places entail a religious experience through interaction with the numinous, manifested in ancestors or primeval divine forces while they also may be places of longstanding reputation for successful healing activity (Gesler 1993).

For the understanding of the historical construction of the healing landscapes it is important to highlight that the continuous long-term use of sacred places with their related rituals in the healing tradition is not to be equated with immutability or inflexibility. While many peoples, especially indigenous peoples, have claimed land rights in terms of their rootedness in the landscape, this does not warrant the conclusion that populations forcibly removed from their lands of origin did not reinterpret their worldviews in new environmental contexts. Halbwachs (1992 [1941]) showed in his *Legendary Topography of the Gospels in the Holy Land* how Jews, Romans, Muslims, and Christians re-modeled the landscape of Jerusalem according to their religious needs, and that memories are often symbolically reproduced when separated from their original space. Similarly, Arawakan groups replicated common sacred places in newly settled areas, inhabited as a result of colonial processes of displacement or socio-political dynamics. Santos-Granero (2002) and Whitehead (2002) have noted that widely dispersed Arawakan peoples share similar toponyms, sacred cartographies, and enchanted

21 For more details on the issue of time in landscape see Overing (2004).

landscapes, which appear to have been reproduced in newly inhabited regions, an indication that their landscape constructions are not fixed in time and place.

Thus, when accounting for the conceptual landscape transformations in the Caribbean we should consider the construction of culturally significant landscape features. Santos-Granero (1998) calls this process topographic writing: historical memory has been inscribed (and is re-inscribed) on the land through sacred narratives and rituals, leaving us (in the Yanesha case) with sites that remind us of past consecration and the more recent desacralization of traditional territory. Bollig and Bubenzer (2009) and Kavarie et al. (2009) are among those who have studied similar processes of inscribing histories into landscape features to memorize significant activities of past on the African continent.

The importance of landscapes lies beyond being just a mnemonic "tool" carrying historical and cultural knowledge. The transfer of the historical knowledge might also be less intentional. The landscape bridges the past and present not only through material human imprints, but also by the continuation and re-adaptation of practices such as narratives and rituals associated with the landscapes that our predecessors were part of. We and our predecessors are connected through landscapes which are essential to our human existence. Their importance and knowledge related to them is culturally encoded in various forms often conveying values and messages from the past, reinterpreted according to the current cultural (medicinal) cultures. The time depth of some of these healing traditions and the role of the landscape often go beyond one generation. This time depth will be assessed with the help of Assmann's concept of cultural memory.[22]

Assmann's (2011) theory of cultural memory focuses on the role of the past in constituting our world and investigates forms where the past presents itself to us as well as motives that prompt our recalling of it. Drawing on Halbwachs notion of collective memory, Assmann (2011) extends the time span of collective memory – some 80-100 years – back towards the time of creation. In short, his cultural memory encompasses collective memory, but also traditions that go back much further than a few generations. Because individual memory is considered to be in a constant interaction with other human memories. The individual memory is registered and communicated in symbols, it is embedded and embodied in cultural frames of reference and stored away in symbolic forms, which may be transmitted (and transformed) from one generation to another. Therefore, memories are stored in landscapes, texts to be learned, feasts to be celebrated, churches and places of commemoration, reflection and devotion, music, theatre and other performances, and especially narratives that contain messages about the world and about life.[23]

22 Places transcend generations and connect the present time with the time of the ancestors. As Morphy shows, the past time is materialized in places as transformation of ancestral beings, representing forever the memory of associated events (Morphy 1995; 188). More specifically, for Yolngu speakers of Arnhem Land in Australia, landscape is not just a sign system that serves the purpose of passing on information about the ancestral past, but it is a referent integral to the message.

23 Assmann sees landscapes as disembodied forms of cultural memory, which is preserved because it does not depend on individual memory – but its reproduction depends on the wider framework of participants through which it is handed down to the posterior generations. He also used the concept of mnemotopes, which are cognitive maps as networks of places, which form a grid to which the collective memories are attached (Assmann 2011).

According to Assmann, placement also plays a main role in the collective and cultural mnemotechnics. The placement has been a popular mnemonic tool in ancient Greece (method of loci) but is also present among, for example, indigenous peoples in Australia. The study of cultural memory should consider the interaction between memory and landscapes or reminding objects, but also pay attention to how these change and how these changes produce memories of their own. Cultural items or landscapes may trigger a beholder's memory because they carry the memories that previous inhabitants invested in them. The transfer of this memory is not dependent on the individual's memories (which tend to fade away easily); through codification it becomes part of the cultural framework shared by the community at large.

The concept of cultural memory was selected in order to examine what the role of indigenous peoples may have been in the becoming of contemporary medicinal cultures. In the case of Caribbean healing traditions it is to be expected that different time dimensions will emerge which might further complicate Assmann's differentiation between communicative and cultural memory. That division is mainly based on the work of Halbwachs (1992 [1952]), which is reinforced by arguments of Vansina (1985) about the value of oral tradition for historiography. Assmann (2011) incorporated Vansina's argument concerning the "floating gap" between generational memory (referring to the closer past) and formal memory (referring to the remote absolute past, the period of origin). In short, the floating gap refers to the limitations of oral tradition for the reconstruction of historical events (Vansina 1985). This issue – the possible historical value of oral tradition – is of obvious relevance for the Caribbean context (see the earlier discussion by Price 1983).

The floating gap might be less important in religious experience or cultural expressions for which the exact date is of less importance than the message that is conveyed. To illustrate this idea in a Caribbean context: the memories of resistance to slavery can be activated when engaging with places and landscapes related to this part of people's history and can also be enacted later in rituals for spiritual or physical health, obviously without regard for exact chronology. In addition, there may be more temporalities involved, which may become manifest in the various cultural interactions of communities with their landscapes.

Assmann's division between communicative or generational and formal or cultural memory may become blurred in healing practices in another way as well. To illustrate this: Hill and Wright (1988, p. 79) explain that the Wakuenai in Northwest Amazonia (an oral society according to Assmann's definition) integrated historical events into narratives about the time of origin, while also weaving events from that primordial time into the historical past.[24] An example of the integration of historical events into narratives of the time of origin is the reference to the white man who is said to have

24 First was the time when no spatial distances had come into being and when beings were still undifferentiated from each other. The spatial distances between places as well as the places themselves were created later by journeys of primordial creators. Today narratives about earlier and later primordial time are also related to places and spatial movements, which are used as metaphors to re-enact past times (Hill & Wright 1988: 87).

also emerged from the rapids of the Hipana river, the place of origin of the Wakuenai (Hill & Wright 1998, p. 91-92).[25]

This brings us to the consideration of the participatory structure of botanical knowledge and healing knowledge transfer in the Caribbean. More specifically, Halbwachs (1992 [1952]) argued that an individual cannot remember without the recourse of group thought. His view on memory as being socially conditioned, in accordance with an individual's involvement in a variety of social groups, led him to conclude that forgetting was caused by the disappearance of the old social frameworks. Bastide (2011 [1978]) argued that by following Halbwach's ideas literally we would not be able to explain the survival of African religions in Brazil where the Transatlantic Slave Trade has destroyed this transmission structure. The process of continuity, according to Bastide, relies on the (religious) structure of the groups rather than on the groups per se. In this sense, he supports Mintz's argument of a shared grammar of African heritage (see Mintz 1992 [1976]). Bastide suggested further that the collective memory does not come into play unless the ancestral institutions have been preserved, which is why survivals of African religions have maintained themselves infinitely more vigorously in towns than in the countryside (Bastide 2011). In the countryside, religions would be learned during the process of initiations, through the inheritance of images from an older generation, or in conversations with a few devotees. If these conditions would not be there, the totality of the liturgical order would disappear. In contrast, Bastide believes that in cities the old structure could easily find many of its actors so that memories could be reconstituted almost in full (Bastide 2011). When assessing African heritage in rural areas the mobility of individuals especially in the period after emancipation should also be considered.

One of the institutions that were crucial for the transfer of the medicinal cultures in the Caribbean context was that of the brotherhoods (fraternities). These were organizations that had an important role in attending to the sick, providing funeral services, and dealing with the inheritance of members of the brotherhood throughout the colonial period in the Dominican Republic and Cuba (see Deive 1988, chapter 5). Besides the brotherhoods, there are clearly more actors who could pass down their knowledge of healing practices and the underlying religious worldviews onto the next generations. Therefore the whole participatory structure in the transfer of knowledge and ideas about healing landscapes is to be examined.

The distinction between communicative and cultural memory has guided Assmann to examine differences in their respective forms of transmission. Generally, communicative memory should be less formalized as to its register and be passed down by non-specialists. In contrast, cultural memory if it is to be carried on has to be formalized, institutionalized and transmitted by an expert, such as the *griots* in West Africa (Assmann 2011). Ethnographic works, however, show that these patterns (derived from the analysis of cases in Ancient Egypt) are not universal across all contexts. The degrees of institutionalization, formality and uniformity may differ as well. Macuil (2017) has described the central role of the *tlamatque*, "wise persons" (fiscales, mayordomos, grandfathers/mothers, and healers), as important indigenous agents in the transfer of

25 For more detailed descriptions of the coexistence of multiple timescapes see Halbmayer (2009) for the Carib speaking Yukpas and Overing (2004) for the Piaroa.

worldview and knowledge through oral traditions and ritual practices, which express the collective memory in Nahua communities (Mexico).

In a similar vein, we find that healing activities and related knowledge in the Caribbean context often is in the domain of both specialists and non-specialists. Specialists such as healers, herbalists or midwifes, but also the public at large have a general knowledge of medicinal properties of certain plants and their religious symbolism. Next to healers, herbalists and therapists (*sobadores*), many other agents such as storytellers, poets (*decimeros*), and agriculturalists express by different means their particular views of the healing qualities of the Cuban and Dominican landscapes. All these various agents pass down meanings, values and behavioral norms that are associated with the healing landscapes and play a role in the general process of enculturation. The traditional healers often possess a type of more specialized knowledge that is learned according to the specific prescriptions of the professed religion, and these are to be situated within the broader cultural landscape symbolism, which might also be evoked during other tasks, for example agricultural activities. Memories of religious significance of the environment are not only meaningful for the patients and healers but also for a broader public in a specific time such as time of patronal celebrations. The broad participatory structure that assures the continuity of diverse medical cultures until today often involves oral means and healing rituals that position themselves on a continuum of variance and invariance.

Based on Assmann (2011) the basic premise is that traditional healing practices have survived until today – although always in a process of improvisation and change – because the previous generations considered them to be meaningful and wished to transmit them as a particular message and valuable knowledge for their descendants. Obviously, there can be tensions between what is considered to be meaningful by people and its institutionalization. The fourth chapter mentions and analyses some discrepancies in the institutionalization of medicinal cultures and their underlying religious systems in a colonial context.

Clearly, the construction of meaning of landscapes does not occur in a socio-political vacuum. The cultural hegemony is an important factor in the continuity of knowledge and worldviews that are being passed down, and may also subsequently affect the character of healing landscapes. When speaking about the memory of specific population groups one of the questions that arises is: whose memory is being remembered and why. The transfer of the knowledge is interweaved with power, or one's ability to *«define what constitutes information… control of this socially-constructed information, and the symbolic mobilization of support"* (Russo 2008, p. 51). Consequently, the continuity of (some aspects of) cultural memory may be limited or restrained due to oppressive power structures.

This institutionalization of the cultural memory may be part of the general process of enculturation, or, in Ingold's words, education of attention through, for example, an initiation ritual.[26] Rituals can indeed be considered a specific form of the education of attention. Rappaport defined ritual as *"the performance of more or less invariant se-*

26 According to theories on cultural learning meanings are transmitted through a process of socialization within a specific cultural context and via individual experiential learning. In a sense, Ingold applied the latter idea to the environment in his description of the process of dwelling, active engagement ...

quences of formal acts and utterances not entirely encoded by the performers" (1999). The fact that performers of a ritual have not themselves encoded all the acts and utterances that constitute their performances begs to clarify its origins. Just like Rappaport (1999) suggests for the case of religious rituals, healing rituals too are rarely considered to be calculated and deliberate inventions. There must be some degree of social consensus on the correctness of the ritual because otherwise it might seem a charade. As in the case of religious rituals, the healing rituals, though often including many new elements, are largely composed of elements taken from older rituals. This produces an internal stratification of the cultural practice in accordance with the complex and layered cultural history (see Chapter 5).

Its relative invariance is precisely the reason for the continuity of certain rituals over long periods of time. The religious rituals are given frequently as examples of practices that involve the most invariant and the most repetitive features. However, even within the most invariant of liturgical orders there is an unavoidable variation between performers at different moments in time (producing the self-referential messages of ritual). The adherence to a specific form, defined by a clearly distinct stylization, repetitive punctual behaviour and a performance in a specific (often liminal) time and place; all these elements contribute to the fixation of the message in collective memory.

Returning to the basic premise of transfer of cultural memory, identified by Assmann (2011) as meaningfulness, Rappaport (1999) argued the main function of ritual is not its physical efficacy: it does not achieve goals through principles of physical causality, but it does so through what he terms occult efficacy, which is founded upon emotions and words. Rappaport continues by stating that efficacious rituals are a sub-class of a larger class of ritual, which is itself one of many modes of communication. Therefore, an efficacious ritual is the one that achieves its effects through the communication of meaning; the efficacy being meaningful rather than physical. One might expect that this aspect will not be essentially different in the case of healing rituals, although a direct physical impact (more than placebo) is likely to be connected to a higher order of meanings as described by Rappaport. Our analysis will, therefore, consider the healing rituals as a form of communication but also as having physical efficacy.

According to Rappaport (1999), there are two broad classes of messages that are communicated. First there is the canonical message, which is not encoded by the participants themselves but is encoded in the liturgy and tends to be positioned on the continuum towards invariance. The second aspect is the self-referential message, concerning the participant's physical, psychic, or social status, which is of a specific nature at each specific occurrence of the ritual and therefore is likely to vary over time.

...with the environment in combination with education of attention. Like Ingold (2013) proposes later in his short reaction to Barrett's work: *"...religious experience does not lie in the perception of a ready-made world, nor does religious practice lie in mastering the skills for engaging with its constituents. It lies rather in the perception of a world that is itself continually coming into being both around and along with the perceiver him-or herself."* And he reminds us that the word education literally means in French: *"to wait"*, and even in English *"to attend to things or persons carries connotations of looking after them, doing their bidding and following what they do."... "So than animism is about attending to other beings, in perception and action, as they attend to you-or, in a word, about corresponding with them... As with animism in particular so religion in general, I would argue, is about neither belief nor direct perception but mutual attention or correspondence. As the philosopher Michel Serres (1995, p.48) puts it, the opposite of religion is not atheism or lack of belief but negligence"* (Ingold 2013, pp. 157-158).

Since rituals represent a social contract of humans among themselves (as the construction of a community) and a covenant between humans and the forces of the cosmos, we must consider how a healing ritual can order healers/patients' experience of the world and how it positions the participants in time and space. As such we will assess also healing practices that engage with the cultural memory of the indigenous past, which is expressed through narratives and rituals at specific places where the indigenous spirits are invoked and participate in the healing process.

To situate this within a broader overview of the healing landscapes (where healing is only a particular way to engage with the past), it is of foremost importance to concede that many worldviews regard the whole environment as a divine creation, which humankind and other beings are part of. Sacredness and numinous agency are therefore qualities that may permeate and manifest themselves in specific places (Santos Granero 2004, p. 102; Santos-Granero 1998; Viveiros de Castro 2002).[27] Different perceptions of temporal aspects within the landscapes (events in sacred or secular history) may motivate the selection of a specific landscape feature for its innate power to heal.

Healing Landscapes

Like landscape, healing (which, in turn, implies a concept of health) is a cultural construct to be understood within a particular historical context and trajectory in the region of study. The following wider theoretical and empirical horizon of the relation between healing and landscape will provide some background for further data analysis of the knowledge and ideas concerning this matter that are present in Cuba and the Dominican Republic.

In general, the concept of health in indigenous communities in the Americas is not restricted to the physical corporal wellbeing but includes a psychic or mental component that implies the need for a harmonious, and respectful dwelling in the world, which has both visible and invisible dimensions. As such, the concepts of illness are closely related to a broader medicinal culture, which is often intimately connected to religion and worldview.[28] The history of studies on the religious experiences of landscapes has been marked by various misconceptions, biases and stereotypes, and this is particularly true in the case of the cultures historically related to the Caribbean. As Perrin (2011) showed, the efficacy of the Wayuú traditional healing practices is

27 According to Taçon (2010), certain landscape features are more likely to be sacred because they are able to elicit feelings in people such as awe, power, beauty, respect and enrichment. In general, these feelings are supposed to occur in response to four types of places. Firstly, it should be places *"where the result of great acts of natural transformation can best be seen, such as mountain ranges, volcanoes, steep valleys or gorges."* In addition, it includes *"...points of relatively abrupt transition in geology, hydrology, vegetation, or some combination of these"* or *"unusual elements such as peak, cave or hole in the ground that one comes upon suddenly"*. At last, the same impact should have vantage points with "dramatic views" (2012, p. 37). Similarly, Tomkins (as cited in Moyes, 2012) confirms that mountain peaks, rivers, monuments, tombs, and caves are often liminal spaces that help to create the sense of distance or otherness that is necessary to distinguish ritual time and space from everyday life activities. However, both approaches are quite ocular-centric. In addition, there might be also other landscapes features like trees, plants, stones, winds, the sun, the rain, which might be conceived as sacred and therefore are also engaged with when seeking recovery.

28 Following Taylor and Case (2013) the term 'religion' is applied to all religious beliefs dealt with in the following chapters. This concerns both institutionally acknowledged and not recognized religious beliefs.

until now ridiculed rather than systemically studied.[29] Similar tendencies have been observed in past reflections upon Cuban and Dominican religious beliefs of historically marginalized groups (see Chapter 3), and are still very influential in the present (see *e.g.* Taylor & Case 2013; Tejeda Ortiz 2013).

In contrast, since the ecological turn in the humanities, the therapeutic function of the landscape returns again to the "Western academic field". Previously to this turn, perhaps the longest and the most widespread practices and beliefs in the salutary effects of the environment in Europe are those pivoting on curative waters (balneotheraphy) or sacred sites of religious pilgrimages. Cultural geographer Gesler (1992, p. 735-6) introduced the concept 'therapeutic landscape' into the academic literature as a *"landscape associated with treatment or healing"*. In his later publications he refined this definition to describe various places that have a long-standing reputation for healing, promoting physical (in the sense of biomedical), mental (psychological), and spiritual healing (inner renewal and wellbeing), such as Epidauros in Greece (a sanctuary of Asclepius, the god of healing), the Spring at Lourdes in France, and the hot springs of Bath in England (Gesler 1993, 1996, 1998). Next to the role of faith and its power to heal, Gesler also argued that some material aspects of these places are conducive to health, for example, as they invite you to remove yourself from daily stress, and that such places lead to psychological renewal by providing a sense of belonging to a community and place. The sense of belonging is considered in social psychology as a fundamental human need, a powerful factor that influences people's health (Baumeister & Leary 1995; Walton & Cohen 2011).

The definition of therapeutic landscapes has been further extended to include places, settings, situations, locales, and milieus that encompass both the physical and psychological environments associated with healing treatments, and the maintenance of wellbeing (Williams 1998). Following Gesler, Palka (1999) suggested, on the basis of surveys of visitors to Denali National Park in Alaska, that here the therapeutic quality of the landscape was the historical link to the spirituality of the indigenous peoples of Alaska: the awareness of this link provided a sense of place, a social interaction between the visitors, an escape to a relaxing and aesthetically pleasing environment, remoteness, and the perception of an authentic setting, which all contributed to a belief in and experience of the park's healing powers.

Wilson (2003) assessed the existence of a therapeutic landscape among First Nations in Canada, arguing that the concept of health of the Odawa and Ojibway peoples has to be examined within the context of their cosmology, which sees Mother Earth as a provider of all things necessary to sustain life and as an essential force for maintaining or restoring health. Such cosmologies imply the need for a balance of reciprocal relationships between humans and earth (referring to earth' overall importance for health, not just to the effects of a specific place).

---

29 This is illustrated by what Pineda Giraldo (1950, pp. 57-58) wrote about the Wayúu perception of disease: *"All that relates to the surroundings of primitive people: rocks, plants, animals, natural phenomena…, are active beings in the best sense of the word, capable of intervention and worthy of the Indian's respect, fear, or admiration. The primitive has not at this stage reached the discernment necessary to establish the logical relation between phenomena and their real causes, but establishes a magic relationship that in the majority of causes does not correspond to any concrete or objective reality."*

In a similar vein, Russo (2008), examining healing landscape from a historical perspective among the indigenous peoples of Pacific Northwest Coast of United States of America, has emphasized the relational concept of health and landscape. In the category of healing landscape Russo included places associated with religious rituals such as those carried out for spiritual renewal or reinforcement. Healing landscapes may be sacred natural places where one may communicate with the spirits (*e.g.* the guardian spirits associated with animals), but also historical places. The latter are considered able to cure long-term negative impacts on health and wellbeing (for example those that resulted from the loss of sacred sites) through their ability to reaffirm the connection between history and place.

Seeking recognition of indigenous worldviews, Russo (2008) compared the roles of landscape in Western worldmaking and indigenous peoples' concepts. According to him, the latter considered space as an extended emplacement, being empowered, and relational to the self, which is spatialized, dividuated, and embedded within the landscape. According to his analysis, the Western conventional making of space is more site-localized and neutral, while people's relation to it has disembodied the personal identity and made it rather autonomous from space. The latter account refers to a Western atheist perspective of a person living in a capitalist system. The fourth chapter will argue that this perspective differs from the Spanish religious view of landscape wherein such a nature / culture dichotomy was not present; instead, the Christian idea of the environment as divine creation was somewhat comparable to indigenous concepts, which may have facilitated the process of transculturation concerning this subject matter.

When trying to understand how the healthy self is embedded in place among one of the indigenous peoples of the Northwest Pacific Coast, O' Brien (2013) argues that to be healthy among Coastal Salish is tied to place through particular resources, through a sense of ancestral connection to particular place, and through personal relationships with the spirit powers that emerge from and are tied to natural landscape. According to that study, the Coastal Salish view healing as restoring wholeness to a person by means of maintaining or re-establishing a balanced reciprocal relation with spiritual, ecological communities in the landscape (nature).

The previously mentioned spiritual link between landscape and health in the cosmology of the Coastal Salish seems to be related to a general awareness of interconnectivity and interdependence of humans and natural resources, which are translated into ritual practices involving crops, animals, and places that are of key importance for the community. This can also be interpreted as respectful treatment of the environment, including animals, plants, and places, which all are considered powerful beings of their own or the abode of such forces, and as such are crucial in maintaining the health of the community. The character of this relation is fundamentally social, which usually is explained by narratives about the shared natural origin of humans and landscape features.

The relational character of health and the surrounding landscape has also been noted among several indigenous peoples of Venezuela. Here, Freire (2011) suggested that health is not just the presence or absence of illness, but a condition that results from relations that a person establishes with the social group and with the physical and symbolic environment. Etiologies as soul loss or penetration of a pathogenic object into the patient's body seem to be triggered by other beings living in the landscapes (see Perrin 2011 for the Wayúu; Wilbert & Ayala 2011 for the E'ñepa; Villalón & Corradini 2011 for the Warao).

In the Amazonian context we find that this relation is often based on the original state of the common condition of humanity. Viveiros de Castro (1998) argued that animal species, which have a key symbolic and practical role, have their spirit masters and are treated as ex-humans in Amazonian Indigenous religious history (for critiques see Halbmayer 2012 and Rival 2012). Some scholars qualify the relationship between humans and other beings in the landscape in terms of predation and reciprocity. Viveiros De Castro (1998), for example, has emphasized the predatory character of this relationship: certain animals are inedible or require their desubjectivization by ritual means before they can be consumed, a ritual that, if omitted, can lead to an illness. However, while indeed many illnesses are considered to have been caused by a spiritual attack, it is not convincing to characterize the whole relationship of humans with the healing landscape as one of a predatory character.

In contrast, Descola (1996) argued that there exist two main variants of Amazonian animistic belief: one centered around predation, as in the worldview of the Jívaro, and another focusing on reciprocity, as in the worldview of the Tukano people. More specifically, Århem (1996) suggested that in the case of the Jívaro the predation is to be understood also as a process of procreation, in which people can be hunted by creator gods, divinities, jaguars, anacondas, and other spirits. Consumption of human souls allows the souls of humans to return to their birth house. In this eco-cosmology, the animals live and behave like people and are linked to humans by acts of reciprocity, concretely by exchanging spiritual aliments (*e.g.* coca, tobacco, and incense from wax) with the animal owners who allot animals and fish to the humans.[30] Similarly to Viveiros de Castro's observations, Århem's account shows the Jívaros' conviction that aliments, fruits, cultivated plants and animals share the forces generated during the time of creation, which are necessary for continuous recreation and must be "blessed", *i.e.* transformed from being harmful and causing illness to being vitalizing factors. By blessing them, the spiritual specialist helps the souls of these to return to their birth house and enables their rebirth by neutralizing the weapons that the unblessed foods contain. Illness is seen as a temporary soul loss, which in the majority of cases comes from improper and unblessed food. This can be cured by "sucking out the weapons," *i.e.* removing entangled objects like spines, and splinters from the patients' bodies (Århem 1996, p. 196). Disease is also often seen as a result of neglect to offer the spiritual aliment to the animal owners, which, therefore, capture human souls and take them away to the rivers and hills, causing the illness or death of humans. Not only the gods and the animal spirits, but also malevolent necromancers have the capacity to slay humans with sickness.

Århem's interpretation of the Makuna people's theory of disease (which emphasizes the relatedness of humans with other beings), expands the notion of health beyond the individual or natural to include a social whole of which the patients are a component (Århem 1996). In other words, by conceptualizing the world as consisting of different living beings, which are interconnected and interdependent, the Makuna

30 Ecocosmologia is defined as *"un modelo cosmológico que estipula una estrecha relación de continuidad y contigüidad entre lo social y lo natural"* (Århem 2001, pp. 270- 271).

link the illness to environmental abuse, and cosmologic mismanagement. In spite of the diversity of modes of nature-human relatedness, this link is, according to Århem, characteristic for the whole Amazonian region. The illness has been considered as a consequence of nature's revenge also among other indigenous peoples worldwide, and should be understood as a cultural codification of ecological insights emerging from the long intimate interaction with the environment (Århem 1996). This approach offers a glimpse into an experience of the landscape not just as a setting or backdrop of healing activities but as an active agent in recovery or curing. Similar observations have been registered in the Circum-Caribbean and West African contexts.

Glimpses into the relation of health and landscape on the South American mainland

There is consensus that the pre-colonial inhabitants of the Caribbean islands had strong cultural and linguistic links with the South American mainland (*e.g.* Rouse 1992; Boomert 2000; Wilson 2007; Keegan et al. 2013; Keegan & Hofman 2017). Therefore it is worthwhile to have a closer look at the way healing landscapes are conceived by contemporary indigenous peoples in that vast region. The Wapishana, for example, consider that the landscape – especially places like big lakes, certain mountains, areas with rock engravings, rocky outcrops and some mineral springs – is populated by spirit beings and keepers that should not be disturbed (David et al. 2006, p. 37).[31] The visit to such an area is possible only when taking ritual precautions in order to not offend the spirits of the place (see also Gomez 2017, p. 201). In addition, each species or family of animals and plants has its own spirit "grandfather" or "keeper" which watches over it and can bring illness or misfortune if it is wasted or abused. Among the grandfathers of animals who are dangerous for health are the grandfathers of aquatic anteaters, anacondas, and boa constrictors.[32] This cosmology is reflected not only in the healing practices but also in other customs such as asking permission from the spirit keeper of the tree or plant before trees are felled, or medicinal and charm plants are collected.[33] Similarly, fishermen are cautious not to provoke the spirit keeper of the fish as well as other water spirits.

The *marunao* ("shaman") can cure the spirit-related illnesses (brought on by a violation of ritual prescriptions or customary law) through the communication with the grandfather spirits of the savannah, bush and mountains (David et al. 2006, p. 37).[34]

31 In their study of indigenous hunting patterns across the landscape, the authors not only took into account the biophysical aspect but also some spiritual factors; they identified more than sixty spiritual places including streams, ponds, rivers, rocks and mountains, which usually have guardians and associated narratives.

32 A variety of beings dwells in the dangerous parts of the river such as land camoudi, anaconda, boa constrictor, aquatic anteaters, tiger-like and giant-like beings. More specifically, aquatic anteaters are able to capture and drown swimmers while anacondas and land camoudis appearing in a dream may cause harm that is felt during the day.

33 Similarly, the Jívaros ensure the successful growth of plants through ritual chanting to the Mother of plants and her sons. Simultaneously, these protect humans and in particular children from the danger that comes from the cultivated plants such as yucca (Århem 1996).

34 While there are less and less specialized shamans who go through an extensive training, there are still prayer specialists present in many communities. Prayers specialists tend to specialize in specific types of traditional prayers, for curing and preventing specific illnesses, but they lack the knowledge to diagnose the source of the illness and to divine the future (Kambel and De Jong, 2013, p. 307).

The traditional remedies for illnesses caused by spiritual entities have different remedies, which may consist of the application of plants, blowing, massages, bathing in ritually prepared water, incense for ritual cleaning or more specialized methods such as blood-letting, soul retrieval, and extrusion (Henfrey 2002).[35]

Similarly, the Kaliña and Lokono teach us that everything that is on the planet has a soul and everything is interconnected (Kambel & De Jong 2006). All kinds of animals and plants, but also stones, creeks, and rivers, have protecting spirits, which have character and individuality just like human beings. If the balance between humans and nature is disturbed, or does not exist anymore as a result of misuse or overuse, there can be negative consequences, such as illness, accidents, and bad luck. The shamans, called *pyjai* by the Kaliña and *semechichi* by the Lokono, play an important role in maintaining this balance. They are the persons who are in contact with the spirit world and are able to find out through their protectors or allied spirits (*jakoewa's* in Kaliña) if someone has committed an error and ask forgiveness – also through the *jakoewa's* – for the misconduct. The balance also has to be maintained by following a social conduct that prevents misfortune and disease. This social norm includes all other human-like-beings and is expressed in customary laws with respect to hunting and gathering. These activities are also social interactions in which balanced relationships have to be maintained by collecting only what is needed, or by respecting hunting taboos.

There are many sacred and spiritual places in the Bajo Marowijne region where hunting and fishing is prohibited or can be entered only by *pyjai* (shaman). Among these places are different creeks, which are abodes of the king rooster, water spirits (*okoejemo*) or other invisible beings, as well as swamps and places where unusual sounds and events occur – some of these places have archeological remains. The hunting of certain animals should be avoided completely.[36] Some trees hold a spiritual and historical importance, and never should be cut.[37] The powers of trees and plants used by Arawakan speaking communities in healing rituals are not restricted to effects of

35 The blowing is an exhalation of air or tobacco smoke in the process of saying a prayer or chant. The blowed water refers to the water that has undergone this ritual.

36 This category includes, among others, the constrictor boas, marine turtles, sea cows, dolphins and nutrias (Kambel and De Jong 2006). Dolphin and sea cows also figure in the origin narratives. Before hunting, the hunter sprinkles some water and talks to the spirits so that they may remove all evil from his path and that he may have good fortune. It is customary to keep the environment clean and not disturb the invisible beings when one goes fishing. Other Kaliña and Lokono's customary laws prohibit the entrance of menstruating women to agricultural plots because this could offend spirits that could cause poor growth of the crops. Women in their period should avoid coming close to the river because this would enrage the water sprits (*okojoemo*) (Kambel and De Jong 2006).

37 One of the trees that helps to remember historical events is the Aware tree (*Astrocaryum vulgare*), which represents the killing of indigenous peoples by runaway enslaved persons. The Kaliña and the Lokono agree that the following trees should never be cut: the Kankantrie (*Ceiba pentandra* L.), the kwasini, the posenterie, the takini, the urewari. Takini and uremari have also an important role during healing sessions. Places with takini and kankatrie are sacred, and can provoke sickness when not respected. It is also custom to make offers before hunting and when gardening. It is said, for example: *'You take a calabash with beteri (sweet cassava drink)* (Kambel and de Jong 2006). *Then you speak and pour it on the land to let your plants grow well and chase away spiritual obstacles'.* Van Andel et al (2015) on the ritual use of plants among speakers of the Arawakan language family in Suriname and Guyana indicate the following species to be prominent*: Caladium bicolor, Maranta arundinacea, Eleutherine bulbosa, Zingiber zerumbet, Cladium schomburgkii, Capsicum annuum, Cyperus articulates, Hippeastrum puniceaum, Xanthosma brasilense, Abelmoschus moschatus, Caladim humboldtii, Lycopodiella cernua, Mimosa pudica, Montrichardia arborescens, Protium heptaphyllym, and Scoparia dulcis.*

their chemical composition on people's bodies but also proceed from an inner force (Van Andel 2013).

In Wayuu belief (Perrin 1987), health is the harmonious co-existence of body and soul. In normal circumstances, the soul only leaves the body in dreams, which may indicate the cause of harm. The immediate cause of sickness is an alteration or departure of the soul, whatever the symptoms, whatever the ultimate causes. Death is the permanent separation of the soul from the body. The healer can travel to another world to discover the causes of the diseases and calamites in the patient's life, and so cure the sickness by reconstituting the soul or bringing it back to the patient's body. Diseases are the consequence of the souls being detained elsewhere. If the person passes away it means that his/her soul has travelled to the Jepira homeland of death souls. The entrance to this place is a small well at Cabo de la Vela, and/or the cavern Jorottuy Manna. Jorottuy Manna is the passage point of the deaths when going to the skyworld and at the same time the site of origin of the Sun (Kaí), the Moon (Kashi) and the Wayuu.

The Wayuu perception of sickness and death is well summarized in the following statement of Makaerü Jitnu: *"To each of us is attached a soul. It is like a bit of white cotton fluff. Like smoke. But no one can see it. Our soul leaves us only when we sleep or when we are sick, we have been pierced by the arrow of a wanülü… Everything that happens in our dreams is what happens to our soul….And yet it's our soul that makes us die. He who dreams that he is dead never wakes up again. His soul has left him forever. He is still alive, he who dreams that knife has been stuck in his chest, but his soul is already wounded. Sickness is there. Death is near. When a Guajiro is sick, it is as thought his soul were a prisoner in Dream's abode. It's there that the spirits of the shaman can find it and bring it back to the sick man. But if he doesn't find it …the Guajiro dies…But already his soul has gone to its homeland, over there, in Jepira, the land of the yolujas. When they die, the Guajiro became yolujas. They go to Jepira by Milky way…."* (Perrin 1987, pp. 8-7).

Health in West African landscapes

For understanding the healing landscapes in the Caribbean it is also important to consider the influence of concepts introduced from Africa. A quick review of ceremonial landscapes in Nigeria, Ghana, Benin and Cameroon shows that they include natural shrines of deities, spirits, and ancestors, which live or are being materialized in physical landscape features such as groves, rivers, trees, rocks, etc. As subjects of ritual activities and social restrictions, these places or natural features are considered sacred. Their long-term protection has led to high environmental diversity in Nigeria, Cote d'Ivoire, Ghana, Benin, and Togo (see for an overview Verschuuren et al. 2010; for Benin see Juthé – Beaulaton & Roussel 2006).

Sacred groves are prominent among the sacred places in West Africa. The most internationally famous example of a sacred landscape is probably sacred grove in Osogbo, Southern Nigeria, which has been declared a World Heritage Site by UNESCO. This sacred grove was probably founded four hundred years ago together with the city of Osogbo, the remains of which are still observable in the forest. Through the forest meanders the river Osun, the abode of the Yoruba deity of fertility Osun. Osun helps the Osogbo people with their physical and spiritual problems in exchange for their worship and respect of the deities' shrines. The waters of the Osun river have healing, divinatory, protective, and procreative powers. This example demonstrates that even when this sacred grove is mainly a domain of Osun, the grove surrounding the body of the deity is full of shrines dedicated to this same deity as well as to other Yoruba deities manifested in sacred trees, stones, metals, mud, animals and temples. All of these are active contributors to the spiritual and physical wellbeing of the Osogbo people. The Ifa Bush in the grove is a place for initiation of priests, known as *babalawos*, who are able to identify the causative agents of diseases. Furthermore, the grove contains shrines dedicated to other deities such as Sango, Oya, Esu, Obatala, Ogun, Ela, and Sopoona (NCMMA 2004).

In a related vein, the sacred grove Jaagbo, a dwelling of Twin Gods, in Northern Ghana is a place associated with fertility where people come to ask help from the deities when having problems conceiving babies, healing the sick and bringing rain. In Coastal Ghana a ceremonial landscape is inhabited by *Kusasi* beings, which are manifested as stones, rocks, large trees, ponds, and forests. These sacred forests are places where ancestors are buried: therefore, their powers also reside there (Chouin 2002). The different spirits of the land are often fused with the spirits of the founding ancestors, and, according to anthropologists, provide the ultimate rationalization for establishing and maintaining reciprocal relations with the land (Chouin 2002). In other contexts, the spirits animating the soil or particular places might not even be considered to be direct ancestors, but people that have been dwelling in these landscapes before the ancestors (Post et al. 2014). The ancestral worship in the Vodoun religion in Benin) is not restricted to the known deified ancestors, but includes also *Toxosu*, the abnormally born, who become spirits of rivers and guard the entrance to the kingdom of death, and are ruled by the king of abnormally born children, as well as the group of *Damabala* or *Dambada Hwedo*, which encompasses powerful unknown ancestors who have entered loko and silk-cotton trees or mountains (Herskovits & Herskovits 1933).

Mathers (2003) suggests that in North Ghana sacred groves are associated with archaeological settlements such as the Asantemanso, the cradle of the Asanti nation. The grove itself has been used for rituals and burial practices since the 18th century (see Bosman 1967 [1705]; McCaskie 1990; both cited in Chouin 2002). Besides the sacred groves, there are several individual plants and trees that are considered to be sacred; each of them has a specific symbolism, which might be replicated in new Caribbean environments.[38]

In the Niger Delta, the Biseni and Osiama peoples perceive their lands and particularly their lakes as the sacred abode of the gods Esiribi and Adigbe (Anwana et al. 2010). Similarly, the Duala, Bakweri and Sawa peoples of Cameroon worship a *jengu* (pl. *miengu*), a water spirit similar to Mami Wata, a water deity honored in West, Central Southern Africa and African diaspora in Americas. The *miengu* are said to

38 Among the vegetal elements used in rituals in Benin are products that can be extracted from the sacred iroko tree *(Milicia excelsa)*, the raffia palm *(Raphia sp.)*, cola nuts *(Cola acuminate)*, Guinea pepper *(Aframomum melegueta)*, products used in offerings such as African palm oil *(Elaeis guineensis)*, maize flour *(Zea mays)*, cowpeas *(Vigna unguiculata)*, and calabashes *(Lagenaria siceraria, L. breviflora and Crescentia cujete)*. Gabonese plant products included: *Pterocarpus soyauxii, Garcinia kola, Aframomum giganteum, Aucoumea klaineana, Xylopia aethiopica, Tabernanthe iboga, Barteria fistulosa, Alchornea floribunda. A. melegueta, C. acuminata, and Lagenaria spp. A. klaineana, T. iboga, G. kola, and P. soyauxii, A. klaineana and T. iboga.* Ritual use in the Caribbean has been documented for the following of plants of African origin: *Newboudlia laevis, Kalanchoe integra, Lagenaria siceraria (Molina), Cyperus Rotondus, Sesamun radiatum, Pennisetum Purpureum, Cola acuminate, Afromumun malegueta.*

be beautiful, mermaid-like beings with long hair, who live in rivers and the sea and bring good fortune to those who worship them. The West African belief in this deity has crossed the Atlantic Ocean and has survived in Suriname, Guyana, the Lesser and Greater Antilles.

Likely the fact that African water deities and spirits have analogies in American environments facilitated a process of symbolic exchange, transculturation and synergy. Water symbolism – and more specifically the figure of a Master of the Water – is well-known in the Lowland South American cosmologies. Rivers are considered the abode of deities or spirits by peoples such as the Arawatés (Viveiros Castro & Howard 1992), Barima (see Gillin 1936), Makuna (Barandiarán 2012), Pemón, Trio, Warao, (Roe 1982; Hugh – Jones 1980), Wayapi (moyo anaconda: Campbell 1982, 1989), as well as Misak, Nasa and Sanemá (Rocha Vivas 2010).

In many cases the subterranean world has an aquatic connotation. The Araweté believe in Iwikahá, the Lord of rivers, who steals women and carries off the souls of children who live in their villages; Iwikahá also controls fish (Viveiros Castro 1992). Similarly, the Makuna venerate Water Anaconda, which is the Spirit Owner of an underwater *maloca* at Maneitara, the mythical birth place and waking-up-house of the Water People. The waking-up-house of the Water People is also the birth-and-dance house of the fish population that inhabits the river system, which defines the territory of the Water People. When death finally comes, the human soul separates from the body and travels to the spirits in the Sky World. Here, according to Makuna shamans, the gods cook and consume the dead person, thereby reconstituting the dead as a spirit person in the birth house of the clan. Reincarnation is evident because the deceased is reborn as a new person.

Previous approaches to healing in Cuban and Dominican landscapes

It is important to acknowledge that for the Native American and African cultures mentioned here the cause of a disease is not necessarily limited to metaphysical agents; physical factors are generally also taken into account in both the explanation and the cure. Also, if the disease is explained in terms of the divine or spiritual agency this does not imply that its diagnosis or cure is not based on empirical evidence. For the Garifuna the concept of illness can be perfectly linked to the agency of the ancestors who feel neglected, the malevolent agency of another person, or the physical contact with a powerful entity represented in a place or object, while many illnesses are also agreed to have "natural causes" (Bianchi 1988). Yet, my attention has focused generally on the religious aspects of illness in order to examine the links with cultural memory and ritual landscapes.

Inspired by previous approaches, this study will examine relevant agents such as ancestral spirits, deities, and other powerful, normally invisible beings, which intervene in human health. These beings often reside in natural places or are manifested as natural entities. At the same time, this study will use the concept of healing landscapes to identify other natural entities that promote physical, mental, and spiritual healing.

Until now the studies of healing landscapes in the Cuban and Dominican contexts have focused on particular facets. Different authors have registered the medicinal use of flora properties (Roig y Mesa 1974; Portorreal 2011; Germosén-Robineau 2005;

Ososki 2004; Roersch 2016), clarified their religious symbolism (Bolívar Aróstegui et al. 1998; Quiroz-Moran 2009), or described healing practices (Brendbekken 1998), either in monographic fashion or as part of a general overview of Caribbean religions (*e.g.* Deive 1988; Tejeda Ortíz 2013; James Figarola 1989).

In healing practices, the religious and botanical knowledge are integrated, the ritual plants are collected at specific places with permission and blessings of the divine entities and later used in baths invoking others. One of the corollary aims of the study therefore is to provide a general overview of different religious associations of landscape features that exist in both study regions in order to define how some of these entities influence individual health.

Among the first Caribbean scholars who addressed the landscape symbolism and its relation to the health was the Cuban author Lydia Cabrera in her book *El Monte* (2009 [1981]). This title is loosely translated, not just as the "mountain", but also as "uncultivated nature" (manigua – bush). For Afro-Cubans (Congo and Lucumí), *"el monte"* is sacred because it is the place where life originated, the locus of the foundation of the cosmos, providing all things needed for life, health and protection of the person (Cabrera 2009). El Monte is equivalent to the land, to earth, as the source of life and the universal mother. One of the contributors to her book compares *El Monte* to a church, *"full of saints and deceased people, we pray to them for everything we need, for our health and for our business"* (Cabrera 2009, p. 21). It is clear that in some Cuban religious practices trees and plants are animated beings, with intelligence and will as everything that grows under the sun, as all natural manifestations and existing things, and even those that are not the abode of a specific deity or saint have their grace (*aché*). As El Monte is the domain of all deities, souls of deaths, saints, and spirits, it is also a dangerous place where both benevolent and malevolent divinities reside in bushes and trees such as jagüeyes and ceibas.

Cabrera defined the cause of the illness according to Afro-Cuban religions as a minor divine punishment for forgetting, offending or failure to comply with a debt to one of the deities, or just their whim.[39] As also pointed out by previously mentioned studies, disease can be caused by the attack of a spirit but trees and plants can help to defend against such an attack: the soul is then to be "*tied up*". Illness can also be a work of *"some bilongo, uemba or morubba, wnaga or ndiambo, of a harm, iká or madyáfara, that is introduced to the body: and one must submit to the evidence that it is the result of the work of some hidden enemy"* (*ibidem*, p. 30). The etiologies and the remedies are based on the hierophanies and symbolism reflected in the environment. The consulted ritual specialist, in whose body a saint, orisha, or other spiritual entity, has incarnated – makes the diagnosis and suggests the remedy.[40] In spite of the occasional presence of biased vocabulary, due to the period of the creation of the book, *El Monte* brings us

---

39 Similar to the Catholic beliefs that certain Saints can cure specific diseases *(e.g. Saint Lucia – eyes, San Bernardo – stomach, San Ramon – birth),* also some Afro-Cuban deities are associated with specific illness Babalú Ayé with smallpox, lepra, Changó of burns, Obatalá blind and *paralizes, Oshún and Yemayá of the illnesses relate to abdomen, and punish by the rain and humidity, and kill in the sweet and salty waters.*

40 Orishas are intermediate beings, which were created by Olodumare, the supreme -being, the owner of all destinies (Edmonds and Gonzalez 2010). For more on the topic see Fernández Olmos & Paravisini-Gebert (1997).

closer to the understanding of Cuban landscapes wherein seemingly inanimate beings (trees, stones, rocks) are filled with *aché*, and of the related worldview in which the divine beings may communicate with humans through their incarnation into human bodies or by influencing the outcome of divination.

Since Cabrera's pioneering work multiple works studied different Cuban religious traditions, especially *Regla de Ocha* (*e.g.* Meighoo et al. 2013; Edmonds & Gonzalez 2010). Cuban and Dominican sacred places are important loci during annual celebrations of popular saints and orishas. Our Lady of Charity (patron of Oshún) is publicly honored with a pilgrimage by thousands of devotees. Similarly, great amounts of pilgrims gathers at El Rincón in Havana to pray to Babalú-Ayé/Saint Lazarus for their health and wellbeing. More detailed studies of particular religious traditions reveal also the symbolism and significance of various landscape features. From this broader perspective pilgrims making their petitions at sacred places as the sanctuary of the Virgen of Altagracia in Higüey or the Virgen of Mercy at Santo Cerro. By focusing only on the officially recognized sacred places we might leave out other important divine entities that are considered to have a powerful effect in the reconstruction of human health and wellbeing.

Also for devotees of *Palo Monte* (Bolívar Aróstegui et al. 2013) the surrounding environment is empowered by different invisible forces. To illustrate this rich symbolism, the Ngurunfinda, the Nature Spirit (in Regla de Ocha: Osain) brings wellbeing and prosperity. The Ngurunfinda can have various names depending on the place from where it proceeds: from *el Monte* (Simbi, or Yimbi), from rivers and lakes (mbuiri, Nkisi Masa, Mother of Water, Nkisi Mbumba), or from *manigua* (Nkisi Minseke), while the one that is the spirit that inhabits the boa is called Niksi Mboma. This spirit is enclosed in a vessel of calabash, turtle shell, head of jutía, with other ingredients and buried this under the silk cotton tree (ceiba) for three weeks. The knowledge of environmental elements representing divine and spiritual forces returns in offerings, amulets, plants and animals that belong to specific divine beings and therefore are an inherent part of the religious life of the devotees and consequently important for their wellbeing.

Dodson (2008) mapped several spaces that are sacred for Palo Monte, Vudu, Spiritism and Muerterá Bembé de Sao in Oriente. Among the various sacred spaces registered were house temples including small ones that were destined for individual devotion as well as large settings for communal performance and reenactment of religious traditions. All these stimulate the communication and communion between devotees and divine / spiritual entities through ritual exchange. In addition, they serve to create meaning and memory, reminding participants of the traditions. Dodson furthermore notes that these sacred spaces include uncultivated environmental features (*e.g.* rocks, stones, seeds, trees) which represent the creative life force.

These previous works raise more questions about the symbolism of the Dominican landscapes and their role in healing practices, and also about how these compare to and interact with the religious traditions of Cuba. In Dominican studies there have only been vague references to the spiritual relation with powers residing in the landscape. In *Talking to the Plant* (1998) Brendbekken briefly elaborates on the social life of the plants, their role in identity construction, and more specifically their *"curative, nutritive, esthetics and magical properties"*. In the testimonies she collected, it becomes clear that at least in Río Limpio (the site of her study) there are ideas about illness that are similar to those registered by the above-mentioned Cuban studies. Here we also find the distinction between illnesses caused by natural causes (including the disruption of the humoral equilibrium) and illnesses caused by a malevolent spirit that has entered the patient's body. This spirit is then paid by a third person that later penetrates his head and body. These causes may also include social conflicts, divine punishments, and not behaving according to ascribed social norms. If the spirit takes control over the patient's body involuntarily it can cause an illness. The spirit (*lwa*) can also enter the head of an initiated healer (*"caballo del misterio"*), who then may establish the diagnosis and the cure.[41] There are indications that some diseases are the results of the soul being "tied up", but Brendbekken does not elaborate on this aspect.

In summary, this is the state of the art that was the point of departure for my dissertation research. Obviously the existing data set needed to be expanded. Therefore, I have carried out ethnographic fieldwork in the Dominican Republic and in Cuba: the results will be presented in Part II. In interpreting these data there is always the question how the ethnographic present is related to the pre-colonial and colonial past. This is particularly complex in the case of the Caribbean, a crucible of cultural influences from diverse continents. The limitations of the historical records make it very difficult to trace continuities, disjunctions and transformations. Furthermore, the colonial encounters implied a series of problems in intercultural communication, which need to be taken into account. In order to create an adequate context for discussing this matter, the rest of Part I will deal with the historical background of the present-day healing landscapes and their social context. First, chapter 3 will briefly review how the European conquistadors and colonizers of the Greater Antilles have interpreted the unknown lands and peoples of the "New World" according to their own cultural and religious framework.

41 *Lwas* or *misterios* are spiritual agents, which intermediate between Gran Dios (Bon Dieu) and the adherents of 21 Division. Lwas can incarnate in persons at certain occasions such as consultations for healing or celebrations of Patron Saints.

3

Natural Man in the Caribbean Paradise: the origins of colonial discourse

The history of healing landscapes is to be understood as a part of a broader landscape transformation, including material and conceptual aspects, which went hand in hand with the introduction of new religions and medicinal cultures into the region. This chapter highlights a few European influential ideas in the first written references to Caribbean peoples and landscapes that are fundamental to the discussion of the complex transformations of healing landscapes in the Caribbean after European conquest. This brief review of the representation of the indigenous peoples sheds light on the role of the colonial sources in shaping people's relation with the landscape, with history and, more specifically, with those who lived on these islands long before the European invasion of five hundred years ago.

The first European accounts of the Caribbean region have traditionally been described as motivated by the economic and political interests of the colonizer. The search for trade routes and ways to extract resources, was accompanied by religious zeal, imperial ambitions and ideologies, which were expressed in colonial discourse. All these motivations were interwoven and mutually reinforced each other, having their impact on human practices and institutions.

When analyzing the first written accounts about the indigenous peoples, the flora and fauna of the Greater Antilles, we should consider the influences of Ancient Greece and Rome, in particular the idea of a Golden Age, described in Ovid's *Metamorphoses*, the Herodotean and Plinian monstrous races, and the Aristotelean argument that some men are slaves by nature.[42] References to the Golden Age are especially prominent in the writings of Italian authors, such as Christopher Columbus, Petrus Martyr D'Anghiera, and Amerigo Vespucci, who depict the Caribbean in conformity with Ovid's rhetoric about happy, simple, naked people without work, law, war or illness, living in a biblical or rather classical idyllic landscape with a vivid and fecund land where men had no adversities or discomforts (Levin 1969). The myth of the Golden Age seems to have been easily fused with the Judeo-Christian idea of Paradise, the same

42 For the influences of the worldview of classical antiquity on the accounts of Americas see Mason (1990) and Haase & Reinhold (1994).

motif that strongly charged the (in)famous voyage of Columbus to the New World (Levin 1969 in Lemaire 1986; Hofman 2008).

According to Lemaire, the West that Columbus was forced to head to (in his wish to arrive in China while avoiding the military presence of Islam in the East), was associated with Atlantis, and the garden of the Hesperides. During his first journey, Columbus (1492) admired Cuba as one of the most beautiful islands that his eyes had ever seen, full of very good ports and deep rivers, beautiful mountains, with calm seas, abundant fruits of amazing flavor, and singing birds. On several occasions Columbus calls the Gulf of Paria and La Vega (Cibao valley in the Dominican Republic) paradisiacal regions (Pérez Memén 2000). His account has traditionally been interpreted in the context of his agenda to promote the colonial enterprise. His explicit comparison of these lands with paradise might be understood as a common expression among believers but also as a real wish of a pious man to locate the Earthly Paradise. By renaming these Caribbean places according to European sacred referents, like Monte Cristi or Montserrat, Columbus clearly projected his worldview and knowledge of sacred European places onto the local landscapes, giving them new meanings by which these until then mysterious parts of the world became integrated into the European concept of Divine Creation.

The European values and beliefs are also displayed in the accounts about the original inhabitants of the islands. Columbus' description of the Lucayos, the most repeated description of Caribbean indigenous peoples, may serve as an example (1961 [1492]). In describing the way, he took possession of San Salvador in the name of the Spanish King and Queen and with a ceremony of gift exchange, Columbus portrayed the Lucayos as poor, naked, friendly, of good will and easy to be converted to Christianity. Since the exotic regions were, according to Mandeville's travel accounts, full of deformed creatures, such as antipodes, sciapods and anthropophagi, which Mandeville supposedly encountered during his journey to the East, Columbus emphasized the well-formed physique of the indigenous peoples of Greater Antilles (Mason 1990).[43] The emphasis on the form of the bodies might be also rooted in the beliefs of classical authors such as Pliny, Aristotle, and Hippocrates in physiognomy, according to which the physical appearance of people was seen as an indication of their character. Unlike D'Anghiera, Columbus viewed "the nakedness" of the natives not as an indication of their uncivilized nature but as a consequence of their poverty (1961 [1492]). Columbus' knowledge of the classical authors' writings about mysterious beings that were living in remote regions is apparent when he describes sirens (later identified as *manatís*) and cannibals (Columbus 1961).

Chanca's report (2011 [1494]) about the anthropophagi, which was based on the finding of four or five human bones in a house of the people called Caribes during the second voyage to the New World, can also be interpreted as having been influenced by Pliny's description of the Chalybes tribe. Pliny had already mentioned the Chalybes as people that feed on human bodies and that lived on some exotic islands centuries ealier. Although the members of Columbus' crew never witnessed anthropophagous practices, they rapidly interpreted the cultural elements they did not understand in

43 Mandeville's accounts are most likely based on Pliny's Natural History written more than a thousand years earlier (Mason 1990). For more on John Mandeville's travels see Macleod Higgins (1997).

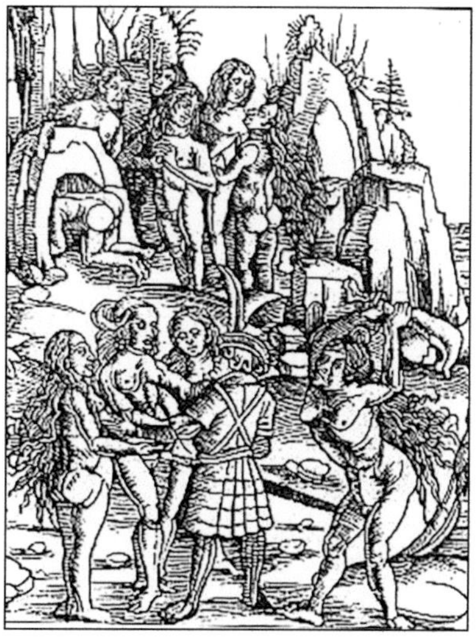

Figure 1 German Illustration from the Mundus Novus of Amerigo Vespucci (1509).

terms of their expectations, formed by such ancient images, and so reinforced their bias, which was later used as a justification for their enslavement. The fact that bones were removed from their original context may be interpreted in multiple ways, varying from secondary burial practices to forms of ancestral veneration. In contrast, the human bones deposited in the European churches were seen as relics of Saints, or ossuaries that contained a moral message.[44] Nevertheless, Chanca's colored portrayals appealed to European fantasies and fears about foreign others and had a lasting influence on subsequent accounts of indigenous peoples of the Lesser Antilles.

Soon after the discovery, the Caribbean islands became the region where all kinds of mysterious beings lived. Cannibals are said to be visiting Amazons living on Madanina, who like those women of Lesbos were dangerous to man, luring Spanish men into their caves (D´Anghiera 1992 [ca. 1505-1511], pp. 73-74, see Fig. 1). Considering the narrative registered by Friar Pané about Matinino as an island where the first ancestor left the first woman, these accounts might not be totally invented but inspired by the oral traditions of indigenous peoples and rephrased according to ancient Greek motives (Pané 2011 [1498]). At the same time, these narratives, as in the case of the *Sirenas*, might reflect more the European imagination than real observances or information obtained from the indigenous peoples of the Caribbean.

The first accounts of the Caribbean were quickly used as a justification for the conquest. Forty years before Columbus sailed to the Caribbean, Pope Nicholas V issued a Papal bull to the Portuguese King Alfonso V that all "saracens, pagans and other enemies of Christ" can be put into slavery, to take all their possessions and property (the bull Romanus Pontifex, Newcomb 1992). Acting on the bull, the Portuguese expanded their colonization in West Africa and enslaved the local inhabitants. Soon after Columbus' report on the Caribbean islands, the Spanish Catholic royals Isabel

44 One of the famous Spanish ossuaries is the one of St. Mary's Church in Wamba, on the pilgrimage route to Santiago de Compostela. The epitaph on one of the walls says: "As you look (now), I (once) looked. As you see me, you will look. All ends in this (form) here. Think about it and do not sin" (own translation).

and Ferdinand were granted possession of these lands by Pope Alexander VI (the bull of *Inter Cetera* 1493).[45] One group of the native inhabitants of these islands – those who welcomed the Europeans in a friendly manner – was described as people apt to be converted to Christianity and to become loyal vassals of the Spanish crown. They were depicted as unclothed, helpless people: their land was not defined in terms of formal ownership and land titles. Another group – the ones who resisted the invasion – were seen as warlike cannibals, enemies of free trade and true religion, and who also did not possess any rights. This dichotomy between peaceful Arawaks and warlike Caribs has been preserved in many historical sources until today (Hulme 1986).[46]

The religious bias towards peoples of different religious systems was often formulated in the rhetoric of Classical Antiquity. Peoples who were *not yet* Christians but were capable of being converted were described as if they were living in another time, in the case of the accounts about the Caribbean: in the Golden Age (see D'Anghiera ca. 1505-1511, p. 79*).*

The dismissal of any values associated with the beliefs and cultures of other peoples was convenient as it automatically justified the expropriation of the lands and later the establishment of the *encomienda* system.[47] The conversion would then also automatically civilize the peoples, and simultaneously give rights to the Catholic King and Queen over these lands. As Esteban Deive suggested, the *encomienda* was, in fact, disguised slavery (Deive 1980). The encomienda that legalized forced labor in the spirit of the salvation of the indigenous souls and became a justification of conquest.

Before the conversion, it had to be determined whether these peoples were even capable of it. The missionaries and encomenderos disagreed about whether the indigenous peoples were capable of being converted to the "true religion", and as such of becoming "civilized". Friar Ramon Pané was assigned to write about the beliefs of the natives in order to see if they could be instructed in the Christian faith. Pané (2011 [1498]) concluded that some of them, under strict supervision would be able to be converted in a mild way, whereas others needed to be persuaded by force. [48] To support his argument, Pané mentioned examples of conversions or miracles, which occurred during his stay with the indigenous peoples of Hispaniola. Distorted by his religious-political agenda and cultural bias, Pané's account is the only known first-hand information about indigenous worldview and origin narratives in the Greater Antilles.

45 See the "Demarcation Bull Granting Spain Possession of Lands Discovered" of Pope Alexander VI, reproduced with English translation in The Gilder Lehrman Collection *(www.gilderlehrman.org).*

46 Hulme (1986) summarized the big narrative as follows: *"The Caribbean islands had been populated first by the gentle agriculturalist Columbus had met on his first voyage, who turn out to have been called Arawaks; and then by the fierce, man-eating and nomadic Caribs, who were renowned for stealing Arawak women, and who over several centuries had chased their enemies up the chain of islands as far as Puerto Rico. The Island Arawak proved too fragile to resist the adversities of the Spanish presence, falling victim to the twin evils of new virus and enforced slavery, and rapidly died out. However the militant Island Carib defended their islands so ferociously that the Spaniards left them alone and turned their attention to Mexico"* (Hulme 1986, pp. 47-48). As Hulme suggests, much of this information is doubtful but it has been consistently repeated.

47 The *encomienda* was a legalization of servile labor, which in practice was very close to slavery (Sued Badillo 2003; Deive 1980).

48 In contrast, Oviedo for example argued that the indigenous peoples could not be converted. He claims that they were far removed from wanting to understand the Catholic faith, and this was conditioned literally by their physical characteristics: "just as their skulls are thick, so is their reasoning bestial and ill-intentioned as will be related further on with respect to those aspects of their rites, ceremonies, customs and other matters of some ilk as may occur to me (*Natural History* Lib.I, p. 125).

The base of the disputes about the ability to convert was disagreement about whether indigenous peoples of the Greater Antilles are slaves by nature or not. This dispute is also illustrative of how man and the environment were viewed by the Spaniards of this period as interrelated. Less than ten years after the Pope issued the first bull for land demarcation and appropriation for Spanish royals, the Dominican friar Antonio de Montesinos challenged the legitimacy of the harsh treatment of the natives of Hispaniola. Montesinos' preaching led to disputes about the legitimacy of enslavement, particularly in the Antilles, with Las Casas as the best-known defender of the indigenous peoples. Montesinos had to return to Spain to explain his position in front of a series of commissions and the Spanish king. There, the royal preacher Gregorio justified slavery by the Aristotelean argument that Caribbean peoples are slaves by nature their geographical position.[49]

The commission produced a document in which Queen Isabel insisted that indigenous peoples should be treated as free men while at the same time endorsing the *encomienda* system. This in the end resulted in the Laws of Burgos, which state that the principal obstacle in correcting the 'vices' of indigenous peoples would be the fact that their dwellings are remote from the settlements of the Spaniards: although they serve the Spanish, they return to their dwellings where they immediately forget what they have been taught and go back to their customary idleness and vices (The Laws of Burgos 1512). Instruction in the Catholic faith was promoted as being essential *"for the health and rescue of their souls"*.[50]

---

49 To summarize briefly, the aim of Aristoteles' argument about some people being slaves by nature was that barbarians were by nature slaves and Greeks by nature their masters. Berbers (name of the same origin as barbarians) of North Africa, the Turks, the Scythians, the Ethiopians, the Irish, the Vikings, the Germanic peoples, and European "pagans" (also Czech) all have been called barbarians. Aristotle's division between real citizens and natural slaves was based on the imperfect spiritual condition of the slave himself: inequality was seen as an inherent aspect of the order of the universe. In his view, the universe was characterized by a duality in which one element naturally dominates the other. In man the ruling element is intellect and the subordinate is passion. Natural man's intellect was dominated by his passions (Pagden, 1987, p. 42). The classic work on how the Aristotelean doctrine of natural slavery was used during this dispute is the book of Hanke (1959). In related vein, John Mair argued that the inhabitants of the Antilles were slaves by nature because they: *"live like beasts on either side of the equator; and beneath the poles there are wild men as Ptolemy says in his Tetrabiblos. And this has now been demonstrated by experience, wherefore the first person to conquer them, justly rules over them because they are by nature slaves. As the philosopher (Aristotle) says in his book the Politics, it is clear that some men are by nature slaves, others by nature free; and in some men there is a disposition to slavery and that they should benefit from it, by nature barbarians and slaves are the same."* (Pagden 1987: 38).

50 The instructions regarding the treatment of the indigenous peoples do not only include information about the position of the villages and the crops cultivated there, but also stipulate that every village should have a building to be used as a church, with an image of Our Lady and a bell where they could pray after the day of (forced) labor. The same document also decrees that the performance of their dances (*areítos*) should not be prevented, or else the indigenous peoples would cause great harm. If we were to interpret *areítos* as a means of transmitting the indigenous religious and historical teachings, this instruction paradoxically supported the continuity of the indigenous beliefs.
The emphasis on the instruction in the Catholic faith led to another directive: that all sons of chiefs from the island should be given to friars of the Order of St. Francis so that they might be taught; thus, after four years when returning to the *encomienda*, they might teach others. One year later it was requested in an amendment that the order of St. Dominicus amend the previous ordinances, that treatment of the indigenous women and children had to be gentler, and that those who became competent to live by themselves and lead a kind of Christian life would serve as Spanish vassals, paying tribute as is the custom in Spain (Doña Juana Amendments, 1513).

With the increasing complaints about the treatment of the *encomendados*, the Hieronymite Interrogatory of 1517 should provide a response to the question of the indigenous peoples of Hispaniola could live as free vassals and be placed in villages close to Spanish settlements for their protection. The testimony of the Hieronymits is unanimous in their agreement about the inability of the natives to govern themselves; their self-government in liberty would mean that they would continue to practice their religious ceremonies and dances (*areítos*), and establish new settlements far away from (and beyond the control of) the Spanish population (Anderson-Cordova 1990). Without a doubt, these "testimonies" were biased by the interest in the benefits that the Spanish would receive from the continued indigenous enslavement. However, it is likely that during this period much of the indigenous worldview was still remembered and was in the process of becoming reinterpreted as a result of religious encounters with other belief systems, including those originating from West and Central Africa. It is also to be assumed that the acceptance of Catholic beliefs varied greatly among individuals and communities, some indigenous people converted to Catholicism (especially those who were instructed in it from early childhood), some went obligatorily to church, while preserving their own worldviews, and others were never baptized.

Following Montesino's appeal for religious conversion and treatment of indigenous ancestors, Las Casas (1556) depicted Hispaniola as fertile and full of natural resources, arguing that these were favorable conditions, in Aristotelean terms, for the natives to have a soul and be rational beings. Following Columbus' idea that somewhere there should be a paradise port, Las Casas states that actually the entire island looks like an earthly paradise (La Casas 1566, Vol. 1, Book 1, Cap. 2).[51] This qualification would create even more contrast with the crimes that the Spanish colonizers had committed in the Indies, the main issue that Las Casas tried to denounce. Later, in 1552, he published his observations and ideas in *A Very Short Account of the Destruction of the Indies.*

The climax in the discussion about the legitimacy of the Spanish conquest was the Valladolid debate (1550 – 1551) between Las Casas, "the Protector of the Indians", and Sepúlveda, a chaplain and defender of Spanish empire's right of conquest. Sepúlveda argued that the natives were natural slaves as defined by Aristotle, and that it is legitimate to save those endangered by human sacrifices, to end and exorcise the crimes of the man-eaters, and to wage war against infidels. Las Casas opposed him in pointing out that Aristotle's model of the natural slave cannot be applied to the indigenous peoples, using Vitoria's argument that natives are reasonable in their own way.[52] In his

51 In contrast, Bernardo de Mesa used the insular position of Caribbean indigenous ancestors as the argument for depicting them as barbarians and therefore natural slaves (Pagden 1987, p. 48). According to Mesa´s view: *"their nature does not allow them to have perseverance in the virtue, which is due to their insular position naturally less persistent, because the moon is the lady of the waters, in whose center they inhabit, this causes vicious habits that they incline to similar acts"* (cited by Las Casas 1986 [ca. 1557], p. 35). The inconsistencies of his argument were easily pointed out by Las Casas (*ibid.*), who argued that, if true, the same should apply to peoples of England, Sicily, Candía, and the Baleares because these peoples also live on islands where the moon controls the waters.

52 Vitoria, theologian, jurist and professor at University of Salamanca states that the hypothesis of Aristoteles about natural slavery cannot be applied to indigenous peoples because even though they seem to be without reason they are still capable of reasoning given that they have cities, laws and ...

opinion, they could not be barbarians because that would be in conflict with nature, as everything in nature was normally perfect as created by God.[53]

As part of his defense, Las Casas tends to overemphasize the characteristics of indigenous peoples being easy to obey, serve, and convert to the Roman Catholic religion. Las Casas (1552) describes the indigenous peoples as the humblest of God's creatures, the most peaceful, who lack hatred or desire for revenge. According to him, they were also a very delicate people, who die easily because of hard work or illnesses, as they were poor people without property, ambitions or greediness. All these arguments fitted in with his plea that these peoples were capable of receiving the Christian faith. Las Casas did not mind whether they themselves wanted to, because as father of the children he would know what was best for them. This argument about the fragile nature of the indigenous peoples together with the harsh treatment under the encomienda system have served as a main reason for the prohibition of *encomienda (New Laws 1542)*, and later also as an explanation for the rapid disappearance of the indigenous population in the Greater Antilles. Even after the prohibition of the *encomienda* system, indigenous people could still be enslaved if they were captured while resisting Spanish authority or accused of cannibalism.

Las Casas' influence is notable in various chronicles, present-day historiography and cultural memory. Las Casas is one of the standard references for those who argue that the indigenous peoples in the Caribbean became rapidly extinct, and his work, frequently used by later authors, forms part of the present-day educational system. Benzoni, in his *La Historia del Mondo Novo* (1565), for example, extended Las Casas' criticism of the Spanish crimes in the Americas; his work happens to be the major inspiration for de Bry's *Grand Voyages* (1590-1634), images from which are frequently used as illustrations in many popular books and museum exhibitions (see Figures 2 and 3).[54]

...commerce (referring to the states of Mesoamerica and the Andes). Even their capacities and qualities were somehow lacking in comparison with Europeans as demonstrated by the (supposed) presence of cannibalism, human sacrifices, sodomy and the lack of literacy, yet they had enough attributes to be called human and as such they could not be natural slaves (Pagden, 1987; Lemaire, 1986). While criticizing the violent religious conquest of the natives, Vitoria still believed that to intervene in their countries in order to exercise the right of guardianship was just. In this way he anticipated the European attitude of later periods treating America (and Africa) as an immature continent (Todorov 1982, p. 149).

53 Las Casas (1552/1966, pp. 33 -34) writes: *"Todas estas universas e infinitas gentes, a todo género crio Dios los más humildes, más pacientes, más pacíficas y quietas: sin rencillas ni bullicios, no rijosos, no querellosos, sin rencores, sin odios, sin desear venganzas que hay en el mundo... "*

54 Different illustrations were published earlier, already since 1565. For the history of the publication of different engravings see the Introduction of the edition of 1979. The accompanying text of the illustration nr. 2 argues that Balboa conquered the prince (cacique) of Esquaragua with his subjects because they were dressed up in women's clothes. He considered it such a sin that he took about forty prisoners and let his dogs devour them *(Bry 1594/1979)*. Fig. 3 illustrates how de Bry engraved Oviedo's description of a religious ceremony on the island of Hispaniola. The accompanying text describes how during this feast a procession led by the cacique was guided to the temple of a behique where the statue of a zemí was located, and accompanied by drumming, singing of traditional songs, festive attires, purging, and offerings. The statement that the being to which these offerings were brought was Cacodaemon, the devil, shows de Bry´s difficulty in understanding the indigenous religion..

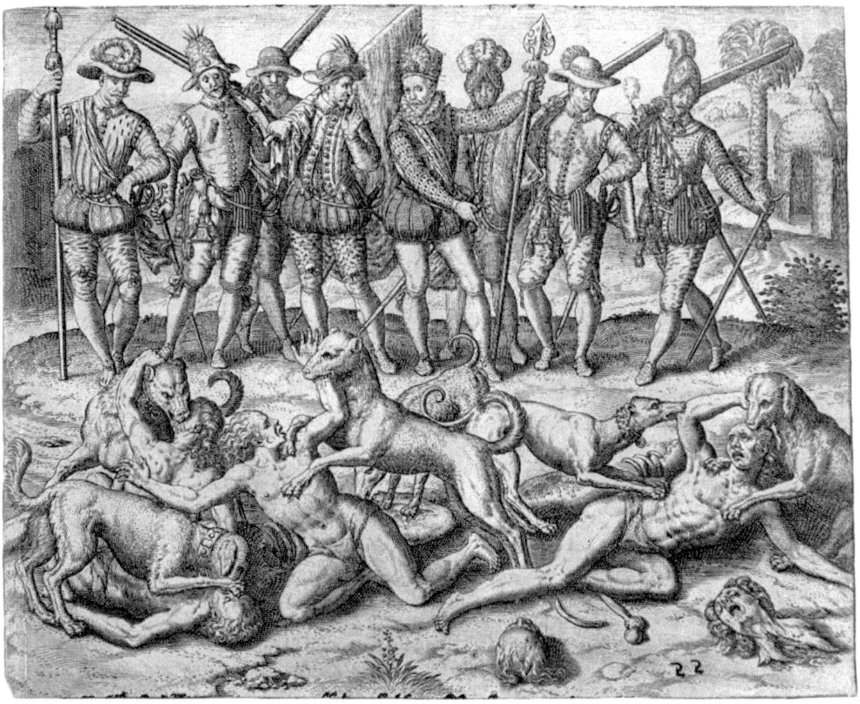

Figure 2 The dogs of Vasco Nuñez de Balboa attacking indigenous peoples by de Bry (1594/1979).

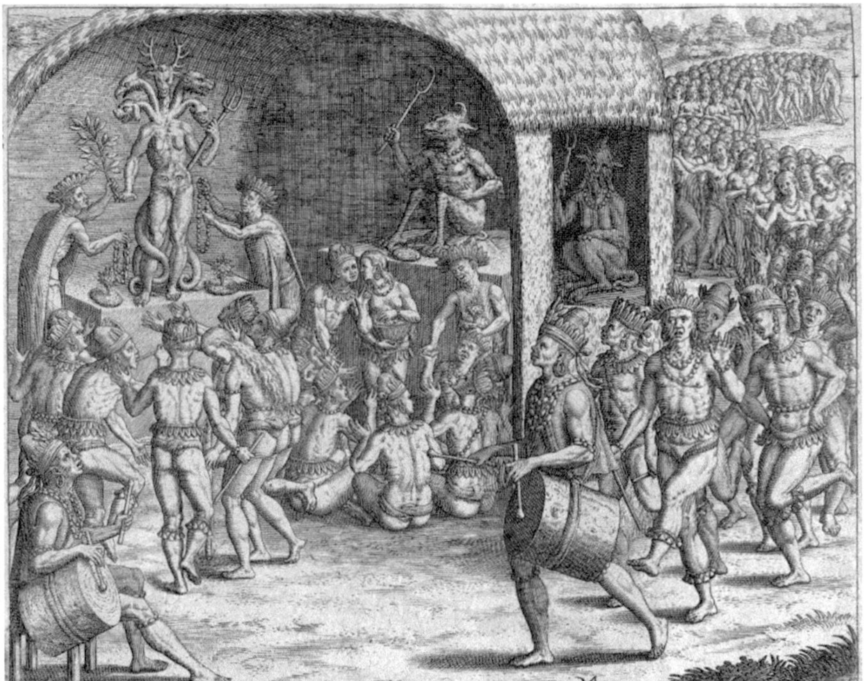

Figure 3 De Bry's (1594-1595/1979) illustration based on Oviedo's treatise about the religion of peoples in the West Indies.

The noble savage idea in Lesser Antilles

While the reports about the Arawak, Carib and Tupi peoples in the coastal area of South America as well as the Aztecs of Mexico and the Incas of the Andean world set the tone for the discussions about indigenous peoples in the 16th century, the encounter with the North American natives was crucial in the next phase of the theorization about the development of human nature and society, and about the relationship between culture and environment (Lemaire 1986; Mitchell & Scheiber 2010). Over the course of the 17th century, the dichotomies barbarian vs. civilized and pagan vs. Christian were replaced by the opposition of natural man vs. citizen. This tendency is particularly characteristic of the works of Hobbes and Locke.[55] Their opinions have precedents in the colonists' arguments in Hispaniola and Cuba.

By the middle of the 18th century, differences among people were explained by schemas that combined long outdated 'conjectural prehistories' with more recent ideas about cultural and biological evolution that brought all humans under one progressivist unilineal historical continuum. The non-European cultures were categorized according to the absence or presence of European technological traits and modes of subsistence (McNiven & Russel 2005, p. 38 – 42). Over the course of the 18th century, depending on the agenda of the author in question, the other is again dehumanized as brutish barbarian or romanticized as a noble savage, which had been earlier described in the rhetoric of a Golden Age. The most prominent writers that applied the latter idea to the Caribbean were Jean-Baptiste Du Tertre (1667) and Jean Jacques Rousseau (1751).[56] Rousseau, drawing on Du Tertre, popularized the concept of the noble savage (see Hulme 1986).

Rousseau's objective – criticizing French society, comparing it to examples from other cultures, in order to improve it – is not as problematic as the way in which the author expressed his arguments. In his view, the indigenous peoples of the Lesser Antilles remained in the past, being at a different stage of development.[57] In evaluating the current promotions of environmental protection, on the one hand, and of neoco-

---

55 Hobbes applied the idea of the savage to North American peoples, which he called natural men who lacked knowledge or morals. Hobbes argued that their character was comparable to that of prehistoric Europeans: both were considered closer to nature than the contemporaneous Europeans. Placed back in time, indigenous peoples in Hobbes' account are like Las Casas', not yet in the same historical phase as the Europeans. This opinion intersects with the first modern ideas about the history of religion, in which animism is often placed as preceding "real religions". Unlike Hobbes, Locke considered the state of nature as a state in which people are placed by God and are free and equal if they behave in accordance with the norms of natural law, governed by reason. In his classic *Second Treatise* (1690) on property, he argued that the earth is the communal property of all humans; every person has a property right when his labor raises the value of the object. Although he admitted that hunting and collecting was a way of modifying the state of nature, he did not consider it to be a proper use. His lack of knowledge about native agriculture (or lack of willingness to investigate this further) led him to legitimize the expropriation of the indigenous lands by European colonizers.

56 Du Tertre described Caribbean indigenous inhabitants as the true youth of the world resembling the earlier Golden Age motif. Du Tetre imagined these as: *"the happiest, the least vicious, the most sociable, the least deformed, and the least afflicted by disease in the whole world. For they are just as nature produced them, that is to say living in great and natural simplicity: they all equal, almost without knowledge of any sort of superiority or servitude [...] they are all of a good build, well proportioned, large and powerful, so energetic and healthy that it is common to see amongst them old men of a hundred or a hundred and twenty [...] who have hardly any white hair, their foreheads marked by hardly a wrinkle* (Du Tertre as cited in Hulme 1986, p. 230).

57 For the most recent insights into complex transformations of indigenous peoples of Leeward Islands see Mans (2018).

lonial exploitation on the other, we should be aware of this long tradition of pervasive colonial discourse, well established in classic works.

During the Enlightenment, colonial knowledge about the indigenous peoples of the Americas contributed to new thoughts about human nature and its development. Using colonial data to support their arguments, evolutionists transformed the biological and cultural divide established by colonial discourses into a temporal and structural divide (Mitchell & Scheiber 2010). Evolutionary developmental schemas referred to other cultures as living examples of the early stages of human development and to Europeans as progressive producers of history (McNiven & Russel 2005, p. 12). Europeans were characterized as literate and civilized, in opposition to the illiterate natives who were bound by their traditions and customs, which, being incompatible with future progress, were forecasting their imminent extinction.

The first academic works about indigenous heritage in the Dominican context were produced in the 19th century and according to them the indigenous peoples were representatives of the first phase of human development (for an overview see Ulloa Hung 2016). Even after Cuban (1902) struggles for independence from Spain, the regions were faced with series of periods of oppression such the neocolonial occupation of the US in Cuba (1899-1902), Platt Amendment (1901-1934), Machado's (1925-1939) or Batista's dictatorships (1952-1959), and others including the US embargo (since 1960 until present). Similarly, after the Dominican (1821) struggles for independence Dominicans were soon faced with the Haitian occupation (1822-1844), US military interventions (1916-1924, 1965-66), or Trujillo's dictatorship (1930-1961). The following examples will show that also revisionist studies of these later periods did not manage to escape to perpetuate of the colonial discourse.

Indigenous past as the beginning of the Dominican nation

References to indigenous ancestors should be seen in the light of the turbulent years of nation-building. The Haitian revolution (1791 – 1804) posed a great ideological threat to the slave-holding states of the Americas. While this historical event was a positive symbol of emancipation and the end of a crime against humanity for many, in the Dominican context this was overshadowed by the Haitian occupation of the Dominican state, which followed soon after the revolution and as such left a profound imprint on the construction of the Dominican national identity.

One of its leaders of the movement for independence, Juan Pablo Duarte, aimed to integrate the Dominican nation, while differentiating the population from the Haitians by extolling its Hispanic identity, its allegiance to Catholicism and its relative whiteness. In their quest for an own national identity, the founders of the Dominican nation drew on the indigenous ancestors as a factor that distinguished them from Haitians and Spaniards (García Arévalo 2008).

The *indigenismo* of this period represented for many a glorification of the extinct peoples which should be recovered and acknowledged as symbols of the real authentic origin of the nation, while others saw *indigenismo* as a movement that obscured – for ideological reasons – the participation of the slaves of African descent, who should be considered more fundamental to the Dominican historical processes (García Arevalo

2008).[58] Both currents in this regard follow the traditional colonial racial categories, which equate race with cultural knowledge, and simplify the intercultural dynamics at the outset of the historical becoming of the Dominican society.

During the Trujillo´s Era (1930 – 1961), the indigenous history was represented in an opposition to the African roots of their Haitian neighbors. The term "indio" was generalized in the Dominican self-perception in a way that changed the category "mulato" into "indio oscuro".[59] Trujillo's discriminatory policies of racial purification, exiling dark skinned Haitians, culminated in 1937 in a Persley massacre of thousands of Haitians. This horrific event is still very much alive in the memory of the people, and is recalled again and again, especially during the statelessness crisis when the official authorities threated with large-scale deportation of peoples of Haitian origin. Trujillo's racist policies were extended by Joaquín Balaguer, president of the Dominican Republic for 16 years until 1986. In his Eurocentric discourse, he profiled the Dominican citizen as a Hispanic Christian white man, and blamed Haitians for "ethnic decadence". In this light, it is clear that the studies on the indigenous history or heritage have been haunted by the social context wherein ideologies were present that do not fit into the value system of a democratic society.

Indigenous ancestors during the formation of the Cuban nation

The reference and identification with Cuban indigenous ancestors was also central in the construction of Cuban national identity as distinct from the traditional colonial masters, as well as from that of the later U.S. occupiers (Catá Backer 2008) or of the US imperial imposition of the embargo after the revolution.

Continuing with the idea noble savages, José Martí (1889) idealized Cuban natives as premature unspoiled fruits of nature and portrayed them as passive, immature, fragile, simple, innocent infants, needy children, without clothes, unable to protect themselves and in need of a protector (Martí 1889).[60]

---

58 One of the prominent Dominican historians Moya Pons (2008) describes this situation as follows: *"By calling themselves Indians, Dominicans have been able to provisionally resolve the profound drama that filled the most of their history: that of being a colored nation ruled by quasi-white elite that did not want to accept the reality of its color and the history of race. Somehow the Dominicans assimilated the romantic discourse of the indigenista writers of the 19th century, and found it instrumental in accommodating their racial self-perception to the prejudices of the elite, by accepting their "color" while denying "their race"* (Moya Pons 2008, pp. 141 -142).

59 Rafael Leónidas Trujillo Molina (1891 -1961) was a Dominican dictator, who ruled the Dominican Republic until his assassination in May 1961. It is estimated that his rule caused approximately 50,000 victims – possibly more than half of them in the infamous Parsley Massacre.

60 The following is a part of the Martí's La edad de oro (1889) Las ruinas Indias: *"Unos [indigenas] vivían aislados y sencillos, sin vestidos y sin necesidades, como pueblos acabados de nacer; y empezaban a pintar sus figuras extrañas en las rocas de la orilla de los ríos, donde es más solo el bosque, y el hombre piensa más en las maravillas del mundo. Otros eran pueblos de más edad, y vivían en tribus, en aldeas de cañas o de adobes, comiendo lo que cazaban y pescaban, y peleando con sus vecinos. Otros eran ya pueblos hechos, con ciudades de ciento cuarenta mil casas, y palacios adornados de pinturas de oro. Y gran comercio en las calles y en las plazas, y templos de mármol con estatuas gigantescas de sus dioses. Sus obras no se parecen a las de los demás pueblos, sino como se parece un hombre a otro. Ellos fueron inocentes, supersticiosos y terribles. Ellos imaginaron su gobierno, su religión, su arte, su guerra, su arquitectura, su industria, su poesía. Todo lo suyo es interesante, atrevido, nuevo. Fue una raza artística, inteligente y limpia. Se leen como una novela las historias de los nahuatles y mayas de ...*

Influenced by European romanticism and nationalism, Latin American *indigenismo* views the indigenous peoples as relics of the past and identified with them in order to distance themselves from a foreign oppressor, and to exalt the beauty of nature, to which the indigenous peoples were seen as being very close (see Fornaris 1862), to compare the situation of the young nation with the oppressed first inhabitants.

The limited access to the archives in Spain led to a reliance on the writings of Las Casas, which were considered the most critical of colonial oppression. Las Casas' critiques of Spanish crimes, together with his account of the Hatuey, proclaiming that he would rather go to Hell than Heaven if the Spanish should go to heaven, have been until now adopted as a symbol of the first martyr and defender of the fatherland against foreign domination (Catá Becker 2008).

After the Cuban Revolution, drawing on the writings of Martí, Fidel Castro used the indigenous resistance as an example in one of his speeches in 1985 commemorating the Cuban revolution. Like Hatuey, the first warrior, first leader, and first martyr of the fatherland, Cubans should fight against these intrusions (Catá Becker 2008).

The indigenous past in Dominican and Cuban History textbooks

Formal education is one of the important building blocks of the collective memory about the indigenous past. Educational institutions provide one of the major mechanisms through which power is maintained and challenged (Preiswerk & Perrot 1978). Together with teachers´ beliefs (see Aguilar 2018) history textbooks are one of the elements of the education systems that perpetuate specific perceptions and representations, presenting them as historical facts.

When reviewing the content of Cuban and Dominican history textbooks (Vargas 2002, 2007, Callejas Opisso 2010, Albelo Ginnart et al. 2011) it is clear that these have the difficulty to move away from the vocabulary and ideas present in the colonial sources or the later works of the 19th century *indigenistas*.[61] In short, these texts often rely uncritically on historical sources (*e.g.* Las Casas) as the only authority with respect to indigenous history. Often they portrayed these ancestors in Eurocentric visions of fixed historical developments and include direct citations of some early sixteen century texts without historical contextualization.

The textbooks should not be considered in a socio-political vacuum and in isolation from the practices of school teaching, and other forms of formal education including the role of museums, literature, monuments, and media.[62] This might include the institutionally driven commemoration but also more private ways how peoples relate to the

---

...México, de los chibchas de Colombia, de los cumanagotos de Venezuela, de los quechuas del Perú, de los aimaraes de Bolivia, de los charrúas del Uruguay, de los araucanos de Chile." Martí's remarks on indigenous resistance are as follows: "*Running away to the mountains where they were defending themselves 'with stone and water jumping the streams from shore to shore firing the spears.*" Martí´s argument was not the same for other Latin American states where he acknowledge the importance of indigenous peoples in the nation-building.

61 For a recent work on the influence of teachers' beliefs on teaching indigenous history and heritage in the Caribbean see Con Aguilar (2018).

62 Some of the problematic aspects of Dominican museology have been addressed by Alvarez (2017). Monuments like the Columbus statue in front of Santo Domingo's Cathedral, Columbus' Lighthouse, and other monumental architecture in Santo Domingo all commemorate in a certain way the European ...

past. The latter can be expressed in oral traditions and other cultural practices within landscapes with many material imprints of the indigenous ancestors. Some of such views are presented in Part II.

The colonial bias has been also influential in studies of and attitudes towards Caribbean religions and medicine. Terms such as witch, evil, idols, superstitions, ghost stories, or backward are often associated with medicinal cultures of the historically marginalized ancestors. The ongoing religious intolerance, adherence to different religious systems and secularization can further help to perpetuate the colonial bias existent in attitudes towards healers, their practices and our ancestral history. The contemporary healing and its history entails a great amount of historical, environmental, medicinal, and knowledge. Regardless own religious beliefs, the medicinal history and ogoing healing traditions offer us great opportunity to learn and reflect upon the ancestral values which are often encoded in religious methaphores and symbols.

The Alienation from Natural Man in the collective memory

In the meantime, several scholars, such as Sued Badillo (1978), Lemaire (1986), Mason (1990), Keegan & Bright (2008), Hofman & Duivenbode (2011), Hulme (1986), Whitehead et al. (1995) Keegan & Hofman (2017), Ulloa Hung & Válcarcel Rojas (2016), have addressed critically the stereotypical image of indigenous peoples of the Lesser and Greater Antilles. While the notion of Carib as warlike cannibals has been discussed on several occasions, the descriptions of the Arawak have been left unchallenged. This might be due to the seemingly positive characteristics of the Arawak as having a peaceful and gentle nature. This picture becomes more problematic when used as an explanation for the rapid extinction, cultural change or uncritical reproduction in the current knowledge system. This image can also lead to alienation from one's own past when phrased according to Eurocentric visions of history as rooted in a particular land and connected to a particular group of people. The past and ongoing archeological and historical research about the indigenous peoples of the Caribbean has been a valid contribution in deconstructing simplified pictures of Caribbean first inhabitants (*e.g.* Hofman et al. 2014; Keegan et al. 2013; Keegan & Hofman 2017). Different community outreach activities have been initiated to address these colonial biases for the indigenous peoples in the Caribbean context (see *e.g.* Hofman & Haviser 2015; Rodriguéz Ramos & Pagán Jiménez 2016; Con Aguilar et al. 2017). More recent studies have begun to provide new insights into complex indigenous cultural transformation in the colonial period (for an overview see Valcárcel Rojas 2014, 2016). These have helped to nuance the big narrative of rapid indigenous extinction, failed transculturation and such have open to discussion of indigenous legacies in medicinal histories. The next chapter summarizes some of the historical sources regarding the medicine in the studied regions, paying special attention to the role of indigenous ancestors.

...colonization but not necessarily those who were colonized. While there are some memorials dedicated to those who offered resistance, such as Lemba or Enrique, more investigations should be conducted into the ways whether and how the life of those subjected during colonialism are memorized.

4

Empty Pages in the Biography of Healing Landscapes

The previous chapter showed how the early colonial European accounts of the Caribbean landscapes and peoples are power saturated. The chapter 4 briefly summarizes some of available information on the indigenous co-authorship in medicinal histories and situates this within the broader colonial material and conceptual landscape transformations. The majority of data in this chapter come from a few of written documents, which are to be complemented and contrasted with ethnographic fieldwork and archaeological information.[63]

The medicinal histories of the Caribbean are not to be reduced to the arrival of the first European graduated physiciants or the establishment of first medical institutes. The rich pool of knowledge of present-day healers has a long history which is clearly power saturated. The Catholicism and medicinal cultures of 16th century were powerful tools for extending the ideologies (be it religious, political or otherwise) of the Spanish state. This power was, however, often far from being fully implemented in practice in the colonies.[64]

The success of colonization was closely related to the health situation in the colonies. Physicians were inseparable members of crews on voyages crossing the Atlantic Ocean. During his first trip, Columbus brought one or two physicians and an apothecary, one of who was left at La Navidad. During the second journey, physician Chanca arrived and stayed for six years at La Isabela. Few years later, Nicolás de Ovando, the governor of Hispaniola (1501-1509), let build a hospital in Santo Domingo where poor people, Christians, and indigenous peoples could be treated together.[65]

Some hospitals such as the one in Santo Domingo or in Habana relied on labor of enslaved people of local and non-local origins (Gómez 2017; Sáez 1997).[66] One of the interesting cases is that of Bernarda Álvarez, a *mulata* from Santo Domingo who was

63 The medicinal history of the Cuban island has been briefly described by Górdon y de Acosta (1894) and López Sánchez (1550-1730).

64 See on this topic also Foster (1960).

65 *De La Instrucción del Gobernador Nicolas de Ovando sobre el gobierno de las Indias.*

66 San Nicolás of Santo Domingo, later Yaguana. Cuban hospitals were located in Havana, Trinidad, Sancti Espiritus, Santa Clara, San Juan de los Remedios, Puerto Príncipe, Holguín, Bayamo (San Roque), Santiago de Cuba, Consolación. More studies are needed to assess the role of the brotherhoods and indigenous peoples in these establishement.

accused in Cartagena of poisoning a man; she was punished with four years of exile and two years working in the hospital of San Sebastian (Crespo Vargas 2011). Another case was that of a *mulata* woman from Puerto Rico who worked in a Havana hospital, and was later accused of instructing other women in Habana: her art consisted in giving herbs for wellbeing, in predicting the future and in bringing good fortune in different manners (Crespo Vargas 2011). Inventories of possessions of hospitals and convents reveals endemic but also exotic plants were used to create cures. Together these references indicate that hospitals as well as convents were also loci of medicinal exchanges.

Medicinal cultures of the 16th century Spanish Caribbean were of heterogeneous character, including a plurality of actors of local and non-local origins. Physicians, surgeons and apothecaries coming from overseas were trained in works from Classical Antiquity and the Arabic world. Greek works such as *Dioscorides' Materia médica* (1st century AD), containing more than six hundred medicinal plants and more than two hundred remedies of animal or mineral origin from the Mediterranean, was very popular in Medieval and Renaissance Spain.[67]

Next to institutional physicians, Spanish healers found their way to the Caribbean. Spanish healers could cure and repel all kinds of misfortune, dissipating storms, combating plagues, and even transforming things and beings (Tausiet 2010). Although belief in their powers varied, even the most skeptical agreed that some men by the grace of God were able to heal through their devotion, by laying on hands and reciting prayers. In addition, 16th century Spain had many enpsalmers, conjurers of clouds, necromancers, but also priests who warded off illnesses, plagues, and hailstorms by using prayers (Christian 1989). Some of these practitioners are still remembered in Cuban and Dominican rural areas in today (see Part II).

In accordance of teaching of Hippocrates it was believed that as illnesses and as such also their remedies were locally specific. Physicians sent to the Indies were instructed to contact other physicians, *herbolarios*, (explicitly said to be both Spanish and Indigenous) in order to learn their art, to write about medicinal flora and to report their observations to the Crown (Real Cédula de Felipe II, Madrid 11 1570). An example is Lic. Juan Mendéz Nieto, who worked as a physician in Santo Domingo, where he observed the flaws of the medicinal care in the colony but also indigenous practices related to childbearing and childbirth, which he evaluated as more suitable than the Spanish practices (1611).[68] In addition, European physicians of later periods such as Sloane (1707), Chateusalins (1854) and other doctors from plantantions recorded oc-

---

67 Among the mentioned plants are: *Arnica montana* L., *Atropa belladona* L., *Cassia fistula* L., *Prunus lauro-cerasus* L., *Ruta graveolens* L., *Zingiber officinale* and many others. Cf. A. Laguna Pedacio, *Dioscorides Anazarbeo acerca de la materia medicinal y de los venenos mortíferos*, Amberes, J. Latio, 1555. Available at https://www.wdl.org/es/item/10632/.

68 On the childbirth of Mariana de Bacán from Santo Domingo, who died because of improper treatment during the delivery, causing overheating and later death: *"Y desta manera no paría en aquella tierra megueres de suerte y ponderosa que no la matava la cura y regalo que le azían, y, si algunas escapaban, eran las que, por más no poder, carecían deste regalo y cura, como las negras e yndias y la demás gente pobre que, por no tener con qué abrigar, no moría ny se pasmava persona de todas ellas. Y con ver esto y con ver que las yndias, ansý desta costa como las del Nuevo Reyno Granada, a donde hace poco menos frío que en España, lavan las madres su hijos y se lavan ellas mismas, en acabando de parir, en arroyos de agua frigidíssima, de las cuales asta oy no se á visto alguna dellas pasmada, no podía acabar de persuadir, ansý al vulgo como a sus médicos, que ellos eran homecidas..."* (Mendéz Nieto 1610, p. 209).

casionally remedies used by the Afro-Caribbean ancestors. In short, the health care in the colonies relied greatly also on healing specialists of both local and non-local origin.

The profound demographic changes triggered by the colonization of the island implied that non-local healing specialists were faced with landscapes of unknown flora, places and peoples. Before discussing specific ways of how the botanical knowledge was circulated in the colonies, I will present some ideas about how the Caribbean predecessors reshaped the contemporary landscapes in material and conceptual ways. The existing medicinal practices discussed in later part of this dissertation should be seen as developed in close relation to these large scale transformations which co-created meanings of Caribbean places, flora and other landscape features which are today employed in the healing practices.

Indigenous ancestors transforming Caribbean Landscapes

In contrast to what the accounts about the existence of a pristine wilderness might suggest, Caribbean landscapes have been altered for millennia before the European conquest (Pagán-Jiménez 2013; Siegel 2015; Fitzpatrick & Keegan 2007; Siegel et al. 2018; Siegel 2018). In fact, the peopling of the Caribbean went hand in hand with the dispersal of plants[69], the cultivation of different introduced plants in *conucos*, clearings of the forests (as early as 5400 – 2500 BP Higuera-Gundy et al. 1999), construction of raised fields (agricultural mounds) and irrigation canals (Hofman et al. 2018; Pagán-Jiménez 2013; Rodríguez Ramos & Pagán-Jiménez 2013).[70] The human migration to the Caribbean has been accompanied also by practices and worldviews which redefined the meaning of newly encountered places (see Pagán-Jimenéz 2007) and implied reevaluation of environmental affordances (including those of religious character) for the health.

Historical sources have left us only fragmentary references to indigenous worldviews, their views of surrounding landscapes and their healing system(s). Modern investigations of indigenous worldviews in the Greater Antilles have until now strongly relied on origin narratives recorded by Friar Ramon Pané. Although Pané's account is a valuable primary source of information, it has considerable limitations as to its documentation of ideas about healing landscapes. First, the main goal of Pané's work was dictated by the assignment to establish whether indigenous peoples had a religion or not. As a result, he produced a sketch of a complex worldview summarized in a few pages. In addition, the author faced various obstacles when writing his account;

69 From historical records it is clear that certain species were objects of inter-island exchanges. To illustrate, D'Anghiera describes that people of Hispaniola exchanged with peoples from other surrounding islands, *aroma* trees for other objects they desired such as ceramic plates, *duhos* (wooden seats), and other items produced from materials that were lacking on their own island, (D'Anghiera, Décadas del Nuevo Mundo, 1494 -1526, Libro VII). The pan-regional mobility of pre-colonial Caribbean ancestors were confirmed by archaeological findings from the pre-colonial period (e.g. Hofman & Bright 2010; Hofman & Duivenbode 2011; Hofman et al. 2007; Hofman et al. 2018; Rodríguez Ramos 2007, 2010).

70 Among the plants brought by indigenous peoples to the West Indies are amaranth (Amaranthus spp.), peanut (Arachis hypogaea), common bean (*Phaseolus spp.*), manioc (*Manihot esculenta*), potato (*Ipomoea batatas)*, cotton (Gossypium spp.) squash (*Cucurbita maxima*), bottle gourd (*Lagenaria siccerraria*) and tobacco (*Nicotiana tabacum*) (Scarre 1999, p. 78). Beans, maize, pineapple, peanuts are not endemic and required systematic cultivation.

there were his own linguistic limitations, which made it difficult to interpret what his interlocutors told him in what most likely was a poetic idiom, full of metaphors and symbolic expressions. As Pané writes, the indigenous peoples of Española had their *"antique songs through which they are governed, like the moros through the script"* (2011 [ca. 1498], p. 94). Secondly, some information was likely to be filtered out by this foreign priest on purpose, because of misunderstandings and other flaws of intercultural communication. Lastly, the fact that the text has only been preserved in later translations complicates its precise reconstruction and comprehension.

However limited, some passages of this text give us first impressions about indigenous ideas about human-nature relatedness, values of certain landscape features and beliefs regarding the illness. Some narratives address situations in which the boundaries between the divine and nature could be crossed and so illustrate their relationality. The sea originated from the remains of Gaigaiel (Arrom´s Yayael), the child of the divine being Gaigai (Arrom´s Yaya). These boundaries are also crossed in references to turtle-women who came forward from a swelling of Demian Caracaracol, children-like-beings turned into frogs-like-animals, or human-like-beings turned into guanin.[71]

Certain sites, such as caves, are said to be places of origin of primordial or divine beings, for example the sun and the moon. The sun and moon are said to have enjoyed great respect. About one of the caves in Hispaniola Pané writes: *"they hold the cave (where the sun and moon came out) in a great esteem, and they paint it all over in their own way, without any human figure, with many leaves and similar things. And in said cave there were two cimini made of stone, half an arm big with the hands tied, and they looked as if they were seating; and they had them in great esteem; and when there was drought they say that they went to visit the cave, and it rained at once. And of said cimini one is called Boinaiol and the other Maroia"* (Pané 2011 [ca. 1498], p. 92). Besides caverns, the category of religiously significant places included sites related to the agency of specific *zemís* (divinities and culture heroes), places where the dead depart, or the house of cimiche where offerings were brought.[72] Pané mentioned all of these only vaguely.[73]

The indigenous perceptions landscape as animated seems to articulated also through various zemís who were said to be represented by, are identical with or control some of the environmental forces like rain, winds or storms, as well as plants: *"there are some zemís that speak, which are shaped like big turnip with the leaves lying on the ground, and as long as those of the caper; their leaves are generally shaped like the elm leaf; and other have three tips, and they say that these make the yucca produce"*(Pané 2011 [ca. 1498],

71 Note that Fernández de Oviedo mentions that the hobo tree was used as a source of drinking water in situations when the water was scarce. This information is stated to have been learned from indigenous people. The baths with the tree bark were noted as very healthy and relaxing, especially for tired legs (Fernández de Oviedo 1535/2000).

72 In Whitehead's translation (2011) keeps the variation of certain words such as cimini, cimiche as mentioned in the original. Arrom (1974) transcribed this word as zemi, this term is also more widespread in the Caribbean literature. In Lokono *semi* means shaman.

73 According to Oviedo (1535/1851) the images of *zemís* were deposited in the houses and dark places that were reserved for prayer. In addition, some zemís are said to depart to places near the village or a lagoon. Zemi Guamorete after his house was burned down went to a place that is a bowshot distant from the village. Similarly, zemí Opieyelguobirán escaped after the Spanish came and went to a lagoon. From the text it is difficult, however, to discern whether these places had any symbolic or sacred meaning. These places could just be referred to because they were loci of the narrative.

p. 111). Pané's multiple references to the plants *digo, güeyo, sacon, guayaba, guanaba/ guabasa/mamey* might indicate both their cultural importance and even ritual significance (*e.g.* guava as one of forms in which ancestors could manifest).

These are only snippets of the pre-colonial worldview, but when his account is read in relation to present-day Arawakan speaking groups from the mainland, we notice that different components of the landscape are likely to be perceived as animated by different divine and spiritual beings (also potentially both beneficial and dangerous), or might be associated with past events, religious history or sociopolitical systems (Santos-Granero 1998, see chapter 3).

Pané mentions illnesses only a few times. Firstly, when he narrates about a man from primordial times, named Guayahona, who was living in a cavern that he left to search for a herb called *digo* to wash himself. He convinced all women to go with him to search for *digo*, and searching this he arrived at Matininó.[74] This led to a transformation of children into small animals resembling frogs, left at the water stream. Guayahona was full of boils that called by Friar *"French disease"*, that he wanted to cure by bathing in a pool.[75] A women called Guabonito puts him into a secluded place (guanara), and then, remaining there, he recovered from the boils. Upon his recovery, he changed his name.

Illness is mentioned it the context of the origin of women. When bathing, (primordial) men saw women descend from trees, but when they went to grasp them, the women fled as (if they were) eels. Because they could not catch them they called a Caracaracol, a man with coarse hands, hands which could hold the women tight. Said Caracaracoli is a disease, like scabies, that makes the body very coarse.

The Caracaracoli personage comes back at another occasion, as one of four identical children (twins). Here again Caracaracoli is said to be scabious: this can refer to the same person/carrier or embodiment of the disease. This person caused a flood that was the origin of the sea and received from Bayamaco, the grandfather who made cassava for bread, a *guanguayo*, which was full of cohoba (identified as Anadenanthera peregrine, see Pagán Jimenéz & Carlson 2014), a ritual plant to communicate with the other world.[76] Caracaracol's swelling grew, his brother opened it with an ax, and from the swelling, a turtle (turle-women), emerge. Afterwards, two brothers construct their house and raise the turtle. This part could be interpreted as an indication that the person representing the illnesses is the one who has a destructive power leading to a creation (flood-sea). Another message of this narrative could be that the illness encounters remedy, which leads to a transformation, a new life.[77] The moral of the second part

74 Matinino possibly is Martinique, where according to Vespucci there were women like in Lesbos, which were dangerous to man, luring Spanish into their caves.

75 Citing work of Harper et. al. (2008), the translator notes these boils should not be identified with syphilis as the syphilis spirochete did not exist in this time, being a result of contact between New World disease, and the precursor of syphilis in Europe. For archeological evidence of tropenamous disease in the Caribbean see Crespo-Torres (2013).

76 In Peter Martyr D'Anghiera's translation of Pané, not cohoba but tobacco is thrown at Caracaracol.

77 This account could also be read in the light of Rochefort's (1666) notes on curing syphilis, and works from Goeje (1928), and Penard on indigenous peoples of Guayanas. Gullick summarizes that a patient suffering from pyans (probably syphilis) had to eat part of the Lamantin or Caret, the consumption of which produced blisters, which were later pierced with burnt reeds and water from the Baliefier tree or by the juice of Genipa Americana or by scarification with agouti teeth.

could be that the personage who has a power to deal with the divine beings, receives (by accident) the plant which enables him to communicate with the divine world in order to diagnose and to cure illnesses.

Friar Pané described also one of the curing sessions. After a patient purged himself he was visited by the *behique* (religious specialist) to consume plants (güeyo), to sing a song and to drink juice.[78] The *behique* cured the patient by sucking out the pathogenic object and spitting it away. Depending on what the object was, the *behique* established a diagnosis. The illness was generally considered to be caused by something that a *zemí* had put in the body of the patient because he/she was neglecting the zemí. If the object is a stone, it might be used later during childbirth, and so it was preserved in the same conditions as the zemí's image. On ceremonial days offerings were presented to zemís.

Another historical account about healing practices of the indigenous peoples of the Caribbean is from Dominica, provided by Father Breton nearly two hundred years later. [79] Breton (1665) writes that the Kalinago in Dominica believed illnesses to have been caused by Mapoya (which he translated as "devil" or "evil"), and sorcerers (from the mainland). Deities could be beneficial by indicating to the healer which plants he should apply helping to cure but could also send illnesses to men.[80] The healer/priest (boyáicou, niboyeiri, bóye) were intermediaries who communicated with the invisible realm in times of need, droughts, and illness or before going to war.[81] In the case of an illness, an offering is prepared and deposited in the ground near the bohío, where the healer, chanting, blows tobacco smoke up to make the god descend, after which the deity is to be seated and to be offered a meal and drink. Sometimes the illness materializes in an object such as a stone, arrowheads, a spine of a fish (Rajiformes sp.), which the healer would remove by sucking it out. As a reward, he would receive a calloúcouli, highly valued precious metal (see for translation Breton 1665). Preventive medicine included relics (*e.g.* light colored green stone as a remedy for kidney stone or an element to help in childbirth), and plants for protection.[82]

Both descriptions find some parallels in the South American context. Several themes illustrate this point. First, the role of religious specialist (*behique,* bóye) in establishing the diagnosis and remedy through their ability to connect with the invisible world (by plant-induced altered state of consciousness, *e.g.* ñopo). Furthermore, the illness can take concrete form as an object in the patient's body, which can be removed by a religious specialist (De Goeje 1943; Beyer 2009; Århem 1996). There is coincidence in the beliefs that the illness is due to an imbalance in the divine/spirit world, to consuming infected

78 This plant, described as a plant used frequently for purging, was identified by Arrom 2000 as Mourera fluviatilis. De Goeje's name for the herb was "abona-gita-hti".

79 With respect to the historical link between peoples of Greater and Lesser Antilles it is interesting to note that according to Breton the Carib pantheon consisted of a God and lower deities, some of whom had (a lot of) children. One of them was Arahuaco, another came from another nation.

80 Breton described that some lizards and birds (called Loumacachítina) belonged to ¨the gods of the buyei¨. Mabuya is until now a type of skink of shiny color in Lesser Antilles (personal communication with Katerina Jacobson, Angus Martin 2017) and for Haiti (personal conversation Sony Jean 2017).

81 *Bóye* means firefly. During my fieldwork I learned that in the Greater Antilles fireflies or *cucuyos* are believed to be deceased persons.

82 One such a plant was taya, mixed with achiote, as a protection against enemies, another one was a small gourd that was filled with birds' remains (caicouchi, Mansfenix) worn around the neck to protect or gain force.

food, or to the acts of a malevolent shaman. Indigenous peoples on the mainland use the same therapeutic techniques: blowing tobacco smoke, ritual purging, taking bathes, accompanied by singing and reciting prayers, charms, and making offerings.

Aforementioned references indicate some aspects of indigenous worldviews underpinning medicinal cultures of indigenous peoples of Greater Antilles in the time of European conquest. In general, it is assumed that these beliefs did not survive the genocide and the centuries of transculturation. Before addressing the circulation of the medicinal knowledge among the historically marginalized ancestors the following section addresses the role of the West African ancestors in shaping of meanings of landscape and an co-authorship of medicinal legacies.

West African ancestors shaping Caribbean landscapes

The post-conquest physical human imprints in the landscape have often been discussed in terms of the ´Columbian exchange´ (Crosby 1972), a model that has focused on the staples of American and European crops. The botanical legacy of captured West Africans brought to the Caribbean has often been neglected (see Voeks & Rashford 2013). The lack of acknowledgement of the West Central African botanical legacy in the Caribbean seems to be prompted by a consideration of the constraints created by the brutal forms of imprisonment, transportation and conditions in slavery. For these captives, opportunities to bring plants were indeed severely constrained, but they could still retain some of their botanical knowledge, healing skills, and religious convictions in their memory. Without doubt, a lot of traditional skills and knowledge did not cross the Atlantic and has been lost together with millions of lives. However, recent studies (*e.g.* Voeks & Rashford 2013; Carney 2003; Van Andel et al. 2015) have shed light on some of the African contributions to the botanical traditions of the Caribbean. The African legacy was identified in the cultivation of several specific crops, in agricultural systems, in handicrafts, as well as in ritual and healing plant use in the Americas.[83] African ancestors transformed the Caribbean landscape physically through their work on field, cattle ranches or gardens for own consumption.

The economic changes accompanied by the cultivation of mono-crops (such as sugar, tobacco), cattle farming, timber extraction or the later introduction of mechanized agriculture has carved into appearance of the Caribbean landscapes until nowadays. Castilla-Beltrán et al. (2018) analyzed paleobotanical record of some of these long term environmental changes in the Dominican Cibao valley.[84]

As the majority of the current population of the Greater Antilles descends from forced laborers or voluntary migrants, a key question for this dissertation is how those

83 One of the extraordinary examples that Voeks gives is the case of a Brazilian enslaved man who after buying himself out of slavery went to Dahomey from where he started to ship palm oil and kola nuts to Bahia in Brazil. The kola nuts were planted and employed in religious ceremonies (Carney & Voeks 2003). Cola acuminata is present also in the Greater and Lesser Antilles (Acevedo-Rodríguez & Strong 2012). According to Quiras-Moran (2009), kola nut has known medicinal use and religious use in Cuba. It is administered a.o. for cardiac problems, digestive problems, migraine, and depressions. In the religious realm it belongs to the *orishas* (spirits) Odua and Orunmila and is used for amulets and rituals dedicated to them.

84 Some of these findings matches and should be further related to the specific historical development of these locations as known from historical records (see e.g. history of La Jaiba in the next chapter).

who migranted to or were brought by force from elsewhere treated illnesses in the new environments. First, some of the plants might be the same or at least resembling the known families and share some of the features of plants from their homelands. Some of the plants floated across the Atlantic independently of human agency and others are believed to have a shared origin that goes back to the time before the continental separation (Carney 2003; Voeks & Rashford 2013). Other plants were quite rapidly incorporated into the local flora as a part of peaceful trade or wars, conquest, and colonization. After the first years of European colonization of the Greater Antilles, American plants such as corn and manioc were planted in Africa, became rapidly integrated in the diet throughout the West African coast and were supplies of the slave ships (McCann 2001). This process facilitated recognition of these crops by later waves of captives over the years.

Enslaved people were likely to recognize certain families and genera that were valued in Africa for medicinal properties (Carney & Voeks 2003; Vossen et al. 2014). Carney (2003) identified 125 plants used by Afro-Americans that have analogous uses in the Circum-Caribbean region and tropical West Africa, including 95 species that were present in Africa prior to the Transatlantic Slave Trade. The African botanical legacy in the Caribbean concerns the dietary staple foods, including (but not limited to) *guineos*, yams, plantains, coffee, palm oil, but also medicinal plants, for instance cundeamor (*Momordica charantia)* or cañafístola *(Cassia fistula)*. Some of the plants used in rituals, such as coconuts and ajonjolí (*Sesamum indicum)* have also been related to the African continent.[85] Other plants were introduced later but became an inseparable part of the foodways and lifeways of enslaved peoples in the newly emerging American societies.[86]

Tropical forests in Africa and the Americas differ substantially, however. People who survived the journey across the Atlantic Ocean also had to figure out how to use unknown plant species in foreign environments. Newcomers were looking for plants that were similar to African families, but they also practiced a heuristic method to discover new plant cures (Vossen et al. 2014).

African captives were severly restricted in ways they could take with them any medicinal plants or images of their deities. However, the rich repertoire of meanings of

---

85 Captives landing in the Caribbean would recognize many plants, such as Raphia Taedigera, bottle gourd, and genera such as *Acacia, Dacroydes, Dorstenia, Euphorbia spp., Quassia, Strychnos, Rauwolfia spp.* (Brent Berlin 1992 as cited in Carney 2002). New crops of African origin that were introduced included: coffee, palm oil (*Elaeis guineensis*), African rice (*Oryza glaberrima*), yams (*Dioscorea cayensis)*, cow (black-eyed-) peas eyed] peas (*Vigna unguiculata*), melegueta peppers (*Aframomum melegueta*), sorrel/roselle (*Hibiscus sabdariffa*), okra (*Abelmoschus esculentus*), sorghum (*Sorghum bicolor*}, and the Bambara groundnut (*Vigna subterranea*) (Carney, 2003). Also medicinal plants of African origin are now growing in the Caribbean. These include Guinea corn, yellow yams, ackees, Phyllanthus amarus, Leonotis nepetifolia, Corchorus spp. and Cola acuminate (Carney 2003; Sherindan, 1972). Ritual use was registered for the following plants of African origin: *Newboudlia laevis, Kalanchoe integra, Lagenaria siceraria (Molina), Cyperus Rotondus, Pennisetum Purpureum, Cola acuminate, Afromumun malegueta.*

86 The history of certain crops reveals how the introduction of new crops into foodways met with resistence. This was the case when the British brought breadfruit (Artocarpus communis) from Tahiti in 1792. The enslaved people refused initially to eat it, and preferred crops that they were more familiar with, such as corn, yams, plantains and manioc. Among the plants associated with the period of slavery, which became a symbol of resistance, is *Poinciana pulcherrima* (Cuban term: Guacamaya, Dominican name: Macata), used by enslaved women to abort offspring and end the life of enemies (Schiebinger 2009).

attributed to the various landscape features in present-day Afro-Cuban religions as earlier discussed by for example Cabrera (1954) testifies how African ancestors were capable of finding the divine and remedies also in these new landscapes. Various colonial sources such as records of Cartagena trials (Gómez 2017; Vargas 2011), physiciant´s accounts Sloane (1707), Chateusalins (1854), as well as other European accounts elsewhere in Caribbean (*e.g.* Merian, Stedeman, or Dalhberg in Suriname, Snelders 2012; Alexander´s observation in Grenada, Thompson in Jamaica in Schiebinger 2009), offer us some insights into the ancestral medicinal practices derived from African continent or the health situation in the colonies (*e.g.* for the Dutch Caribbean see Oostindie 2013).

When trying to envision how the African ancestors have redefined the Caribbean landscape it is clear that we should need to get a better grasp on the role of cultural memory as a flexible process of emplacement, individual role of healers but also of ancestral institutions such as brotherhoods (fraternities). The latter are generally acknowledge to be an important preservation mechanism of West African ancestral belief systems and medicinal cultures in the Caribbean. Brotherhoods were organizations, which had an important role in attending to the sick, providing funeral services, and dealing with the inheritance of members of the brotherhood. One of the historical accounts that provide some details about the brotherhoods in Santo Domingo is the work of Alcocer in 1650. His account indicates that these brotherhoods were organized according to the regional origins, others were composed of peoples of distinct colonial categories, and might be also means for preservation of own worldviews.[87] Similarly, also Cuban brotherhoods (cofradías or cabildos de naciones) show how the process of transculturation went beyond genetic exchanges.[88] Cuban brotherhoods suggests not only the constitution of a shared religious tradition among freed peoples of color, but also indicates that the kaleidoscope of fragmented societies was organized around established models of "colonizer institution", which were consequently reinterpreted

87 The brotherhood of San Juan de Bautista was organized by people of West African origin who were born on the island (*negros criollos*) but many of Spaniards cooperated with the brotherhood. This Saint John brotherhood existed until the beginning of the 19th century. Biafaras and Mandingas were members of (poor but very devoted) brotherhood of Señora de la Candelaria with own chapel, celebrated the Virgen every year with processions. The popularity of saints and existence of brotherhood like the one of San Miguel protecting Santo Domingo from smallpox is also related to specific historical smallpoy epidemics. Zapes had brotherhood dedicated to Santa María Magdalena and Aradas were organized as brotherhood having as patron Saints Cosmas and Damian. Among present-day Dominican healers Saints like Cosmas and Damian, are patrons of physicians, and represent Divine twins in Dominican 21 Division. A similar parallel could have been drawn by people shipped from current Benin, where Ewe-Fon-Gbe and Yoruba ancestors also today twins have a special place in local pantheon. As such details of religious expression of this brotherhood of that time in Santo Domingo are unknown, parallels between past and today's identification remains points of speculation but also possible points of nexus and creative reinterpretations of Catholic symbolism according to own religious system.

88 One of the first registered brotherhoods, Señora de los Remedios in Havana (1598), was organized by a group of Temne (Zapes) (Guanche 2011). In addition, we find also brotherhood of Santísimo Sacramento and Animas del Purgatorio in Santiago and in Bayamo (Alonso Enríquez de Armendáriz 1620 in Portuondo Zúñiga 2012a). Brotherhoods from the second half of the 17 century, such as Divino Paraclito and Espiritu Santo, were organized along the colonial categories like "*morenos libres*", and those of Candelaria, Nuestra Señora de Consolación, San Francisco, and Santa Catalina were composed of "*pardos libres*". Another brotherhoods further to be studied are Santísimo Sacramento and Ánimas del Purgatorio in Santiago and in Bayamo.

in a creative manner according to individual religious and other cultural practices in relation to the surrounding landscapes.

European ancestors reshaping Caribbean landscapes

Like African ancestors also European predecessors have left profound imprints in the Caribbean landscapes. As the colonial expeditions into the West Indies were driven by the quest for gold and spices, it is not surprising that the colonial accounts described the Caribbean flora and fauna in terms of their economic potential. Following Columbus, different authors, such as Martyr D'Anghiera, López de Gómara and Fernández de Oviedo, praise the lands for their fertility and flora.

The latter, Gonzalo Fernández de Oviedo y Valdés (1478-1557) collected information about endemic plant use, for alimentation or practical utilitarian use (Fernández de Oviedo 2002 [1535-1557]).[89] He provides us with a valuable insights on the cultivation and preparation of native plants like *yucca, ajes, batatas, yautía, maní* and *maíz*, as well as the knowledge transfer to other groups.[90] The information on medicinal properties of plants (*guyacan, palo santo, manzanillos, perebenuc, yaruma, hobo*) provided by Fernández de Oviedo is informative but rather limited. In the case of guayacán he clarified that it was used to treat syphilis, and that it is consumed through infusion.[91]

The exact identification of the plants as described by the above-mentioned authors in order to assess the indigenous contribution in the local medicinal cultures is complicated by the great diversity of the medicinal plants, their uses, and the change of names over time as well as the fragmented and limited character of the historical information in general.

As for material landscape modifications, the Europeans also introduced medicinal plants to the Caribbean. Early chronicles did not only register the plants used by indigenous peoples but also newly introduced plants (Echagoian, 1568; Fernández de Oviedo 2002 [1535-1557]).[92] Popular Old World herbs used in the Americas included: rue, rosemary, pennyroyal, sweet marjoram, mallow, artemisa, and vervain (Foster 1953).[93] Some of the local species were associated with those known from Europe. Fernández de Oviedo lists many plants that were similar to plants from Spain but were already present in Hispaniola before the arrival of the Christians and many of

89 For more on the life of the author and his work consult e.g. Gerbi (1978) or Myers (2007). There are several editions of Oviedo's work. The first edition of the first part was published in 1535, the second and third part successively in 1544 and 1549. Here I use the version transcribed by the Royal Academy and published in 1851, referenced as Oviedo 1535/1851, and the excerpts about his description of flora as republished by Deive in 2002, which is referenced as 1535/2002.

90 For more about the introduction and cultivation of the crops important for the Dominican colonial economy see Del Río Moreno (2012).

91 Oviedo mentions also other herbs for sore (*llaga*): perebecenuc, used to wash, and another one called curiá. Another medicinal plant of interest might be hicacos, which is described as purgative, or goaconax (árbol se hace bálsamo), which is useful for *humores frios e pasiones que de frialdad proceden* (Oviedo 1535/2002).

92 Among the introduced plants were grapes, wheat, *palms, cañafístola, fruit trees (especially citruses), vegetables (aubergine, cabbage, radish, lettuce, onion, parsley, carrots, turnips and cucumbers, beans,* celery, *zabiras, coriander cucumbers.*

93 European medicinal plants brought to the Caribbean included remedies against witchcraft and evil eye: *Allium sativum L., Centaurea ornate Willd., Cynodon dactylon L., Genista hystrix, Laurus nobilis, Lavandula pedunculata, Magudaris panacifolia, Olea europea, Ononis spinosa L., Peucedanum officinale L., Rosmarinus* (González et al. 2011).

them receive european names, a fact that can lead to confusion (Fernández de Oviedo 1535/2002, Lib. XI: II).[94]

The exotic species of sugar cane and ginger, along with endemic woods such as *brazil, bálsamo, cañafístola, guayacán* and also tobacco, soon became an integral export commodity, as did cowhides (López de Gómara 2002 [1552]). Some of Caribbean remedies like Villasante's balsam became popular trade items in European markets. Also *guayacán* as its Latin name suggest *Lignum vitae* or Wood of Life gained wide spread popularity as a marvelous remedy in Europe. In spite of the initial disapproval of tobacco, tobacco quickly gained popularity amongst Spaniards and the enslaved peoples from Africa and their descendants, and it soon became an important trade item in Europe. Its medicinal properties were acknowledged as beneficial much later (Las Casas *History of Indies*, Ch: XIV; Monardes 1580).

Next to the clear extractionist focus of many of first European account of the Caribean landscapes these texts reveals some of beliefs of that period. Fernández de Oviedo's history displays Catholic interpretation of the environment, beliefs about enchanted places, the doctrine of signatures and humoral links to geographical locations. Fernández de Oviedo believed that the Caribbean landscapes were the results of God's creation, and that the medicinal plants encountered there are divine. When describing medicinal plants, he sees them as a gift to the faithful and the infidels from Jesus Christ as the pious protector/curer of human illnesses. In different parts of Oviedo´s work the author expresses his gratitude to God, as the true doctor of our health, life, and souls. The doctrine of signatures was an important aspect of medicinal cultures, based on the idea that God had provided a natural cure for every illness, and marked the cures by giving them an appearance resembling the infected organ (*e.g.* the eyebright plant serves for eye ailments).

European belief about enchanted places is displayed in his story about a Spanish visit to a mysterious lake in the mountains of Jaragua. During the reign of Nicolas de Ovando a Spanish crew accompanied by indigenous people went to the lake, which appears to be an enchanted place.[95] At last, the Hippocrates' humoral theory about how the environment had an impact on human health has been preserved in his evaluation of the medication of *guayacán* that was considered to be specific to the climate of these

94 Among these are listed: chicoria, cerrajas rostrum porcinum, berdolaga, berbena, hierbamora, llantén, pan y quesillo *(biusa pastoris), altamisa, escudre (nenúfar), albahaca (azimum gariophiolatum), lengua cerval (scoloprendia), culantrillo de pozo (capillus Veneris), poleo montesino, persicaria (herva maculata), salvia (lilifagus), girasol (helitropia).* Also *malvas, mastruerzo and culantro*, the latter two just have different leaves than the Spanish variants.

95 Oviedo writes: *"Y estuvo mirando este lago tanto espacio cuanto se podrían decir tres credos. Dice Pedro de Lumbreras que eran tanto el ruido y estruendo que oía. Que él estaba muy espantado, e que le parecía que no era aquel estruendo de voces humanas, ni sabía entender qué animales o fieras pudiesen hacer aquel horrible sonido. En fin, que, como estaba solo (los otros españoles y indígenas no quisieron subir) y espantado, se tornó sin ver otra cosa."* (Oviedo 1851 in Deive 2002, pp. 63-64).

islands and patients in the Iberian Peninsula were warned to protect themselves from airs (*aires* or bad spirits).[96]

The idea about a close link between the complexion of human bodies and those of plants, and the different effects of the application of remedies at various geographical locations is evident in later European writings as well, when Breton (1665) writes that Kalinago people of Dominica cured their syphilis easily and without danger because the temperature of the air was "even", and because the powerful remedies were considered to be growing in "*the Torrid Zone*". Some believed that Caribbean remedies that were taken to France lost their potency. Others believed that the cure for syphilis in Spain was only possible with the *guayacán* because the illness itself originated in the Caribbean. Also, Sir Hans Sloane, a physician living in Jamaica in 1680s, discussed a fever that every newcomer got before being accustomed to the climate and constitution of the air in Jamaica but also acknowledged that this illness occurred all over the remote Eastern parts of the world.

The European colonization implied also desacralization and resacralization of Caribbean landscapes. The indigenous religions were demonized in the same rhetoric as Christian beliefs had been demonized in the Roman imperium and traditional non-Christian beliefs were often considered witchcraft and persecuted as such in Europe at the very same period that the Europeans invaded the Americas.[97] In the Americas, like in Europe, non-Christian sacred sites (*e.g.* see on a Dominican cavern Morales in D'Anghiera 2002 [1494-1526]) were portrayed such as and believed to be haunted by the devil.

Catholic orthodoxy and Counter-Reformation zeal in Spain during the 16th and 17th centuries did not favor a renaissance of influences from classical "paganism", nor of other non-Catholic religious expressions (Godwin 2002, p. 17). However, purifying

96 Hippocrates, the father of Western medicine, applying inductive reasoning, expressed in his work *Airs, Waters, and Places* (± 400 BC) his firm conviction that there was a relation between the geographical location and one's character and health. Hippocrates opposed the idea that illnesses were caused by divine intervention that could be cured through appealing to the deities. Instead, he argued that illness is a result of humoral imbalances. He distinguished four humors: blood, phlegm, black, and yellow bile, each of which had its own complexion (characteristics). An illness was diagnosed by determining the complexion of the illness, and its cause. The cure consisted of restoring the balance in the body by changing the diet, the humoral imbalance of the body, or the environment. Physicians following Hippocratic teaching believed in deterministic relations between seasons, waters, prevailing winds, physical geography, the soil of a place and the humoral balance, which all together influenced human health. Hippocrates and Galen's teaching were influential at important medical centers such as Sevilla, Salamanca, and Alcalá de Henares during the Renaissance. The humoral theory seems to have also been prominent in popular medicinal cultures in Spain. Spanish healers were said to heal with their breath, saliva or even touch, thanks to their natural complexion, because of a balance of the four humors (Castañega 1529).

97 The conquest of the Caribbean took place a few years after the publication of the main manual for the persecution of witches (Cohn 1975).The *Malleus Maleficarum* (Hammer of the Witches), written by Dominican monks, was published as a handbook for witch-hunters and inquisitors in 1487, five years before Columbus's first voyage. As Jansen and Perez (2017) noted, some of the 16th century famous persecutors of Mexican indigenous beliefs were active in the Spanish inquisition just prior to their arrival in Mexico. Although the Spanish witch hunting was said to have mainly been preoccupied with the expulsion of Jews and repression of *conversos* and Protestants, there are different cases such as the Basque witch trials of the 16th and 17th century where many of people were accused of witchcraft. This was largely based on misconceptions about folk beliefs, healing practices, and celebrations of the solstices in a local cave (Caro Baroja 2003).

medicinal cultures completely from non-Catholic associations was not a realistic option for different reasons. How ineffective the official policy was in practice is clear from the records of trials in Cartagena in the 17th century (Crespo Vargas 2011; Moret 2017). There were many persecuted people of Spanish, West Central African, and Caribbean origin (including indigenous, *criollos* and people of mixed descent) who displayed knowledge and beliefs that were quite different from orthodox Catholicism. The lack of Catholic religious instruction or supervision further enhanced the diversity of medicinal cultures in the Caribbean, which, combined with ideas and practices of indigenous and African origin, led to new religious expressions.

The human tendency to draw parallels between concepts and observations was somewhat obscured in the religious realm of the colonial Caribbean by the justification of colonization and slavery, which created an overemphasis on 'otherness', and so further enlarged the existing differences between beliefs regarding man's position in the creation of the world.

The theoretical dualism expressed in binary oppositions of natural/supernatural and nature/culture should not be indiscriminately projected onto encounters of different worldviews in the Caribbean where this dichotomy was not present. Catholic interpretations of the environment and its importance for health in this period did not separate men from nature. In one mode of interpretation of Roman Catholicism, people were seen as a part of the divine creation, acknowledging that even lower levels of created species are blessed and precious. Francis of Assisi and Thomas Aquinas both preached about the manifestation of God's grace in nature and their teachings are influential until today (particularly with respect to ecological degradation). Saint Francis (called the 'Saint of ecology' by pope John Paul II) stressed humanity's kinship with animals, stars, and plants. As is well known, he referred to Brother Sun, Sister Moon, Sister Water, Brother Fire, Mother Earth and Sister Death, also addressed a wolf as Brother Wolf, and sought to reach God through asceticism in caverns. Secondly, there was a tendency to structure the beings created in the universe hierarchically, with humans dominating over the rest, arguing that God had created humanity uniquely in His image (*imago Dei*).

Both Catholic interpretations did not separate man and nature. This is not to say that all people were seen as equal. Some people were considered to be the head and others to be arms and feet of the body that as a whole was the divine creation.[98] Based on this hierarchy and out-group bias, slavery was justified. Again, we see that economic gain trumped religious morals about loving your neighbors as yourself.

The various interpretations of the Holy Scriptures should be seen in conjunction with various degrees of inclusiveness of some Catholic theologists toward pre-Christian beliefs, which also varied according to the period. As Saint Augustine declared: *'It is*

98 Santos Granero argues that the Franciscans in Peru imposed their religious symbols (cross, churches) on the sacred indigenous places in order to demonstrate their power (2004, p. 109). This does not apply to all regions across the centuries. Similarly, Jansen et al. (2008) writes that the position of a chapel on top of the precolonial pyramid need not be understood as a military victory over one religion over the other, but rather should be viewed as a cultural synergy, which implied profound respect. They also points to the approach of contemporary German Capuchin monks, active in part of the Mixtec region, Mexico, who valorizes and incorporates pre-colonial sanctuaries as sacred sites from the conviction that God has manifested Himself in all cultures, also in pre-colonial America.

the same with sacred forests as with Gentiles, one does not exterminate the Gentiles but one converts them, changes them; in the same way one does not cut down sacred groves; it is better to consecrate them to Jesus Christ' (Belmont 1992). Saint Augustine's teachings demonstrated that it was often easier to fuse non-Catholic views with teachings about God's grace in nature than to eradicate previously held beliefs. One strategy to convert was to incorporate the old ("pagan") into the new (Christian) belief system. The legacy of this process is visible today in many important European traditions such as Easter, Christmas, and other Catholic Saint Days. The fusion of different religious traditions is displayed in the Spanish Marian cult which venerates a Virgin of the Moon (Los Pedroches, Córdoba), Virgin of the Sun (Adamuz y Montoro in Córdoba); Virgin of the Star (in Espiel Córdoba), and many others. It should be considered that at the time of conquest of Americas, Catholic sacred landscapes were composed of sacred places like Eden, the Holy Land, the Jordán River, and the Mount Calvary, but also of sacred shrines that were not officially consecrated. Spanish landscapes counted numerous local sacred natural sites such as the previously mentioned caves, trees (Our Lady of Salceda, Our Lady of Madroñal), and water sources (*e.g.* Our Lady of Grace, Our Lady of the Baths, Our Lady of the Holy Spring).

In his study entitled *Local Religions in 16th Century Spain*, Christian (1989) examined particularities of this two-level Catholicism in reports based on a questionnaire sent on orders of King Philip II to villages and towns of Nueva Castilia in 1575 -1580. Local expressions of Catholic beliefs are typified by particular sacred places, images, relics, locally chosen patron saints, individual ceremonies, a unique calendar built on the settlement's own sacred history. Sacred places were often related to or reinterpreted as places of the manifestation of Saints, and they were often created as consequences of vows after natural disasters such as hail, floods, droughts, pestilences, and insect infestation. Many of the hierophanies shared a similar script of returning miraculously to the site of their first appearance (Christian 1989, p. 76). This phenomenon also displays similarities with the manifestation of the Virgin in the Caribbean (Virgen of Charity in Cuba, Virgen de las Mercedes in Hispaniola), whose reappearance has been earlier interpreted as a remainder of indigenous worldviews (Tricando 1997).[99]

The success of the Spanish spiritual conquest was being constantly proved by different Marian manifestations. The famous manifestation of Virgen Altagracia at Santo Cerro, was an obvious institutional power display. Preceding the appearance of Virgen of Charity from El Cobre, the Virgen Altagracia from Higuey caused several miracles. Like the Virgen of Charity the Virgen Altagracia manifested herself in an orange tree and disappeared when it was ordered that her statue should be sent to Santo Domingo (Alcocer 1650, p. 48). The manifestation of Virgins and Saints have led to creating new holy places, relics and objects that were in physical contact with divine forces. The great esteem for such objects was also manifest in the belief in their power to protect and cure. The cross at Santo Cerro was dismantled until the last nozzle because its wood had miraculous effects for devotees. This fits into the general religious tradition of that period, in which relics and holy images were taken out in processions in Santo Domingo to invoke divine favor in times of pestilence/plague, droughts, hunger, or in public works at the

99 The link between the Cuban patronal Virgen and indigenous inhabitants was discussed earlier e.g. by Portuondo Zuñiga (2008),Oliver (2009), Peña et al. (2014) but see also work of Corbea Calzado (1996).

turn of the 16th to the 17th century (Alcocer 1650, pp. 43-44, p. 50). It was also believed that the dust of the cross could alleviate a fever if taken with a liquid.[100]

Plants that were symbolic representations of the associated Saints or miracles were important elements of European healing landscapes. To illustrate, Verbena, a sacred plant from the Monte del Calvario (Golgotha), which cured Jesus Christ, is an important ritual plant currently in Spain. Until today, Spaniards gather branches of palms, olive trees, laurel, and rosemary that are blessed on Palm Sunday, and then placed on windowsills to protect people's homes. The date palm (*Phoenix dactylifera*), given its ability of quick regeneration, stands as a symbol of the resurrecting soul after death. There were many other sacred plants, like Rosa de Jericó, olive, pines and others that stand as symbols for the divine (clover for the Trinity, lily for the Virgin, palm for victory, olive or pine for the Holy Spirit). In 16th century Spain, many of these plants and other objects were used in protecting against evil, or in curing the evil eye, against bewitchment, and other ailments (see Foster 1956).[101] The plants were connected to different beliefs, like those with the inner force, had to be activated by prayer or by uttering secret sentences. Finally, plants collected on the day of Saint John were deemed to be extra powerful (Foster 1956).

The early modern Spanish landscapes were full of dangerous and enchanted places, which often included demonized pre-Christian sacred sites and therefore expressed a fear for divine punishment (Tausiet 2014). Witches, devils, spirits and beasts such as sirenas, zitirons, hydras, pheonix, arpías, or dragons, along with mysterious anthropomorphic plants like mandrake, magical trees such as the Árbol del Bien y del Mal and Árbol del Conocimiento de la Vida from the Book of Genesis (see *Sanitatis Ortus, Garden of Health* 1491, Langham 1597) add to the richness of symbolism of European landscapes.

When discussing Spanish ontologies related to the environment, it is important to include the Canarian influences. The Canary Islands were an intermediary place in the exchange of plants, animals and peoples between both sides of the Atlantic Ocean. Like in the Caribbean, the Canarian healing landscapes were profoundly altered by the Christianization of the indigenous (Guanche) population. The Virgen de la Candelaria had initially a shrine in the Cave of Achbinico, which was considered already sacred before the religious conquest. Also the figure of Nuestra Señora del Pino, who revealed herself in a miraculous huge pine tree, surrounded by three dragon trees (*Draco Palma canariensis*), and led to the discovery of a healing spring, suggests a synergy of European and Guanche beliefs.

The combination of a place where the Virgin has manifested herself and the belief in healing effects of a visit to this place is not unique. On the contrary, Catholic sacred places in Spain were often shrines for healing since the early medieval period (Christian 1989). Their curative powers were derived from the Saints' manifestations that had taken place there, connected to the miraculous powers of images, relics, and ex-votos. Among the sacred Catholic shrines that were frequently visited for healing in 16th century Spain were those dedicated to the Virgin Mary, Saint Anne, and other Saints,

100 For more traditions from this period in Cuba see also Lampe (2001).

101 González (2011) registered as plant remedies against witches and the evil eye: *Allium sativum L., Centaurea ornate Willd. Cynodon dactylon L., Genista hystrix, Laurus nobilis, Lavandula pedunculata, Magudaris panacifolia, Olea europea, Ononis spinosa L., Peucedanum officinale L., Rosmarinus.*

which are utilized in curing specific illnesses.[102] In addition, in Galiaca healing could take place at crossroads (Foster 1953). Spanish healing places are part of the broader European medicinal cultures where multiple sites, varying from Asclepios' temples in Greece to the Cave of Lourdes in France, and the springs of Bath in England have been popular healing places for centuries. The manifestation of divine powers in such places led to pilgrimages in search of cures for body and mind.

The Spanish fathers, physicians or healers could find analogies about the divine power of nature and its healing aspects in their own worldviews. The constant emphasis on difference in order to be able to justify the enslavement and colonization blinded and silenced possible similarities. In some cases, especially in the context of general poor health care in the colonies the newcomers were more dependent on those knowledgeable of the local flora. In conclusion, Catholic, Hippocratic, and popular medicinal teachings do not separate man from the environment. Some of the previously mentioned etiologies continue as legacies in contemporary Spain, where illnesses have been classified according to material, human, and invisible spiritual causes (Kuschick 1999). Among the invisible immaterial causes mentioned were: possession by an evil spirit (bad air), evil eye, or divine punishment for violating a moral code (Kuschick 1999).

The multidirectional circulation of the medicinal knowledge in the Greater Antilles

The dynamics of exchanges of green medicine are unclear but the general context is marked by conquest, colonial violence and slavery. Some historical references suggest that indigenous peoples did not share their knowledge with the colonizers on purpose as a means of resistance. Antonio de Villasante, when asking to obtain a license for exporting *bálsamo* from Hispaniola to Europe, explained that he obtained this recipe from his indigenous wife, cacique Leonora (Alonso de Zuazo 1518 in Deive 2002). He emphasized the uniqueness of this knowledge because in general indigenous people concealed this knowledge as a way to resist the Spaniards.[103]

Although the early colonial exchanges meant in practice often a one-sided exploitation of the indigenous intellectual property also the indigenous population seems to have also incorporated some plants that were introduced from across the Atlantic Ocean. Chanca claimed to have seen in La Isabela: "*a root of ginger which an indian was wearing around his neck*" (Chanca 2002 [1494]). Although it is unclear if Chanca confused ginger with some other, endemic plant (*e.g.* arrowroot, *Maranta arundinacea*), it is possible that ginger was already brought to the island during the first Columbian

102 The most popular were Saint Lucy and Saint Christopher for curing eyes (based on hagiography), Saint Matthew for throat ailments, Saint Babiles for hernias, and Saint Martin for fevers (Christian 1989, pp. 93-94). Also based on miracles related to their biography, San Ramón Nonato is often consulted for birth, and San Cosme and San Damian are seen as the patrons of physicians. This specialization in curing of ailments was present also centuries later, when people seeking cures for the throat prayed to San Blas, for ailments of the breasts to Santa Agueda, for toothache to Santa Apolonia, and for the plague to San Roque (Foster 1956).

103 *Relación acerca del Bálsamo de la Española que hace Antonio de Villasante,* as published by Deive in his *Antología* (2002). From Oviedo we know that some said that he learned this from his wife, others that he learned it from an Italian doctor, Codro, who later passed away in Tierra Firme. See also the study by Mira Caballos (2000), who discusses the bálsamo fever.

voyage in 1492 and shortly after became incorporated into the local flora. At least, by 1570 ginger was planted for commercial use in various fields (López de Velasco 2002 [1571]), and later indigenous peoples planted and used ginger (see the chapter 4). In present-day Kalinago communities on Dominica the ginger plant (as well as other plants from the zingiberacea family) is cultivated as a spice and as a cure for stomach aches, and its leaves are used as a charm during ritual baths and also to repel misfortune from canoes (Hodge 1957).

The botanical exchanges among the colonized strata of the populations are poorly documented and also not very well studied. Deive (2002) mentions the case of a healer of African descent from Santiago de Caballeros, Hispaniola, dating to the 1550s, who seemed to have obtained some medicinal knowledge from indigenous healers and was said to have practiced *san*, which is translated as *indigenous witchcraft*. Such transfer of botanical knowledge likely varied according to particular circumstances and was probably as diverse as the multiethnic societies during the colonial period. The pioneering study of Gómez (2017) of trial records from Cartagena (1613-1721) revealed that Afro-Caribbean healing experts used plants that were native as well as plants that were exotic to the Caribbean.[104]

If current healing practices are to be considered heritage of a long history of exchanges of botanical knowledge and worldviews, the ritual context of plant use reveals that many new world plants have been integrated into religious realms that were brought from oversea. Studies from Suriname explain that more than four hundred species, many of which were native to Suriname, are used in rituals, bathing, and potions among the Maroons (Van Andel 2013). Similarly, Cabrera (1954/1993) and Quiros-Moran (2009) recorded such native plant use among devotees of Regla de Ocha and Palo Monte. Moreno Rodríguez' study (1995) on plant use in Crossed Spiritism (based on the teaching of Kardec influenced by Regla de Ocha) illustrates how spiritual expressions from different origins are complementing each other within the medicinal tradition in East Cuba.

Comparative studies confirm that ethnobotanical knowledge is time and space contingent as well as a reflection of different sociocultural histories. Moret's (2013) study of Cuban ethnobotany demonstrated that people living in what historically were sugar regions preserved the knowledge of African plants more than that of Mediterranean species, and that the reverse was the case for the tabacco regions which were occupied more often by Iberic and Canarian migrants. It is also evident that, even if there were significant differences, the inhabitants were knowledgable of species of both Mediterranean and African origin. Similarly, cross-cultural comparisons of the Maroons and Trio of Suriname point out that while the Maroons use less medicinal plants than the Trio, the Maroons did develop a robust utilitarian knowledge of native plants (Hoffman 2013).

104 His overview of plants used by Black Caribbean ritual specialists included the following plants: anamú, ariajua, buevera, cañoco, capitana, carara, carcoma, cayaya, de Santa María, escobilla, grango, guano, limpiadientes, orejom, pantailla, pullón, rodo de alacrán, rompesera, tuatua, achiote (*Bixa Orellana*), basil (*Ocimum basilicum*), bejuco (*Mikania guaco*), bottle gourds (*Lagenaria siceraria* or *Agenaria vulgaris*), caraña (*Bursera graveolens*), chamomile (*Asteraceae*), culantrillo (*Adientum canillus-veneris*), guamo (*Inga Feulleei*), guayacán *(Guaiacu spp*.), lulos (*Solanum quitoense*), palm hearts (*Euterpe oleracea*), palo de fraile (*Couepia poliandra*), pringamosa (*Urtica dioica*), tobacco (*Nicotiana tabacum*) (Gómez 2017).

The transculturation of medicinal cultures is not just a matter of learning about the properties of the flora but also depends on broader conceptual transformations related to the demographic changes of the colonial period. These changes and in particular the role of the indigenous ancestors therein merits more research.

Contrary to the general assumption about the rapid ethnocide of indigenous ancestors, Dominican and Cuban indigenous healers continued to exercise their skills in the period after the *encomienda* system. Deive (2002) discusses a case of Puerto Plata in the Dominican Republic, a town that had around 150 inhabitants of mixed origin (including *mestizos* and *mulattoes*), where healers from European, indigenous, and African origin were present. One of them, *cacica* Leonora Torres, wife of Torquemada, was accused of poisoning a local philander. Supposedly, she reunited in her house with another indigenous woman called Inés Estrada in the morning or during siestas in order to practice "witchcraft". Inés had previously been accused of having poisoned her husband and her lover with herbs. Depicted as an indecent lustful woman (in terms reminiscent of Martyr D'Anghiera's account), she was said to enchant various lovers. According to Maria de Velasco, one of the neighbors complained that all *cacicas* or indigenous women of this country knew the "*herbs to harm or to cure.*" Another indigenous female healer, and again wife of a Spaniard, who lived in Santiago de Caballeros, specialized in "*concoctions and potions*" still after the encomienda period. The continuity of the indigenous knowledge in Greater Antilles is suggested by for example Nicolás Monardes.

The *Medicinal History* written by Nicolás Monardes (1580) is one of works that appropriated some of the knowledge of the indigenous peoples from Mexico and Peru, and in lesser detail also from Greater Antilles. Monardes relates how in the 1580s a great amount of guayacán from Española and palo santo (considered to be a variety of the former) from Puerto Rico was transported to Europe to cure syphilis.[105] From Santo Domingo and Puerto Rico cañafístola was brought (said to be better than those brought from Italy, which were known from the work of *Dioscorides´ De Materia Medica*), good to be used as purgative, evacuating cholera and flegma from the veins and intestines, purifying the blood, as remedy against rheuma and high fevers. From Cuban indigenous peoples the Spaniards learned about the medicinal properties of *bitumen*, which was used by natives for "cold illnesses".

Also in Cuba healers of indigenous background exercised their function longer then assumed. In 1609, Mariana Nava received the official authorization to provide medical services in Santiago de Cuba (Górdon y de Acosta 1894; Ortiz 1959). The case of Ms. Nava is not unique. Another person of indigenous descent (*mestizo*) graduated from the medical academy of Cuba in 1760 (Górdon y de Acosta 1894). The

105 Monardes, N. 1580. *Primera, y segunda y tercera partes de la Historia medicinal de las cosas que se traen de nuestras Indias Occidentales*, Sevilla. This account also explains how syphilis had been introduced to Europe and adds some – according to its author – common but incorrect opinions about the origin of this disease (melancholism and bad diet which were burning the blood, the influence of Saturn or Mars) and that the remedy not only works for mal de buas but also for all illnesses caused by cold humors and hydropesia. Monardes also mentions the complexion of the plants. For example, tobacco should be warm and dry and is used for headache. In contrast to the account of Villasante, guayacán is said to have been discovered thanks to an indigenous doctor who gave it to a Spaniard after he had been infected with syphilis from an indigenous woman.

name Mariana Nava also appears in a Cartagena lawsuit, when a black healer Francisco Mandinga from Cuba stood trial there in 1664. He was said to have cured María Navas (said to be an indigenous woman from Cuba), who suffered from abdominal ailments by prescribing a purge made from *pullon* and honey (Gómez 2017). It is a matter of further investigation whether this was the same person and not just a coincidence of names, and then what the possible link may have been with the indigenous woman who received her title to cure much earlier, and how she got to Cartagena.

In the Greater Antilles only few accounts reflect upon the medicinal practices of the enslaved strata of population. Some of the early botanical knowledge transfer among the enslaved strata was discussed for example by Fernández de Oviedo (see part *e.g.* corn, ñame, palm, *perebecenuc*). From the historical sources available it would seem that occasionally the people of African descent learned some of the indigenous medicinal skills. Analogies with surrounding islands provide us with more details on the exchange among the colonized and enslaved inhabitants.

Sloane´s recompilation of the botanical and medicinal knowledge of Jamaican people (1707) also indicates exchanges between enslaved peoples of West African and New World origins. The enslaved people of New World origin are described as composed of indigenous people that were not native to Jamaica but came from different parts. Some came from Florida or Musquitos, and others were Spanish slaves that had been captured by the English.[106] They are described as very good hunters, fishers, and fowlers, but useless for work in the field or other menial tasks usually done by enslaved persons. Besides some details of their lifeways, Sloane (1707) mentions the use of common remedies such as bleeding, purging, blistering, cupping, and scarification among the indigenous peoples in Jamaica. Similarly, among the enslaved peoples of African origin the cupping with calabashes, the bandaging with a mixture of clay and water over parts of the body, were popular cures.[107]

Enslaved peoples of African origin were said to use very few decoctions of herbs, distillations, and infusions and powdered herbs.[108] Other remedies mentioned were baths prepared from the decoction of bay-leaves, wild sage, after which people make a bundle from these plants and sprinkle them with water. The same source adds that both enslaved and indigenous peoples bathe themselves as much as they can. The data from the Cartagena trials (Gómez 2017) adds more on common therapeutic methods such as cupping, cutting, massages, potions, prayers, and application of power objects among ritual specialists of African origin. Gómez (2017) concluded that the results of these methods resembled each other at an experiential level despite differences in origin and in explanation of the relationship between human health and the natural world.

---

106 The Musquitos could refer Mosquito County of Florida but also to the coast of Nicaragua. Sloane also refer to Mosquito when speaking about the King Jeremy who came to Duke of Albemarle, Governor of Jamiaca to seek his help in their fights against Pirates and Spaniards. On this occasion Mosquitos are said indigenous peoples near the Provinces of Nicaragua, Honduras and Costa Rica (Sloane 1707).

107 Cupping consisted of applying heated calabashes on an affected place of the body. When the calabashes were pulled off, the place was cut and the calabashes cupped again.

108 "*For instance, in a Clap, they grind the roots of Fingrigo and lime tree, between two stones, and stir them into lime juice till it be pretty thick, and so make the patient take it evening and morning for some time. This is the same method of preparing medicines, with what in the East Indies is practiced, for I have seen many simples for them, and all, or most, are to be ground on a stone with some simple liquor, and so given the patient*" (Sloane 1707, p. 54).

Sloane (1707) calls some of the cures effective and others less so; mostly he considered those based on other (*i.e.* non-Christian) belief systems ineffective. This evaluation seems to be based on his conviction that those Others did not even have a religion.[109] Later he adds that some of the cures might come from "the Indians", as they were used for the same diseases in Mexico and Brazil, referring to authors such as Piso, Marcgrave, Hernández, and Ximénes.[110]

As the indigenous people considered by Sloane (1707) included persons who were not native to Jamaica or were already Spanish enslaved subjects, this situation suggests a great diversity of healing practices and botanical knowledge coming together and being exchanged. The properties of some of the herbs were learned from indigenous experts of the mainland via European accounts. In relation to this, Sloane suggests that Jamaican colonizers knew how to use a herb called *contra yerba* for the treatment of wounds caused by poisoned arrows, because it was revealed by indigenous people from Guyana to the Spaniards who wounded an indigenous man with a poisonous arrow to find out what herbs they would use to cure it (Sloane 1707).

Likewise, Sloane testifies how Europeans learned many healing practices from enslaved peoples. African captives had the advantage of recognizing some of the tropical diseases and flora. Just one example: the properties of the leaves of the balsam/goaconax tree were taught to Europeans by a man of West African origin who used these herbs to cure himself. A large group of plants used by Afro-Caribbean practitioners was recorded in 17th century documents that show both endemic and exotic plant species.[111] Although these medicinal skills were recorded rather by accident, more in-depth studies like the one by Schiebinger (2017) reveal some of the secrets of the enslaved population in the context of colonial struggles in the West Indies. One of her examples illustrates that what it is registered as European appropriation of slaves' cure for yaws might indirectly transmit an indigenous remedy.

The knowledge of the enslaved persons of West African origin is by no means to be explained *only* as learned or adopted from indigenous peoples. Enslaved people avidly collected, cultivated, and tested medicines to find effective cures to their problems in new environments. The records of the Cartagena trials show that different healing specialists managed to bring their expertise as well as their views and practices across

109 In this respect, he says: "*The Indians and Negros have no manner of Religion by what I could observe of them. This true they have several ceremonies, as dances, playing but these for the most part are so far from being acts of adoration of a God, that they are for the most part mixt with a great deal of Bawdry and Lewdness.*"

110 Willem Piso and Georg Marcgraf of *Historia Naturalis Brasiliae published in 1648. For the most recent work on this work see project BRASILIAE of* Dr. Françozo on https://www.universiteitleiden.nl/en/staffmembers/mariana-de-campos-francozo#tab-1. Francisco Hernández was a physician of Philip II and author of *Historia natural de Nueva España,* important work including some insights from Nahuatl medicine on Mexican remedies, flora and fauna. Francisco Ximénes from Huaxtepec edited Hernández´ work and added his own notes and experiences.

111 Plants used in the healing practices in 17th century by the black Caribbean ritual specialists were: Anamú, Ariajua, buevera, Cañoco, Capitana, Carara, Carcoma, Cayaya, De Santa María, Escobilla, Grango, Guano, Limpiadientes, Orejom, Pantailla, Pullon, Rodo de Alacran, Rompesera, Tuatua, Achiote (Bixa Orellana), Basil (Ocimum basilicum), Bejuco (Mikania guaco), Bottle gourds (Lagenaria siceraria or Agenaria vulgaris), Caraña (Bursera graveolens), Chamomile (Asteraceae), Culantrillo (Adientum canillus-veneris), Guamo (Inga Feulleei), Guayacán (Guaiacu sp/), Lulos (Solanum quitoense), Palm hearts (Euterpe oleracea), Palo de Fraile (Couepia poliandra), Pringamosa (Urtica dioica), Tobacco (Nicotiana tabacum) (Gómez 2017).

the Atlantic Ocean and re-established them in the Americas (Gómez 2017; Vargas 2011).[112] Gómez sketches some of the perspectives of the forced migrants in new societal and environmental contexts. One of the trials discussed was that of Antonio Congo, originally from West Central Africa (possibly of the Congo nation), resident of Cartagena, who confessed to having engaged with the spirits of the indigenous people during healing practices. He testified that his *bohío* (hut) was built on the burial place of an ancient indigenous community and for that reason he commemorated their spirits by sharing his food and the payments of his patients in the hope that they would favor his healing practices (AHN Inquisición, L. 1023, Fol. 482r in Gómez 2017). This is a fascinating illustration of how forced migrants perceived the newly inhabited landscapes.

Although several later works such as that of Chateusalins (1854) sheds some light on the life, illness and remedies of the enslaved population in Cuba during the first half of the 19th century, the majority of their knowledge as well as their history remained undocumented. Chateusalins`s account (1854) deserves further analysis. It reveals practices like *cachexy* or the consumption of clay, which has been observed among enslaved populations in other Caribbean contexts (Kiple 2002). Chateusalins explained this consumption as a consequence of malnutrition, which was rooted in grief because of the enslavement, harsh treatment and homesickness of the former captives. Descriptions like this provide insights not only into the medicinal knowledge but also into the coping mechanisms of the captives at the peak of the sugar revolution in Cuba. At last, there are more sources illustrative of past medicinal traditions (see Fig. 4 and Fig.5).[113]

It would be beyond the scope of this study to review all available resources regarding the medicinal history of both islands. However, when examining some of these sources again the multidirectional character of the ethnic mobility and of the knowledge exchange called my attention. With regard to indigenous and Afro-Caribbean interactions, the locales of the exchange of botanical knowledge should be considered in a more flexible manner. With regard to Afro-Caribbean ritual specialists it is clear that these were sometimes more mobile than generaly assumed. Healer Luisa Sánchez, identified as a *mulata*, is said to have travelled around the city of Bayamo in the 1620s. Paula de Eguiluz moved from Santo Domingo to Puerto Rico, from there to Havana, and later to las Minas del Cobre before going to Cartagena. In another of the Cartagena trials, a healer of African origin, Alonso Venero, born in east Cuba (Villa del Vaqueres), testified in the court at Cartagena in 1686 that he learned his healing practices from

---

112 To mention just a few names: among the healers who were persecuted in Hispaniola in the 17th century were Jusepa Ruiz, Paula de Equiliz, Bernarda Alvaréz, Ana María de Robles, Luisa Dominguez, and Ana Jiménez. Prosecuted Cuban healers included: Luisa Sanchez, Antonio García, Mariana de la Peña, Catalina de Molina, Teodora de Salcedo, María de Tapia, Catalina González, Tomasa de los Reyes, and Ana Ramírez (Gómez 2017; Vargas 2011).

113 Fig. 4 and Fig. 5 are images by Spanish painter Victor Patricio Landaluze y Uriarte (1830 -1899) who illustrated *Tipos y Costumbres de la Isla de Cuba* (1881), edited by Miguel de Villas, with introduction by Antonio Bachiller y Morales. This work was influenced by Costumbrismo, a literary style combining the Romaticism and artistic realism of the end of 18th and 19th century.

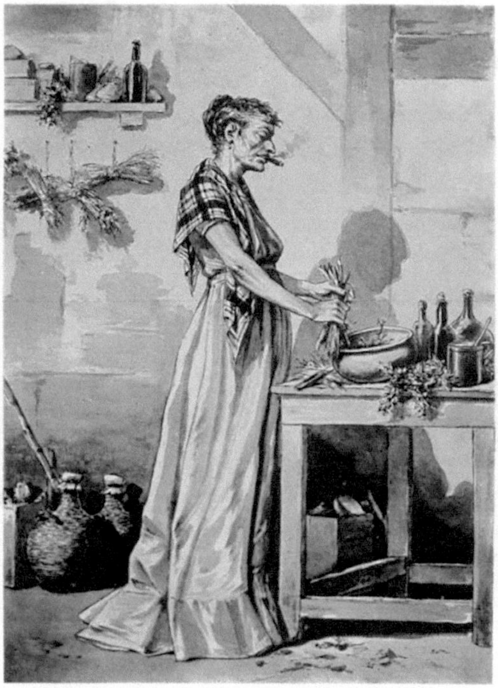

Figure 4 The Cuban Healer by Landaluze (1881).

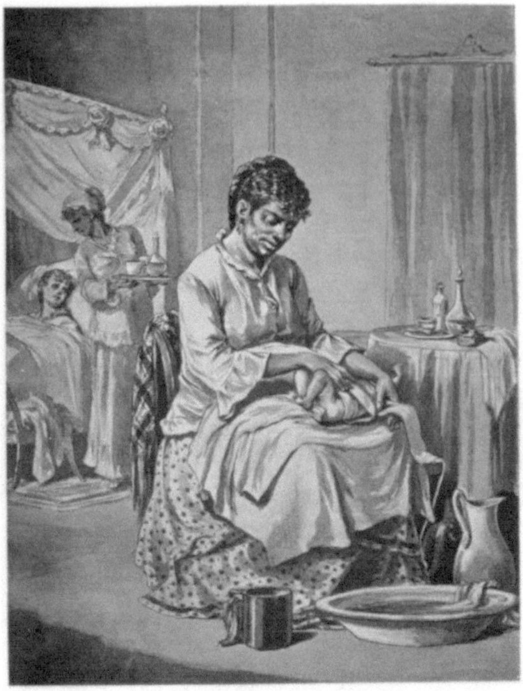

Figure 5 The Cuban midwife by Landaluze (1881).

people in the countryside and from a Spaniard from Jamaica (Gómez 2017).[114] Also some indigenous individuals and healers are likely to be in some occassions more socially and geographically mobile. At last, colonial hospitals, convents, mines or cattle ranches created settings for learning and observing each other´s medicinal skills in the colonial society. To known more about how character of the contemporary healing practices was created we need to first also understand the demographic history of the region and particularities of the local development.

Concluding remarks

"For a colonized people the most essential value, because the most concrete, is first and foremost the land, the land which will bring them bread and, above all dignity" (Fanon 2014 [1961, p. 34]); this quote from the Caribbean classic, reminds us how colonialism has alienated the colonized and the colonizer from the land, constructing it as commodity, point of violence and enslavement. Even though the natural environment and its relation to the body were central to the justification of oppression and colonial exploitation, the land remained a means for survival through subsistence, being a green pharmacy and an agent or mediator in medicine and in the healing process both for the colonized and the colonizer. We have seen that the medicinal history of both regions

114 According to the trail report this healer had a reputation of being able to control the movements of snakes, to tame bulls with his words and to cure people from numb stomachs with *tuatua*. In his testimonies he told the Inquisitors about his encounters with Maroons and dead ancestors (Gómez 2017).

under study was marked by broader profound conceptual and material transformations, which were triggered by the European arrival in the Caribbean.

From historical sources, it is clear that the role of indigenous healers lasted longer than generally assumed and that they received recognition and had contacts and engagement with other healing specialists. The contribution of healers from across the Atlantic Ocean and even from the American mainland should equally be considered. The healing specialists of non-local origin quickly were forced to become acquainted with the properties of the plants in the new surroundings, as these were often the only available remedies available. Their study of the plants, based on recognizing similarities with the flora they knew from their own country and further on a trial and error method, likely integrated occassionaly also information received from the original inhabitants. Although the indigenous people have been said to keep medicinal properties of some plants in secret, the dynamics of the changing colonial society, the coexistence of different strata of population in the same spaces must have led to knowledge transfer. Overall, however, our knowledge about the indigenous medicinal contribution is handicapped by the limited and fragmentary nature of the historical sources, which are only to be (even if only partially) remediated by more systematic and interdisciplinary studies of this topic. The demographic history of both regions summarized in the next chapter approximates us further the context of this medicinal transfer.

5

Crossroads of Cultural landscapes: the indigenous base of demographic changes

1515 Naborías the Names of the Captives
They were not cacicas.
They were not heirs to yuca fields.
There were no concessions made to their status.
They were not "queens."
Their names are recorded in the lists of work gangs
Sent to the mines, the conucos, the kitchens, the laundries
of the Spanish invaders.
Macaney, field hand.
Franciscquilla, cook.
Ana, baker.
Catalina, pig woman.
Morales (2001).

The early colonial encounters of the Old and New World profoundly influenced the composition of the existing population of the regions under study.[115] The following pages summarize that demographic history with focus on its indigenous element. The colonial history of indigenous ancestors is followed by an overview of the demographic history of each island and by a clarification of the historical background of selected locations from which the data originated. This review will bring us closer to an understanding of the role of indigenous ancestors within medicinal history.

Morales' poem reminds us of some of the forgotten figures of Puerto Rican history, the indigenous women who occupied low-status positions in the early colonial society. The invisibility of the colonized strata of the population has always presented obstacles to the quest for identity and to the dignification of one's own heritage, while creating severe gaps in the demographic history, also in other Caribbean contexts. The recons-

115 For studies about pre-colonial societies in Hispaniola and Cuba see among others: Keegan & Hofman (2017), Hofman et al. (2008), Ulloa Hung (2013), Ulloa Hung & Valcárcel Rojas (2016), Curet et al. (2005), Veloz Magiolo (1993).

truction of population records within the colonial context is in need of a deconstruction of colonial worldview, but is also problematized by the selective and fragmented content of the colonial archives (see *e.g.* Roque & Wagner 2012).

In general, scholars agree upon the fact that the primacy of the colonization of Hispaniola and Cuba led to irreversible destruction of the indigenous populations. The great narrative is as follows: colonial rule led to a demographic disaster before the colonizers realized the negative impact of their doings; countless indigenous people died because of violence, germs or labor exploitation. The indigenous disappearance was considered by some authors as an unavoidable, logical step in unilineal cultural and technological development. Overwhelmed by the cruelty of Spanish rule other explanations seem to underestimate the indigenous agency and various ways of resistance. These scenarios were later nuanced by combining various factors, among which the lack of resistance towards exotic germs, the insular environment and labor exploitation were the most decisive. Many of these explanations, however could not escape the dichotomy between the rebellions/resistance or peacefulness/disappearance (Valcárcel Rojas 2016). Later attempts highlighting the indigenous agency during the early colonial period were faced with gaps in the available data on the extent of the impact of 1492 on the indigenous population, the general demographic history, and the cultural transformations in the colonial context.

The estimates of indigenous population in colonial Cuba and Hispaniola are biased and often seem to be intentionally manipulated for economic, ideological (*e.g.* ethnic origin obstructing social mobility), and legal reasons (*e.g.* the illicit slave trade, the prohibitions of enslavement of the indigenous population) (Guitar 2002; Ulloa Hung 2016; Paulino Ramos 2008; Moya Pons 2010; Valcárcel Rojas & Pérez Concepción 2014; Valcárcel Rojas 2016). Briefly, the first problem with the population registers in the following sections is the general invisibility of the lower strata of the population, especially enslaved indigenous people, women, and children. The growth or decline are difficult to estimate as various methods of counting and categorization were used (vecino vs. church categories).[116] To illustrate this point: the provincial council of Santo Domingo in 1623 ordered the separation of the register of the indigenous people in provinces where these people were present, and later in 1673, they issued the order to keep all registers for Hispaniola in one book, including baptisms of enslaved people (Saez 2008). In contrast, in Cuba this distinction seems to be maintained until the 19th century (Vega Suñol 2014). The bias in these registers becomes even more apparent when the same registers are contrasted with other references from the colonial archives.

---

116 More specifically, parochial censuses focused on different segments of society (people of confession, those being baptized, or just those coming regularly to mass). In contrast, general population estimates counted individuals with *vecino* status, according to whether or not they could be employed in war, or just in general as a person. According to Torres in 1577 in Santo Domingo *vecino* referred to a person who had a farm, small farm, or sugar mill. Neither slaves nor their families were counted as part of this category (Rodríguez Demorizi 1945). Alejandro de la Fuente argued that only the head of the household or family was counted as *vecino*. This is also the case of the census of Osorio in Hispaniola. In general, historians focusing on colonial Spanish Americas calculate the number of population by multiplying by five the number of the *vecinos*, but there have been obvious differences in the estimates and critiques of this methodology as it did not include other nationalities or freed peoples of color, which were practically absorbed into the Spanish population (see Wheat 2016).

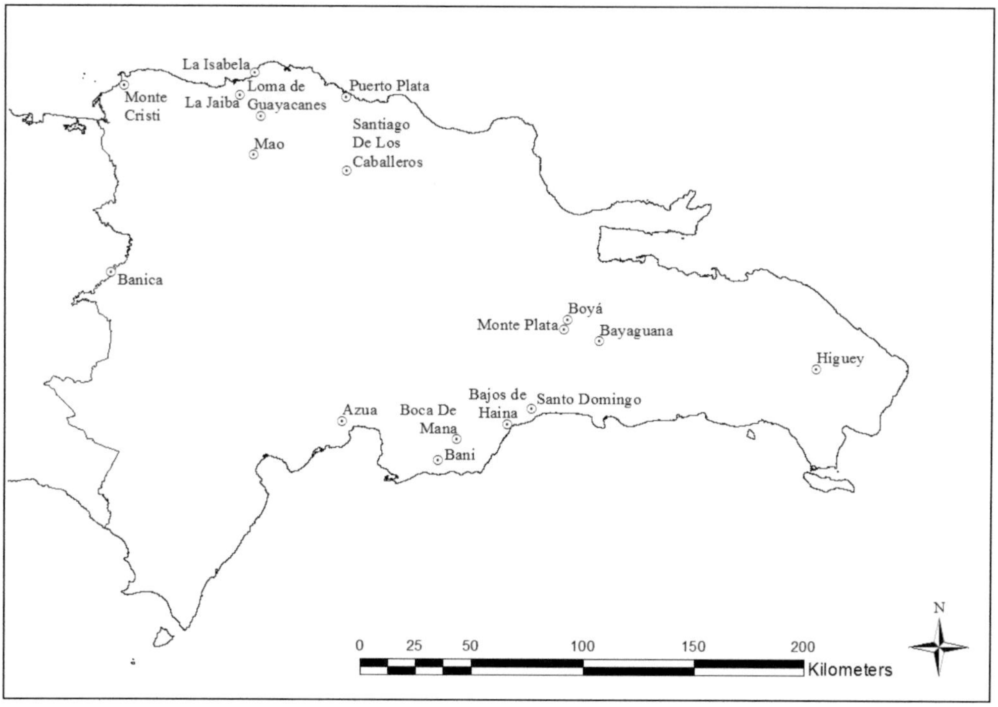

Figure 6 The Dominican locations mentioned in the historical overview.

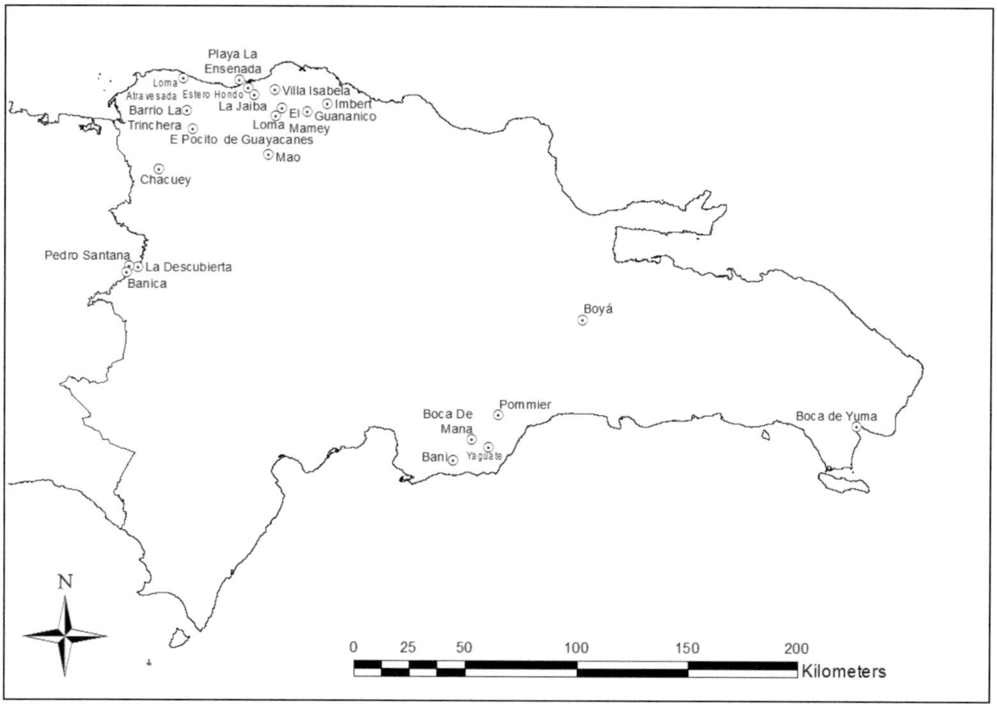

Figure 7 Dominican fieldwork locations.

Brief account of indigenous ancestors in colonial Hispaniola

Different scholars (Anderson-Cordova 1990, 2017; Guitar 2002; Deagan & Cruxent 2002; Deagan 2014; Ernst & Hofman 2018; Hofman 2018; Herrera Malatesta 2018; Mira Caballos 2009; Moya Pons 2010; Samson 2010; Ulloa Hung 2016) have addressed the early colonial history of indigenous peoples in Hispaniola. Until recently, it has been generally agreed that the Spanish conquest and colonization of Hispaniola led to a total genocide of indigenous peoples or at least to their decimation by the 1550s (*e.g.* Moya Pons 2010). Some historians like Guitar (2002) have argued against the rapid disappearance of the indigenous population. While her suggestions were received with skepticism, prominent historians like Moya Pons (2010) called for more research on this topic.

The early demographic development of colonial Hispaniola starts with considerable differences in estimates of indigenous population at the time of the conquest. These estimates have been debated for several decades and ranged from 100,000 to 8,000,000 (Moya Pons & Flores Paz 2013). The idea of a huge decline in number of indigenous people may have resulted from an unclear image of the original population to start with. In 1512, the Spanish population of Hispaniola was reportedly about ten thousand (Moya Pons 2010). The *repartimiento* of 1514, the only surviving document of the early colonial period that provides us with more accurate number of allotted indigenous people, counted 26,330 allocated individuals, which were divided among 3585 Spaniards (see *e.g.* Anderson-Cordova 1990, 2017).[117] In 1516, influenced by Las Casas' critique of the *encomienda* system three missionaries of the Hieronymite´s order were sent to Santo Domingo to dismantle the *encomienda*. One year later, the Hieronymite friars estimated the number of indigenous people to oscillate between fifteen and sixteen thousand individuals (Mira Caballos 2009). This suggests that the indigenous population decreased within one year with ten or eleven thousand. In spite of great opposition from the Spanish colonizers, the Hieronymites reallocated the indigenous people into new villages of their own. In 1518, the smallpox epidemic is said to have reduced the population to only three thousand. This implied that the number of originally planned settlements was reduced to seventeen; of only fifteen of these the location is known.[118] These villages are considered to have been slowly depopulated as a result of continuous Spanish attacks, and the mistreatment by *majordomos* (Mira Caballos 2009). Within this context, details about the lives of indigenous inhabitants of these settlements and their integration into the early colonial society are lacking. By the 1520s, the Spanish and other European population of the island decreased as a result of the huge scale of emigration to the mainland. In 1528, Hispaniola counted little more than one hundred *vecinos* (Moya Pons 2010).

The interpretation of events such as the smallpox outbreak may greatly have influenced the following estimates. In contrast to the Hieronymites' claims about the large population decline, a document from one year after the epidemic suggests that

117 This document has been discussed earlier by various scholars, among them Rodríguez Demorizi (1971), Mira Caballos (2009), and Moya Pons (2010).

118 Among them were Xaragua, Baní, Yaquimo, Verapaz, Santiago, Santa Ana, La Mejorada de Cotuí, Santa Maria de la 0, San Julian, San Juan Bautista and Santo Tome, and three more villages at Minao and el Coco (Mira Caballos 2007). However, the exact location of these settlements should be studied further because there are some discrepancies among the different authors (see later the Baní case).

the population could even have been twelve thousand (Anderson-Cordova 2017). Authors and readers seeking to highlight the possible indigenous continuity in this period might immediately see this figure as a sign of the colonial manipulation of the registers. In this vein, Hieronymites could have exaggerated the impact of smallpox to protect this population and/or to justify the trafficking of humans from West Africa. In the end, the introduction of enslaved African men appeased the anti-*encomienda* critics and satisfied the increased demand for labor in sugar mills. A similar manipulation has also been observed in other colonial regions like Mexico. These revisions could further lend support to the argument that the above mentioned number of three thousand do not include all indigenous inhabitants of the island, for example those who might not have been known to colonial authorities. In contrast, other researchers could doubt the accuracy of these estimates, disregard those twelve thousand recorded by Hieronymites and point to the general inconsistencies in the records. Both interpretations are likely to influence the readers´ diverse conclusions about the genetic and cultural continuities of indigenous society.

These estimates are to be complemented by data (from European colonial sources) about various indigenous responses to the initial contact, conquest and *encomienda* system, which were summarized by Anderson-Cordova (1990, 2017). The initial contact was followed by flight, exchange, and conflict (*e.g.* at El Golfo de Las Flechas and La Navidad). The indigenous people accommodated the colonial exploitation by following the official demands requiring them to pay tribute. At the same time, they resisted by quitting the cultivation of *conucos*, which led to starvation among the Spaniards, and by fleeing to marginal areas or to other islands. For some, the inhumane treatment and the life in captivity were only to be escaped by ending their own life and also the life of the unborn children. Lastly, the conquest was answered by the military defense of the territories of Higüey (using Spanish weapons) and Jaragua, and by a serious resistance that continued on a smaller scale until the 1550s.[119] This resistance went in hand with good knowledge of both cultural environments.[120]

After the establishment of different Spanish settlements close to the indigenous villages, the Spanish *encomienda* became one of the important factors shaping indigenous responses and consequently also the cultural change. Indigenous people were divided among the colonizers three times. From the data about the second allocation, it is clear

119 Leaders such as cacique Enrique and warriors like Hernandillo, Murcia and Tuerta resisted the Spanish occupation for a substantial period of time. In Enrique's case, it was at least fourteen years. But also later in the 1550s, there were around 20 to 25 insurrections in the region between Vega and Santiago. The accounts about these resisting groups indicate their extreme mobility. An army of indigenous warriors from the Bahoruco, led by a leader who previously fought together with Dieguillo Ocampo, was causing harm to Spaniards in the surroundings of Santiago and La Vega (Letter from Licenciado Grajeda to his Majesty, 23.6.1549). The mobility is also evident from the fact that indigenous people from Hispaniola went to warn those of Cuba. During the Kalinago´s attack on Puerto Rico also Caribs from Tierra Firme, who communicated with Kalinagos from Dominica, came to Puerto Rico and took from the estates the enslaved black people and everything they found there.

120 Cacique Enrique or Enriquillo was raised in a Franciscan convent. After several attempts to pacify his uprising he surrendered himself voluntarily in 1533 in exchange for some land, legal status and the lives of other insurgent people, including fugitive Africans.

that indigenous people had to work in mining and agriculture.[121] The allocations seem to have facilitated more contact among people who belonged to various ethnicities, including the Spanish. More specifically, sixty-two of the *encomenderos* were married to indigenous women.[122] The number of the illegal unions and the children resulting from these is estimated to be much higher. While among the *encomenderos* (in total at least 3,585, according to Mira Caballos 2009) were also apothecaries and surgeons, some indigenous people are likely to have served in the hospitals, monasteries, and churches of the first towns. This situation must have created a setting where distinct medicinal cultures circulated and were appropriated.

The Hieronymites left behind not only their estimates but also some insights into later indigenous responses to colonialism. Based on the Hieronymites´ Interrogatory of 1517, Anderson-Cordova (1990, 2017) suggested that in spite of the colonial oppression, indigenous people maintained many of their own cultural traits. This interrogatory examined whether indigenous people were capable of living on their own and of handling freedom. It is no surprise that most Spanish settlers argued against indigenous freedom. Some of them even claimed that when having freedom indigenous people would return to their own religious practices and life-ways. Among the traditional elements were: the knowledge of the *behiques* how to prepare poisonous concoctions, the ritual cleansing and feasting, and the *cohoba* rituals. This indicates that nearly twenty years after the European invasion, at the time when the early colonial societies were established, certain indigenous medicinal practices continued to exist. An unwanted effect of the reallocation to indigenous settlements was the shifting of the villages by the indigenous people themselves. Like in the pre-colonial times, they would take all of their possessions and establish new settlements somewhere else. In this period there were still many indigenous villages, some of them quite removed from the Spanish population, even two large villages with their own cacique. Also, the more distant the settlements were from a Spanish town, the larger their population. Indigenous house servants who spoke Spanish and believed in Catholicism were given as an example of why the indigenous peoples should be located as close as possible to the Spanish settlements (Anderson-Cordova 1990).

Many of these arguments were clearly colored by the economic interests of the Spanish colonizers who opposed the freeing of the subaltern. In spite of this bias, it is indeed possible that some of these opinions were based on observations of the continuity of indigenous life-ways and worldviews. At the same time, there were clearly many indigenous persons who assimilated to the colonial society. This can be seen in the case of mixed marriages, and in the re-education of indigenous children in Spanish convents, which seem to have formed a whole group of bilingual people like Enrique,

121 Alberquerque's *repartimiento* of 1514 showed that the vast majority was located in mining cities like Concepción, Santiago, Santo Domingo (minas de Haina), and Buenaventura. The remaining groups were located in Puerto Plata, Higüey, Azua, Puerto Real, Bonao, Guahaba, Maguana, Verapaz, La Sabana, and Yáquimo.

122 Note that such marriages were already prohibited at this time because in the past they had become a means for common Spanish men to receive more *encomendados*, which endangered the distribution of wealth among the colonial elite. The average of legal marriages with indigenous women varied according to the region: in Puerto Plata up to 27%, in Azua 13%, but in San Domingo only 2% of the total legal marriages (Mira Caballos 2009).

or cacique Rodrigo, who were knowledgeable of and most likely also converted to Catholicism. Lastly, the further coexistence of different groups in later periods, in both urban and rural contexts, led to interactions and mutual influences between the culture of the colonizer and the culture of the colonized cultures: a form of transculturation under the colonizer´s domination.

In spite of strong opposition from the Spanish *encomenderos*, the Hieronymites decided to reallocate the indigenous peoples to their own new villages. The later history of these indigenous settlements is unclear. After the exodus of Spanish people to the American mainland (New Mexico, Florida, Peru etc.), the discovery of the correct route to the Indies, and the exhaustion of some gold mines, the interest in agricultural production renewed. That shift in local demography and economy was decisive for the roles played by the indigenous people. Indigenous ancestors were to continue the production of crops for subsistence, but later they started to export crops like ginger, sugar, tobacco, cacao, *zarzaparrilla*, and *ají*, and to extract precious, colorant or medicinal wood like *cañafistola* and *guayacán*. Indigenous people were also documented as being employed as cattle herders and were valued as huntsmen.

Dominican indigenous ancestors after the New Laws

The history of the first inhabitants of Hispaniola after the New Laws issued in 1542 has not been adequately studied.[123] However, various primary sources mention indigenous individuals and communities that were integrated into the colonial society after the New Laws.[124]

Some of the indigenous villages escaped the gaze of the colonialists for a long time. In 1556, Spanish settlers were searching for runaway captives and found four villages previously unknown to them, one in the neighborhood of Puerto Plata, the others on the coast in the former province of Ciguayos, in the province of Samana, and in Cabo de San Nicolás (Blanco Díaz 2009). Because the inhabitants of these villages were distributed among the Spaniards (against the prescriptions of the New Laws), an appeal was made to free them and to put them in the villages where they should not be disturbed, or at least to leave them in the places where they were found. Similarly, Friar Juan de Ortega found later many indigenous peoples "hidden" in the province of Ciguayos, the Cape of San Nicolás and the cape of Tiburón. In an attempt to convert them to the Catholic faith, this friar concentrated them in settlements. Where the friar reallocated those indigenous people remains unclear. It is possible that he created new

---

123 It should be remarked that the New Laws issued in 1542 were received differently in Cuba and Hispaniola. Although there were some protests against them, *vecinos* of Hispaniola issued less official complains than their Cuban neighbors did. In the context of Hispaniola, this could be interpreted as a consequence of the demographic decline and/or by the fact that the Hieronymites had taken indigenous laborers away more than twenty years before. In Hispaniola the indigenous laborers had since been replaced by enslaved individuals from Africa and the Lesser Antilles. In fact, those laws made that enslavement official.

124 As it was not in the scope of this study to review archival records in Spain, Cuba and Dominican Republic I limited myself to existing literature on the history of the indigenous peoples in the colonial period and primary documents which were transcribed and published by scholars from the National Archive (as early as the 1950s). Additionl aim of this chapter is to highlith the importance of existing bundles of colonial documents which contain important references to historically marginalized peoples but are often not cited by heritage experts.

settlements but he may have also brought them to an already existing one. According to Mira Caballos (2009) San Juan de Ortega, Cayacoa, and Villaviciosa should be some of the indigenous villages that remained after the experiments of the Hieronomites (Blanco Díaz 2009).

In more detail, the royal decree of 1563 instructed that indigenous people found on the island in this period should serve only to the King, and that the friar who concentrated the indigenous people in villages should not be further persecuted by the Spaniards, but should be supported in his attempts to convert them. All indigenous people who were found after this date should live in liberty (Blanco Díaz 2009).

Some indigenous people stayed in urban areas. In 1551, Licenciado Zurita (in Rodriguez Morel 2011) answered a Royal request to educate the indigenous people in a monastery in Santo Domingo by justifying that there were almost no "*naturales de la tierra*" left and those who were living in the city were "ladinos", and knew the Spanish language already. Zurita contrasted this group with those who were enslaved individuals and later were given liberty: they were said to have gone to live inland because the company of Spaniards was "loathsome" for them. In his view, to collect them all for the purpose of conversion was too difficult, unnecessary and disadvantageous for them *"because none of them have the capacity to make ranches or to have a fortune, and what they earn is spent quickly on their bad habits: drinking and eating and other similar things, and if there are some who are not so ladinos they are in their cattle and sheep ranches, and other haciendas far away from this city*" (Rodriguez Morel 2011, p. 124). This reply could be read as a lack of interest in remaining indigenous descendants on the part of some religious authorities, but also as a testimony of their integration into the colonial city, and of the withdrawal of others to rural areas.

The invisibility of the indigenous segment of society in the later colonial period might be due not only to the process of transculturation, but also to its employment in agriculture in areas more remote from the towns. Historical references to this sector proceed from complaints or from extraordinary situations rather than from the interest of the colonial authorities. In this way, we know that indigenous peoples of Mona were cultivating batatas, cassava, and melons in great quantities between 1557-1564 and exchanging them with the French (Echogoian 1565). Mona inhabitants were compared to other indigenous peoples from Ayaguana and La Vega neighborhoods, which were said to live without a village and without being converted (Echogoian 1565). The early 17th century indigenous inhabitants of Boyá are said to have owned different *hatos,* which were producing cassava and ginger (see below). Yet, Boyá inhabitants are given as an example of conversion.

Indigenous descendants lived in rural areas at the time of the evacuation of the North. The North was evacuated in order to end the large-scale contraband trade in which the northern towns were engaged. In 1604 complaints are registered about the negative impact that this policy might have if put into practice. Before the actual devastations, an appeal was sent to consider that the majority of the *vecinos* and inhabitants of this area were "*commoners, mestizos, mulatos and blacks*", who did not have estates, had nothing or very little to lose, and lacked transport (Rodríguez Demorizi 1945). According to this command, many of these people only had a small farm with which they sustained with their own family, and while others might have had one or two enslaved persons, their help was not sufficient for such a relocation. Another danger of the whole removal of the population was that people might choose to stay there and later appropriate other people's properties. One of the people who signed the documents was Antonio Ruiz, an indigenous man who seems to have occupied a high social rank (Rodríguez Demorizi 1945).

Although these requests may have been a bit exaggerated because they were aimed at convincing the authorities to reconsider the evacuation of the North, from later complaints it seems that some of these fears came true. Among later complaints from *vecinos* about how the evacuation impacted their lives, was that the cattle that was left behind was eaten by the people of mixed and West African origin ("*mestizos, mulatos y negros*"), and other people hiding and staying in the North (1609). Although it is not totally certain whether the text refers to local or nonlocal indigenous persons, it is possible that, like in other contexts, the authorities took them away exactly because they were locals and as such, were officially free in this period. The violation of the New Laws was not a unique case when compared to the situation in Cuba or Mexico.

Unwillingly following Osorio's mandate, Spaniards, and some *"peoples of color"* from Bayajá and La Yaguana moved east and founded Bayaguana. Small settlements from Cibao were relocated closer to Santiago, La Vega and Cotuí. Similarly, former inhabitants of Monte Cristi and Puerto Plata constructed Monte Plata next to the indigenous village of Boyá. The establishment of these new settlements also led to land struggles (see later history of Boyá).

The evacuation of the North seems to have generated space for those who wanted to be out of sight of the colonial authorities, the population that became invisible in the historic records. Sometimes, troops were sent to capture the escaped enslaved men, but it is clear that different people stayed, and continued to live from agriculture, cattle raising and most likely continued trading contraband with the enemies (see the later history of the Northeast).

The devastation of the North reinforced the process of transculturation, which seems to have taken place early after the first indo-afro-hispano encounters. The indigenous influences seem to have been visible in the material culture left from these early encounters in both urban areas and in rural areas.[125] With respect to the latter, Ulloa Hung (2016) has suggested that the process of mestizaje and creolization is apparent in the material cultures of rural areas and supports this by referring to a royal decree of 1538 about Buenaventura and Santa Cruz de Acayagua, where there was a population of more than one hundred Spanish people, and six hundred individuals of indigenous and west African origin. After more than seventy years, the population of this region seems to have remained the same. The region still had many small, very dispersed settlements at riverbanks and valleys in the Buenaventura and Acayagua regions, where congregations of Spanish people, hundreds of indigenous people, and people of West African origin (the words used are: "Black and Indians") were working in agriculture, cultivating crops and raising cattle (Gil-Bermejo García 1983).

125 The urban areas have been studied in the archaeological research of sites such as La Isabela, Puerto Real, En Bas Saline, La Vega, Santo Domingo, and Cotuí.

Enslaved indigenous population

When speaking about the indigenous component of the population, it is important to acknowledge that this component in itself was composed of a great diversity of indigenous cultural elements, stemming from pre-colonial and colonial times (for pre-colonial times see *e.g.* the Ulloa Hung 2016, as well as Hofman et al. 2018). The inter-island mobility and engagements between communities were already occurring on a pan-regional scale in the pre-colonial period (*e.g.* Hofman & Bright 2010; Hofman & Duivenbode 2011; Rodríguez Ramos 2010).

Columbus' diary (1961 [1492]) suggests the existence of regular inter-island mobility. More specifically, Columbus observed an indigenous man who travelled from Santa Maria to Fernandina, people who knew how to navigate from the Bahamas to Cuba, and furthermore, he based his knowledge about the population of other islands on the hearsay of the inhabitants whom he had already met. During the later colonial period there are multiple references to – often forced – contacts among indigenous individuals. First, different enslaving voyages were organized to Cuba, and the Bahamas, and continued on other Caribbean islands and Tierra Firme throughout the colonial period. D'Anghiera estimated that between 1508 -1513, approximately 40,000 people were brought from the surrounding islands (Moya Pons 2010). Justifying their colonial invasion by allegations of cannibalism against the native inhabitants, in the context of a theory of "just war", the Spaniards captured even those who were initially reported as being very friendly and welcoming them.

Anderson-Cordova (2017) has provided an overview of the legislation that regulated the indigenous slave trade on Hispaniola.[126] In sum, from the legislation issued between 1495 and 1547, it is clear that slave raids were organized in the following locations: Caribbean islands (Lucayos, St. Croix, Dominica, Martinique, St. Lucia, La Ascensión, Barbados, Tobaco Mayo, Trinidad, San Bernardo, Fuerte Island, and Barú island), Cartagena port, Paria, Venezuela, Honduras coast (Guanajos), Pánuco, and New Mexico (Anderson-Cordova 2017). In addition, people were generally enslaved in zones of conflict and war, or where people rebelled against or attacked the Spanish estates, and in areas where there was no gold. Colonial authorities also requested to bring people from New Spain because they were skilled at searching for sources of silver, and working with silver. These orders suggested to bring them to be sent over with their families *"to make them feel well"* (Yaremko 2016).

The distribution of enslaved non-local indigenous individuals needs further investigation. In 1578, Doctor Gregorio González de Cuenca, president of the Audiencia Real de Santo Domingo, asked His Majesty King Philip II to send a declaration to free the indigenous peoples from Hamana, Maricapana and Cumanacoa, Cariaco and

126 In 1505, provisions were issued to bring 'cannibals' from San Bernaldo, Fuerte, the ports of Cartagena, and the Vany islands. In 1508/1509, colonizers in Hispaniola were asked to maximize the production of gold and to build villages next to the mines. The regions from which the peoples could be captured and enslaved under the excuse of cannibalism varied over time. In 1520, basically all islands where Christians did not live, were declared to be inhabited by Caribs, the only exceptions being Trinidad, Lucayos, Barbados, Gigantes, and Margarita. In 1530, the enslavement of indigenous peoples was prohibited under any circumstances, because of large-scale abuses. This prohibition was lifted only four years later, however, probably because of the rising demands for enslaved workers related to the sugar industry. In 1543, a royal prohibition was issued to transfer indigenous peoples, whether free or enslaved, outside of their province, but this legislation was also periodically violated.

other provinces of Caracas, La Nueva Andalucía, Margarita and others who had been brought as captives to Santo Domingo. In contradiction to the Real degree issued in 1564, the captains did not treat them well and did not release them. Dr. González is said to have made a village for them approximately six leagues from the city, with at least twelve Indians and a friar to indoctrinate them and make them Christians and free them from captivity (González de Cuenca 1578 in Rodriguez Morel 2015). The location of this village is not clear. In fact, the historical foundation of certain settlements is not clear. As late as in 1628, one small village on the bank of the river Yguamo was "discovered" by colonial authorities, being inhabited by around 150 indigenous descendants. As it was considered that these men were without work, they could therefore be used as workforce for planting medicinal plants. In two years, the population dropped to only 18 men and 15 women. The reason of this decline might be that the indigenous inhabitants just moved further away in order not to be harassed by the outsiders, and because their lands were taken away from them. As in other cases, the Spaniards started to claim the land as their own property, because, like in the case of Boyá, these lands were considered uncultivated (see below).

The lives of these enslaved indigenous peoples in the colonies have had the same destiny as those of other enslaved laborers. Since 1518, it was officially allowed to enslave those who were captured during the rebellions in Hispaniola. With the exception of accidental references, indigenous enslaved individuals were dehumanized and homogenized under the label of "slaves".[127]After the number of enslaved people from Africa increased, enslaved indigenous people were sent to search for new sources of silver and gold, clearing savannas and forests, cultivating the land, and taking care of estates, while the women were making cassava, and serving those working in the mines. In the 1520s when the gold profits were invested into sugarcane production, nearly all the owners of sugar mills also had indigenous captives. They were employed in all tasks necessary for the operation of such estates, including domestic tasks, taking care of livestock (also butchering), and cultivating the crops. The Crown also employed indigenous enslaved peoples in the lime kilns, forts, road building, and boats (Rodríguez Demorizi 1957; Mira Caballos 1997; Exquemelin 1971 [1678]; Anderson-Córdova 2017).

Rural and urban areas were the settings where colonized individuals had space and opportunity for mutual exchange of knowledge, while working in construction or as household servants, at markets, churches, and hospitals, but also outside in gold mines, fields, ranches, during military operations, rebellions, and in small rural settlements of freedmen or maroon communities. The changes of indigenous cultures within these settings have taken a place under the Spanish colonial rule, yet where ancestors of West and West Central African origin started to create a substantial part of the colonial societies.

---

127 Enslaved indigenous individuals from Hispaniola were sent to search for pearls in Cubagua and Margarita; together with Lucayos (according to Las Casas Caonabo was also Lucayo), they were shipped to the coast of the pearls, Cabo de Vela, Río de la Hacha and other places. In the first years, *naborías* and enslaved people from the Lesser Antilles were extracting the gold.

African ancestors in Dominican demographic history

The decline of the indigenous population should also be situated within the broader context of large-scale movements of Europeans, intensified by the colonization of Cuba, Darién and Tierra Firme as well as by the later Transatlantic Slave Trade. During the initial voyages, the *conquistadores* were likely to be accompanied by their enslaved men from North Africa (officially maximum four per person). The importance of the Transatlantic Slave Trade and plantation society for both Dominican and Cuban history cannot be overemphasized. In the second half of the 16th century, thousands of African men and women were kidnapped, and shipped in horrible conditions to the Caribbean. Those who survived the terrors of the passage still had to overcome the hardships of life in slavery.

In the first half of the 16th century, the majority of the inhabitants of Hispaniola originally came from the African continent (12,000 Africans vs. 5,000 Spanish in 1546, Hernandez Gonzalez 2010). In 1568, the total population was estimated around 24,550 of which 20,000 were of Sub-Saharan origin (Echogoian 1565). In the 1580s, epidemics affected the territory, resulting in a huge death toll among the population of African ancestry. In 1609, the census after the devastation of the North approximates 9648 enslaved persons (Rodríguez Demorizi 1945). Of this number, only eight hundred worked in sugar mills (twelve at the river Nigua, Haina, including the famous Cepicepi), and the majority occupied different roles as domestic servants or farm workers raising small cattle and planting ginger, yucca and corn.

At the beginning of the 17th century, a considerable number of inhabitants were of mixed origin, among them quite a few freedmen with increased social mobility. Around 1606, different people of mixed origin ("negro", "moreno","mulato") and freed persons received the status of *vecino*. These *vecinos* were owners of estates and farms, which produced cassava, corn and vegetables.[128]

The influx of enslaved laborers to the Spanish part of Hispaniola is displayed in Table 1. The inter-and-intra-island human trafficking should colors these estimates. At the same time, the process of transculturation continued and the number of the free people of color increased, soon becoming an important component of the new society. In one of the descriptions of the islands from 1679, people of color formed the vast majority of a total of 7,500 inhabitants. In 1862, the Spanish crown issued an order to bring families from the Islas Canarias to the island as a human shield against the French intrusion (Hernádez González 2006). Two years later, the first families from the Canary Islands arrived, and were sent to the border between the Eastern (Spanish)

128 The census made in 1606 monitoring the situation in the town after the destruction of the north, counted *vecinos* of the remaining cities, sometimes mentioning their names, race, occupation, marriages and children. This gives us estimates: Santo Domingo had 620 *vecinos* (the majority having family) and 27 representatives of church, Santiago 150 *vecinos*, and 4 clerics, La Vega 38 *vecinos* and 2 clerics, Bayaguana 115 *vecinos* (among them Juan Tamayo), Monte Plata 83 *vecinos* (incl. 1 moreno libre and 1 cleric), Boyá 13 *vecinos* (incl. 1 cleric)" Higüey 22 *vecinos*, Seibo 7 *vecinos*, Azua 46 *vecinos*, in Cotui 24 *vecinos* (incl. 1 priest). More specifically, among the registered persons there are 18 "blacks", 18 "morenos" and 20 "mulatos" (in majority women). For the category *morenos* known examples of baptisms of enslaved people are Antón de Juanes *moreno libre*, Francisca de Moronta, *morena esclava* and also clearly from African continent Pedro Biafara, *moreno libre*. The denominations "mulato/a libres", "moreno/a", "moreno/a libre" "moreno/a jorros", "cimarron", "negro/a libres" are marked by the colonial categories and hierarchies of race (Rodríguez Demorizi 1945).

part and the Western (French) part, as well as to the previously depopulated North and South. At the same time, enslaved individuals escaping from the French area were seeking refuge in Hispaniola, and were granted their freedom.[129]

Tracing the origins of the African ancestors

After a general overview of the origins of the African ancestors of the Dominican and Cuban population this section will proceed to shed light on the ethnic hyper-diversity of African descendants, which contributed even further to the emerging Dominican composition. The identification of the origins of the African peoples in the Caribbean is conditioned by the history of the Spanish slave trade.[130] The methodological difficulties related to the determination of the exact ethnic origin of the enslaved people have become proverbial, and have already been discussed by many authors (Deive 1988; Guanche 2011).

The persons that were captured and trafficked, belonged to various ethnic groups from regions of West, Central and later also East Africa. The majority of African people coming to Spanish America until the 1630s seemed to be from the region of Upper Guinea (Rawley & Behrendt 2005 [1982]; Wheat 2016).[131] Upper Guinea includes present-day Senegal, Gambia, Guinea Bissau, Guinea, and Sierra Leone, with many peoples whose descendants are *i.e.* the Wolof, Serer, Biafaras, Mandinga, Malinké, Mende, Joola, Fulani/Fulbe, Susu, and Temne (Zapes). Also inhabitants of Cape Verde islands and later (1590 and 1640) of Angola (São Tomé island and Luanda being an important embarkation ports) were shipped to the Caribbean (Transatlantic Slave Voyage Database 2017, further only SVD).[132] Some Cuban and Dominican ancestors proceeded also from the mouth of the river Congo and from present-day Gabon

129 In the 17th century the French were bringing most people from Senegambia, later from Bight of Benin, West Central Africa, less numbers from the Gold Coast and Bight of Biafra (SVD 2018). For more on the topic of tracing the African origins of Haitians see the work of Fouchard (1979).

130 The demarcation line that granted large part of the Americas to the Spanish Crown also caused the colonial society to be dependent on the Portuguese, Dutch, English and others for the source of their workforce. In the 16th century the Spanish bought persons from the Portuguese, first shipping them from Sevilla and Madrid, and later from African ports. During the 17th century the slave trade was affected by the raise of other European countries and conflicts restraining the official means to purchase enslaved peoples from the sub-Saharan region. By the mid 17th century the Portuguese lost their monopoly in West Africa and Caribbean to Dutch (Curaçao, Goreé island, El Mina), English (Barbados, Jamaica, Gambia, Ghana) and French (St. Kitts, Senegal). Portuguese maintained their posts from Senegal to the Angolean post in Beguela, including large parts of Upper Guinea, and in the Cape Verde islands. Together with the Independence of Portugal (1640), the Dutch revolt and 80 years war against Spain (1568-1648) and the continuous seizing of African and Caribbean Spanish colonies by Dutch, French and English formed obstacles to official trade and led to large-scale contraband from Barbados, Curaçao, Jamaica, which supplied legally and illegally the Spanish speaking Caribbean (Rawley & Behrendt 2005). At the beginning of the 18th century Spain was forced to grant England the right of Transatlantic Trade (Rawley & Behrendt 2005). In the 1740s, the Spanish Crown returned to domestic trade and gave *asiento* to the Havana company. After the English occupation of Cuba and the Haitian revolution in 1791 the sugar industry expanded and with this also the demand of labor.

131 The ships from this region boarded at the Cape Verde islands, Buguendo (present-day Sao Domingos Guinea Bissau), and unknown ports at Grande River (Wheat 2016). Also captives embarked from Banjul at the mouth of Gambia river.

132 The Trans-Atlantic Slave Trade Database can be consulted on slavevoyages.org. The present-day peoples were identified using the People's Atlas of Africa by Felix & Meur (2001), and its adapted and georeferenced version as published on https://worldmap.harvard.edu/.

(Rawley & Behrendt 2005; SVD 2017).[133] For overview of regions from where African ancestors were shipped to Santo Domingo see Table 1 and for Cuba see Table 4. The high estimates from 16th century of captives shipped to Santo Domingo reflect the fact that from there people were shipped onward to other regions of the Spanish Americas.

In the first half of 18th century people from present-day Ghana (Gold Coast, port Ardra), Angola, Nigeria (Calabar) were enslaved and brought to Spanish Americas. In 1778, when Spain established its trading base in Fernando Po (Bioko) more Caribbean captives originated from the Bight of Biafra, which is situated in Equatorial Guinea.[134] The regional history showed that especially in the later period the French exchanged captives (most likely from regions Angola, Bight of Benin, the Windward Coast, and

the Gold Coast) with the Spanish for goods and other merchandise (Rawley & Behrendt 2005). In the 18th century the import of captives to Cuba significantly outnumbered those imported to Hispaniola (68,033 vs. 2057). In addition, the number of the African ports included in the trade also increased significantly.

Between 1821-1843, people were carried away from Western Guinea, Bight of Benin, Bight of Biafra, Congo, Angola, and Mozambique. In this period, captives were mostly shipped from the rivers Gallina, Manna, Pongo (Rep. of Guinea), from Bonny Island, and from posts like Lagos, Old Calabar (both in Nigeria) and Whydah (Ouidah in Benin). In the 19th century Cuba was much more dependent on the workforce of AfroCuban ancestors brought in great numbers. In fact, the number of captives that were brought to Cuban during 19th century is more then twenty seven times higher (710,172 vs. 28507) then the total amount of captives shipped to Dominican Republic during the whole colonial period (SVD 2018).[135]

With respect to the tracing of the Dominican roots, Deive suggested that the Bantú, Guinean, and Sudanese cultural areas were the most represented in the local historical documentation of this part of Hispaniola (Deive 1988).[136] These three areas incorporate a rich diversity of identities. In the Bantú group, Deive included peoples denominated Ambos, Angola, Bamba, Casanga, Congo, Lemba, Malemba, Manga, Matamba, Mondongo, and Sambú. The area of Guinea comprises the Ewe-Fon family, to which the Arará, Ardá, Tarí, Yoruba, Bañol, Bervisí, Biafara, Biochos, Carabalí, Mina, and Zape peoples belong.[137] Lastly, the Sudanese cultural area was said to consist

133 These peoples were most likely shipped from the ports in São Tomé and Principe and Bioko/San Fernando Poo. In the 17th century also the French established their slave trade companies in Gabon. Among the biggest ethnic groups in Gabon are Ndzabi, Fang (Okak), followed by Kota (Mahongwe, Mbaamba), Eshira, and Punu.

134 This region is inhabited today by the Bubi people, but also by different Bantu peoples such as the Fang of Rio Muni.

135 There are considerable differences SVD data that are presented gere and database and Rawley & Behrendt (2005).

136 His analysis was based on different documents like ordinances, reports on slave revolts, maroons, Osorio orders, baptismal and matrimonial records in the period 1547-1821. See also the work of Saez (2008).

137 Ellis´work (1894) includes a brief (although biased) description of Yoruba speakers.

Period	Senegambia & offshore Atlantic	Sierra Leone	Gold Coast	Bight of Benin	Bight of Biafra & Gulf of Guinea islands	West Central Africa and St. Helena	Other Africa	Total
1501-1600	8715	279	0	0	3658	643	3839	17134
1601 -1700	0	0	0	1201	380	5565	2170	9316
1701 -1800	0	0	412	0	0	736	909	2057
Totals	8715	279	412	1201	4038	6944	6918	28507

Table 1 Overview of Regions from which captives were brought Hispaniola. Data are retrieved from the database of slavevoyages.org. The estimates concern disembarked individuals in ports of Hispaniola. Note that some of captives brought in 18th century might be brought to Saint Dominique not Santo Domingo.

of Bambara, Barva, Chambá, Fula, Mandinga, and Wolof peoples (Deive 1988).[138] At last, it is worthwhile to remark that the hyper-diversity of the African ancestors was often accompanied by multilingualism (*e.g.* among Ghe language group), and occasional common cultural traits (their religions including Islam and Catholicism[139]), factors that could facilitate the transfer of cultural information, including medicinal knowledge and beliefs, among the enslaved population.[140]

The interactions among the colonized strata

The arrival of the Africans to the islands gave rise to hyper-diverse communities, whose composition diversified even further through the interaction with the local population.

---

138 As clear these don´t correspond with contemporary ethnic group names with which the people self-identify in the present. The group denominated "*mina*" proceeded from San Jorge Elmina castle in the present Ghana but sometimes it referred also to Golden Coast or Mina de Oro (probably ancestors of Gen people). Biafaras referred to the region Bight of Biafra, Arará (Aradá) from Allada current Benin, Carabalí from Old Calabar in present-day Nigeria, and Zape were most likely Temne. Matamba was a kingdom at Cuango river in present-day Angola. About more details on the 17th century knowledge about Zapes or other peoples see Sandoval (Sandoval 2008).

139 The missionary activities in West Africa started nearly in parallel to the Portuguese and European colonization. Enslaved people, therefore, may have had knowledge of Catholicism and Protestantism religions prior to their arrival to the Americas.

140 The hyper-diversity is evident when looking at the present-day panorama of peoples (generally called ethnic groups) in the enormous regions of Africa. Felix 2001 registered around 1,900 distinct ethnic groups, based on how these groups self-identified. This hyper-diversity together with the complex dynamic societal situation during the European colonization of West (Central) Africa has complicated endeavors trying to trace the places of origin of Caribbean ancestors. One of the historical documents that brings us a little bit closer to understanding the complexity and hyper-diversity of the cultures and healing practices that were brought to the Caribbean, is the work of Jesuit Alonso de Sandoval (1576-1652), which provides a wealth of information about the enslaved persons brought in the first half of 17th century to Cartagena. Sandoval described over 300 ethnic groups, or nations, their linguistic skills, bodily markings and sometimes how colonizers perceived their value as a laborer or ability to convert (Sandoval 2008 [1627]). Thus, for example, ethnicities belonging to the Ghe language group, representing approximately twenty languages, including Ewe, Fon, Aja, Gen (Mina), and Phla-Pherá spreading from Ghana to Nigeria, were said to be able to communicate among each other (Sandoval 2008). In addition, several groups from Senegambia had Islam or Catholicism as a shared religion.

The cultural interaction of the life-ways of subaltern classes seems to have occurred as early as 1503, when the Spaniards warned people against the influences of enslaved men on the indigenous population. While there is some historical and archeological evidence that has started to shed light on these types of interactions (Pereira Pereira 2007, 2008; Valcárcel Rojas 2012; Ulloa Hung 2016), more research is needed. Concerning the written documentation, Cerrato writes that in 1547, Spanish people who were searching for revolting black Cimarrons, led by Lemba in the mountains of Bahoruco, found some indigenous men and women living with the Cimarrons (Rodriguez Morel 2011).

The colonized peoples of different origins cooperated together (Rodriguez Morel 2011). In 1577, indigenous and enslaved people gave information about the Spanish to the Portuguese and the French in the surroundings of Yaquimo and Sabana, in exchange for wine and trinkets (Exquemelin 1971 [1678]). The exchange of information continued in other regions in the early 17th century. Before its evacuation, Yaguana inhabitants sold cowhides to the French and the Portuguese. Inhabitants of this region, described as being of local, West African, and mixed origins, were informing the other parties about the location of Spanish troops in exchange for textiles and other goods (Rodríguez Demorizi 1945).[141]

During the second half of the 17th century, locations like Azua, Tortuga, Boyá, and Bánica all are said to have had a population of indigenous and West African descent, who were not only likely to have children with each other, but also to influence each other in cultural ways. More specifically, around the 1670s, indigenous laborers (probably paid) worked alongside those of African origin in La Tortuga and in Azua (Exquemellin 1661). Azua´s population counted inhabitants of mixed origin; among the "*mulato*" inhabitants were also "*mestizos*" and "*alcatraces*" (descendants of indigenous and West African persons). All groups had their own racial preferences concerning marriages, which reflected the social status of the respective groups (Exquemelin 1971 [1678]).[142] During the last allocations, approximately eight hundred indigenous persons were brought to this town (Mira Caballos 1997). Therefore, the origin of the indigenous descendants might be both local and non-local.

The subsequent historical development of Dominican society

Further insights into the evolution of the Dominican population come from the study of Moya Pons (2009). The Hispaniolan population grew around 2.3%, reaching a total of over 18,400 persons, between the years 1681 and 1716. Since this period, the population and economy continued to grow throughout the 18th century. The mutual influences among Canarians, West Africans and other groups intensified and the process of transculturation continued. In the first half of the 18th century, in the majority of towns the "people of color" were more numerous than the "white population" (Baní being the only exception). In 1740 Álvarez de Abreu described Santo

141 Mixed origin in this case refers to the colonial category "mulato", "mestizo", and local to "indio".

142 Azua, together with Santo Domingo, maintained their populations and grew even during the period of heavy emigration towards the mainland. Azua´s population remained numerous because it had still gold and copper mines and quickly transitioned to the sugar industry (CepiCepi sugar mills).

Domingo as having 1,800 inhabitants, among them there were only twelve or fifteen Spanish families, and the rest were free, liberated persons and captives (Rodríguez Demorizi 1957). Around that time, the total population was more than thirty thousand, the majority of which were people of color and of different social strata. The annual growth of the population maintained a relatively stable rate of 2.5% throughout the 18th century. In the 1750s, the total population of Santo Domingo was around 70,626 persons. About 12% of this population was enslaved, and the large majority was more or less equally divided between *"white and of freedmen of color"* (Moya Pons 2009). In 1792, the Spanish part of Hispaniola had around 125,000 inhabitants. This growth was maintained until the 1795 Basel Treaty, when France gained control over the island. Two years before the Haitian revolution (1791) slave trading was made free in Cuba, Santo Domingo and Puerto Rico. The Haitian revolution, followed by Toussaint Louverture's abolition of slavery, its reestablishment under the twelve-year Spanish rule, and the twenty-two years of Haitian occupation, produced economic and demographic decline. This period was marked by massive emigration and internal migration. Moya Pons estimated that between 1795 and 1812, 100,000 persons emigrated from the island towards Cuba, Puerto Rico, and Venezuela. Among them were elites who were deprived of their lands and their enslaved subjects, and also Dominican families without great possessions. The arrival of Boyer and his troops provoked further waves of migration.

The first decennia's of the 19th century are marked by significant population decline 1819 (71,223 persons) (Moya Pons 2009). During Boyer's reign, many people from the French areas had married Dominican women and established themselves there as agriculturalists. Since 1844, the annual growth rate was approximately 2.6%, which remained stable through the first republic (1844-1861), the annexation of the Dominican Republic to Spain (1861), and the war of restoration (1863-1865). In this period, immigration from Spain and Cuba (independence war 1868-1878) seems to have contributed significantly to this growth. In 1888, the second republic counted around 382,000 inhabitants. Twenty years later a population of around 638,000 persons was registered (Moya Pons 2009).

By the beginning of the 20th century, a large proportion of the population was living in rural areas.[143] In addition, around 10% of the inhabitants on the island were foreigners, the largest group being Puerto Ricans coming to Santo Domingo after the American occupation. Between 1920 and 1935, the annual growth rate reached 3.4%, a percentage that reflects the immigration related to the sugar industry and the provoked European migration (Jewish and Spanish exiles). The US occupation, which broke up the communal lands and dispossessed thousands of peasants, is likely to have also caused internal migration. The annual growth for the subsequent periods was, on average, around 3.06% (varying from 2.4% to 3.6% according to Moya Pons 2009).

One of the political events that shaped the Dominican demography and identity was the dictatorship of Trujillo (1930-1961). In 1937, the Haitian population living in the Dominican Republic was expulsed and killed on a large scale. It is estimated that between one and twelve thousand died in the Parsley Massacre. During this dicta-

143 To describe the general tendencies of demographic development we follow the insights put forward by Moya Pons (2009).

torship, the national statistics were falsified in order to "whiten" the Dominican population, denying the West African origin of the majority of the Dominican population. In order to avoid calling Dominicans *"mulatos"* the censuses of 1920, 1935, 1950, and 1960 used the term *"mestizo"* and *"indio"*. Although the last census registering race was the one from 1960, to this day the category of *"indio"* has replaced the category *"mulato"* in official documents like ID cards. Moya Pons' analysis of electoral registers shows that 82% of the Dominicans have been registered as *"indian"* while only 4% were registered as *"black"*, 8% as *"white"* and 2% as *"mulato"*. These proportions most likely reflect long-term discrimination within Dominican society.

In 1960 the population was around 3 millions, and since then it increased rapidly until the present, when the country has over ten million inhabitants. Since the 1970s, industrialization, urbanization, improvement of health care, and education, together with programs directed at the regulation of birth rates, seem to have stabilized the population growth. The urbanization was reinforced by commercialization of agriculture producing rice, sugar, coffee or cattle on large scale. By 2010, 25.6% of the Dominicans (2,421,332 persons) lived in rural areas (Moya Pons 2009).

Dominican demography has been shaped also by emigration to the United States that increased during the Trujillo era and by 2015 was close to one million. The previously mentioned law 169-14 that retroactively revoked their citizenship of thousands of peoples seems to have had a long term impact on the immigration from Haiti and as such also on the composition of the future Dominican nation.

A brief overview of demographic background of selected Dominican sites

Based on this summary overview of historical references to the indigenous peoples of Hispaniola, we may conclude that the indigenous population lasted much longer than is generally assumed. These ancestors in many cases seem to have been exposed to the long term cultural influences from the newcomers. The next section briefly summarizes the history of the locations where the fieldwork was conducted. Again, following the objectives of the overall project, where possible the emphasis is laid on the colonial history of the indigenous populations.

Boyá

Boyá is a small settlement situated six kilometers from Monte Plata in the province of Monte Plata. No archaeological surveys of this province have yet been published.[144] Local inhabitants reported three sites, which may be related to the pre-colonial history. It has been suggested that its founding was related to it possibly being the last resting place of cacique Enrique, one of famous leaders of indigenous resistance, but verifi-

144 According to Ortega (2005) in the neighboring provinces Hato Mayor, SaMana, Santo Domingo, Sanchéz Ramírez, and San Pedro Macorís some archaeological sites have been registered. The province Monte Plata is not included in that overview but possibly the data will be published in the future, in the second volume of that publication.

cation is problematic because of the symbolic character of that status and the scarce research on this topic.[145]

The first direct written reference to Boyá is given by Fray Andrés de Carvajal, in his letter to the king (1571): *"there is another village, of Indians, eights leagues from this city, which is called Boyá, it has twenty five neighbors, all old and poor without children. This place is new, created by a member of the Saint Augustin order who brought the Indians here from those mountains and made them a church with a thatched roof"* (Blanco de Diaz 2009, pp. 470 – 437).

The founding of Monte Plata and Bayaguana led to a land conflict. In 1610, newcomers issued an official complaint that the inhabitants of Boyá were hunting cattle on their properties.[146] Indigenous residents opposed that and argued that in fact the newly established settlement prevented them from hunting. The official response was clearly partial, and even contradictory, arguing that the indigenous inhabitants did not use the land properly while those who had signed were owners of yucca and ginger farms (Rodríguez Demorizi 1945; Gil-Bermejo García 1983).[147] This dispute is comparable to complaints about usurping lands from Cuban Caney (1562), Trinidad (1514), and Jiguaní (1700). Altogether, these disputes indicate that, like in other indigenous communities of the Americas, in the indigenous Caribbean the land was considered communal property.

Later, Boyá is mentioned during pastoral visits, which yield some demographic estimates and some bits of information about local religious life. According to church statistics, the population (of believers) in Boyá seems to have been small and to have fluctuated over time. Alcocer (1650*)* writes that Boyá slowly became depopulated, because the indigenous inhabitants went in search of a new life in other locations, and, as a result, only six houses remained in the location. Despite this, the church was well-built (from guano) and decorated with nice ornaments and lamps gifted by devotees of Nuestra Señora de Agua Santa. According to Alcocer, the origin of the image of the Virgin is unknown; he stated that, as far as was informed, this image had been brought by Antonio Moiano, but he acknowledged that it could also have been brought by another Dominican priest. The only certain thing was that the image was deemed to be miraculous among the population at large. Twelve years later, the depopulation of the village was said to have reached such an extent that it was decided that approximately thirty indigenous men would be brought over from La Tortuga (Rodríguez Demorizi 1957).

During his pastoral visit, Francisco de la Cueva y Maldonado (1666 in Gil-Bermejo García 1983) compared Boyá to other eastern villages like Higüey, El Seibo, Bayaguana,

---

145 Some authors (e.g. Vega 1988) have argued that cacique Enrique rests in Sabana Buye, close to Baní, located near Azua, much closer to the place where the treaty was negotiated. It is perhaps worthwhile to mention that a few kilometers from Boyá is a municipality called Sabana Grande de Boyá. His properties were inherited by Doña Mencía (his wife) and Martín de Alfaro (his cousin), who later appealed fir and received a confirmation of their status as caciques of the indigenous peoples from the Royal Court.

146 AGI Santo Domingo, 54, Cartas del presidente al Rey (3 deciembre 1610), published in Gil-Bermejo Garcia (1983).

147 The following persons were registered as owners of yucca and ginger estates around 1609: Tomás Aquirre, Antonio Gato, Domingo González, Bartolomé Pérez, Francisco Ortiz, Pedro Jorge (Councilor), Juan Hernández, Pedro Rubio, Cristóbal Santa Ana, Andrés Hernández, Mariano Hernández, Amador Hernández, Diego de Céspedes (Presbyter) (Rodríguez Demorizi 1945).

and Monte Plata, which were all nearly depopulated. In his comparison, Boyá was doing much better: it had twenty families, increasing in number, and a sanctuary that was taken good care of.[148] The subsequent pastoral visits inform us that many of the inhabitants officially declared to belong to the Catholic faith, and later, other authors even give examples of successful conversion.[149] In his attempt to reunite and baptize enslaved persons that had run away from the French, Friar Domingo suggested nominating a "protector" and leaving them in their village, and from there the maroons would work for the Spaniards once a week: *"if the indigenous village Boyá is governing itself and does not cause difficulties for anyone, and is not being harassed by the Spanish, it seems that the blacks could also govern themselves"* (Fray Domingo 1679 in Rodríguez Demorizi 1957).

Later news about the demographic development of Boyá is less positive: there are no more than two descendants left, one "*mestizo*" and one "*castizo*" (Fernandez Navarrete 1680 in Rodríguez Demorizi 1957). Navarrete´s successor wrote that Boyá was the only indigenous village that had 37 persons of communion and 6 of confession (Friar Fernando Carvajal y Rivera 1690). Fifty years later, the population was reported as being composed of 65 persons, "Yndios," with eleven "slaves", and 24 men of arms (Álvarez de Abreu 1740 in Rodríguez Demorizi 1957). In the late nineteenth century, Boyá's population is described as being of small size and composed of indigenous descendants (Monte y Tejada 1890 evaluated them as "mestizos"). Monte y Tejada (1890) sees the great devotion to the Virgin as the reason that indigenous descendants persisted in this location. Some of his ideas might be influenced by the novel *Enriquillo* (Manuel de Jesús de Galván 1882), published ten years earlier. According to this novel Boyá is the last residence of cacique Enrique and his subjects. The 1888 parochial census counts 450 devotees.

In general, rather than monitoring precise population growth or decline, the sporadic visits of church officials give us a picture of the small size of the population.[150] The process of transculturation seems to have been reinforced by the size of the population and later exponential demographic grow. If at the end of 19th century, the population was deemed to be of mixed Spanish and indigenous origin, their descendants would probably have less and less indigenous ancestry in each generation if marrying outside of the location. The close proximity of Monte Plata, and its position on the royal roads between Santo Domingo and Higüey are just a few factors that may have contributed to further demographic diversification.

---

148 Carta del arzobispo don Francisco de la Cueva y Maldonado, dirigida a S. M., sobre haber hecho la Visita pastoral de la villa de Higüey, Santo Domingo, 15 de enero de 1666, as published in Blanco Díaz (2015b).

149 Nine years later, Fray Domingo Fernández Navarrete, archbishop of Santo Domingo in his description of the island stated that Boyá had: "*14 bohios, 43 are of confession of faith, indios and indias and some mestizos, hermitage of the Lady of Holy Water, which is now in reconstruction*" (Rodríguez Demorizi 1957, p. 15).

150 This fluctuation may be partially due to how the census of that time was constructed. To determine the population growth through these estimations remains a difficult task, because different sources use diverse categories for counting, such as the number of houses or families, of persons who made their confession or who received communion, the number of enslaved persons, or simply use very general estimates. A considerable amount of the population may have been left out, especially the inhabitants of areas surrounding the small settlement or the enslaved persons.

According to the most recent census, Boyá has, at present, 5267 inhabitants, of which 61% are living in poverty and 14% in extreme poverty.[151] The present-day economy is, in general, restricted to public services and agriculture, including small scale cattle raising, and cultivation of yucca, peas, yautía, coconuts, and more recently cocoa.

Current inhabitants are aware of the historical link that Boyá has with indigenous people. According to oral history, the settlement was founded after the Virgin of the Holy Water manifested herself in an orange tree to hunters searching for cattle in the area.[152] At the same place a chapel – and later a church – is said to have been built by indigenous ancestors. The remains of cacique Enrique are believed to have been buried in the yard in front of the church. Among the holy relics of the church, indigenous ceramics are displayed. The fence protecting the church includes pillars with statues that have indigenous faces. This historical consciousness is further reinforced by Mr. Zambrano and his family, who have made a collection of material culture related to the history of Boyá, including some indigenous artefacts. Mr. Zambrano also published an overview of the local history, arguing against the hypothesis that Enrique is linked to Boyá. One of the residents of Boyá claims to be the last indigenous descendant, and her neighbors support this claim: Mrs. Ramona González Moreno self-identifies as being of indigenous descent on the basis of the oral tradition of her family, which includes a narrative about her own mother, a midwife who was able to communicate with indigenous ancestors. A preliminary research in the baptismal book could not verify this genealogical link, although it is possible that Mrs. González descends from the González family mentioned in 1609s as one of the owners of the estates (Rodríguez Demorizi 1945). According to oral tradition, the González and Moreno families, together with the Zambranos, Luises, and Alcántaras descend from the founders of Boyá.

Bánica

Bánica is a municipality situated at the bank of the Artibonito river on the Haitian border. This region has not been archaeologically investigated, with the exception of the work of investigators from the Museo del Hombre in Santo Domingo, such as Glenis Tavares and Rafael Puello Nina, who has registered the rock art in the cave of Saint Francis. Moreau de Saint-Mery (1796) suggests that Bánica was founded by Diego Velázquez in 1504. In the parochial statistics, the founding of San Francisco de Paula de Bánica is indeed dated to 1504. According to Benzo de Ferrer (2005), Bánica is one of the villages founded by the Hieronymite friars in 1516 and one of the last six indigenous villages that remained after the government of Rodrigo de Figueroa (Ferrer 2005).[153] However, a transcript made by Mira Caballos (2009) mentions only Baní and not Bánica among the remaining villages. According to Benzo de Ferrer, the remaining

---

151 The number of people living in extreme poverty is even larger when the rural sections belonging to the municipality are included.

152 The original settlement of Boyá, according to tradition, is situated in a place called El Horno, where the bricks for the church are said to have been made. From there it was moved to its current location because of a huge plague of ants. The holder of the statue of Señora de Aguas Santas is dated 2 march 1533, the same year when the peace treaty with Enrique was signed. However, the holder itself seems to have been made much later. Las Casas mentions a great ant plague around 1511, but plagues tormented the region more frequently also throughout the posterior centuries.

153 Others were Jaragua, Mejorada, and Puero Real, all being under the Hieronymite friars of Rodrigo de Bastidas (Ferrer 2005).

population disappeared soon afterwards. The founding of Bánica and its further demographic development might be related to the history of La Hincha, Guaba, and St. Tomé, as in historical maps these appear on the road between these locations. However, further study of primary historical resources is necessary.[154]

In the 17th century, conflicts with the French led to immigration from Villa Guaba and according to Moya Pons the fear of the French was the main motive for founding this town in 1664 (Hernández González 2006; Moya Pons 2010). Canarian families arrived in Bánica in 1687, the same year the church was built. At the end of the 17th century, Friar Fernando Carvajal y Rivera (1690) reported more than 160 devotees and a small number of black refugees (24), who had fled from the French mines.[155] Around fifty years later Bánica had four hundred faithful men, the church of San Francisco de Paula was taken good care of, and it had five brotherhoods one of them dedicated to San Miguel (according to Archbishop Álvarez de Abreu 1739 in Demorizi 1957).

During the 17th and 18th century, inhabitants of Bánica seem to have been involved in contraband with the French, selling them cattle and horses in exchange for enslaved persons and different items (Rodríguez Demorizi 1946; Ferrer 2005). With respect to the demographic situation, Moreau de Saint-Méry (1796) states that, like in the case of Boyá, the people of Banique continued to identify with their indigenous ancestry in the cases in which a historical link could be proven. Saint-Méry is skeptical about those who identified as indigenous descendants in other locations. As he argues, there were many *criollos* who claimed to be of indigenous descent and who had the corresponding physical characteristics, but unlike the situation in Boyá and Bánica their historical link could not be proven. In the same period, Bánica was famous for its mineral spring, which became very popular and was visited by people from even the French areas for curing different illnesses (Paulino Ramos 2008). As a post on the Dominican-Haitian border Bánica has been involved in different military confrontations. As a consequence of Toussaint Louverture's taking control of the French speaking part, inhabitants of frontier posts like San Rafael, San Miguel and Hincha moved to Bánica. Soon after, his troops also occupied Bánica, which was followed by an English attack on Toussaint Louverture. Like other regions, Bánica was occupied by the French in 1856. In the parochial census of 1869, the Catholic population of this town amounted to more than 1000.

The present-day municipality has around 2112 inhabitants. The vast majority of Baniqueros – 75% – are facing poverty, and 44% face extreme poverty. This reflects the regional provincial trend in which Elías Piña has for many years had the highest score on poverty rank (Morillo Peréz 2014). The main economic activities are trade with Haiti and agriculture.[156] The study of Puello Nina & Tavarez (2013, 2016) has dealt with some aspect of local healing and religious practices.

---

154 For a map see caribsmaps.org (Title: Saint Domingue. Year: 1742. Maker: Covens et Mortier; Lisle, Guillaume de).

155 The church was built with clay walls, and a guano roof; it had no income and only one priest who had passed away that year. Later registers of pastoral visits provide similar information about the amount of believers and church properties but do not contain further references to the patronal feast (and do not clarify whether it was celebrated in the cave). One of the interesting details is the reference to the use of *canoas* in the river in 1765.

156 Interviews with local inhabitants indicate that the traditional crops are batatas, peanuts, corn, peas, rice, yucca, yautia and fruits (incl. plantains, bananas).

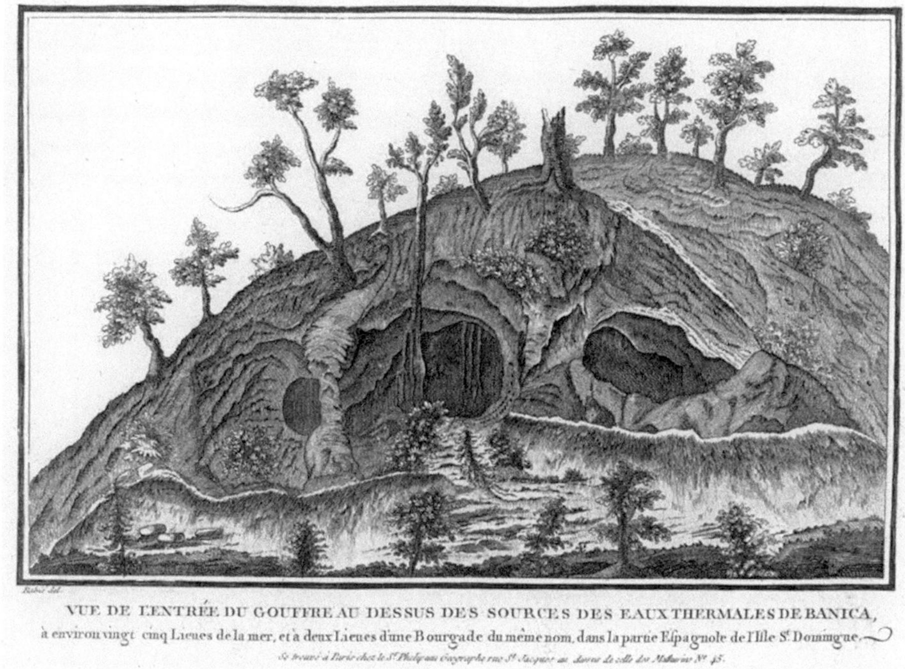

Figure 8 View of limestone caves in Bánica on the island of Hispaniola, by Ponce, Nicolás in Moreau de Saint-Méry (1791).

According to oral history, the founders of the village were the Alcántara, Fernández de Oviedo, Llanes, Moreta, Mora and Ramírez families.[157] One of the most prominent events in the oral history is the appearance of Saint Francis, the local Patron Saint, who manifested himself in the cavern on the hill with the mineral spring, overseeing the municipality. Historical consciousness of the indigenous past is present in the belief that the church of this Patron Saint was built by indigenous people. In addition, the cavern where this Saint was manifested is also a place where indigenous ancestors may manifest themselves. In contrast with Boyá, there are no individuals who would identify as indigenous descendants. Some inhabitants, however, feel a strong spiritual link with the indigenous ancestors. One of the contributors to this research indicated that in the past, there lived a woman, Ms. De Los Santos, who was said to be of indigenous descent. This association was made on the base of her physical appearance and weaving skills.

Boca de Mana

Boca de Mana and Monte Bonito are sections of the municipality Yaguate at the bank of the Valdesia damn, which is situated on the border between the provinces of San Cristóbal (the capital of which is San Cristóbal) and Peravia (capital Baní) in the South of the Dominican Republic. The few known references about of municipal history will be situated to the provincial histories. The relationship between Baní and San Cristóbal is important because according to oral history, the founder of the section of Monte

157 Interview no. 160957.

Bonito, Bibiana de la Rosa, came from Baní and an influential healer, important in this study, came from Haina, which is closely related to the history of San Cristóbal.

The local history reaches back to the time before the conquest. The study of López Belando (2011) registered multiple caverns with rock art. Based on testimonies of inhabitants more archaeological sites are likely to be found when a systematic survey is carried out. The first written reference to Yaguate is dated to 1504, when Pope Julius II in his Bull declared Hayaguata the first Archdiocese in Hispaniola, though this bull was never implemented (Peña Herrera 2006, p. 20). The name of the archdiocese of Hyaguata could refer to the province and to the village.[158] Later records from the beginning of the 17th and the 18th century mention Mana as a small-scale farming region.[159] At the end of the 19th century, the new sugar mill Italia was established. Until now, this sugar mill contributes to the local economy.

Both provinces are historically agricultural regions focusing on farming, cattle raising, and sugar production. Baní figures as one of the names among the indigenous villages founded by the Hieronymites during the infamous reductions of the years 1517-1519 (Mira Caballos 2009).[160] In 1609, various farms holding cattle and sheep were registered. At the end of 17th century, the Baní population was reinforced by Canarian migrants (Carvajal y Rivera 1695 in Demorizi 1953). The foundation of the town around 1763 is related to an attempt of the authorities to facilitate inhabitants of the Baní valley access to religious services.[161] The period of the official foundation was also characterized by prosperity generated by the trade of livestock in exchange of slaves with the French part. In the second half of the 19th century the population increased to 1,500 inhabitants exporting guayacán, colorant wood (Campeche, guatapaná), sugar, coffee, tobacco, and turtle shells (Tejeda Ortiz 1978).

---

158 Bull *Illius fulciti praesedio* of November 15, 1504. With respect to this, Blanco Díaz (2009) writes: "*En 1504 fueron creados por el Papa Julio II un arzobispado y dos obispados en la isla, aquel en la provincia de Hyaguate en la que está el puerto de Santo Domingo y "la propia ciudad Hyaguatense" y estos en Lares de Guahaba y Concepción de La Vega. Accedió a ello el Santo Padre pero sin resultado; y anulada en 1511 la erección efectuada el 15 de diciembre de 1504, de la silla metropolitana Hyaguatense y de los obispados sufragáneos de Maguá y Bainoa, fueron creadas dos Iglesias, una en la Concepción de La Vega y otra en Santo Domingo, a las cuales se donaron los diezmos, quedando asegurado el Patronato Real*". Pedro Suárez de Deza, was assigned to be the bishop of Hyaguata, but was later reassigned to the Diocese of Concepción de la Vega. The diocese of Santo Domingo was erected in 1511 and is situated in the province Hyaguata.

159 The 17th century records mention a farm named Mana, owned by Luis Alonso, and a farm named Yaguate owned by Capitan Juan Tello de Guzmán (Gil-Bermejo García 1983). Yaguate was acquired forty years later by Juan Rivera y Quezada and in 1648 the farm was donated to the Jesuits who owned the farm and its herd until 1767 when the Jesuits was expelled from Santo Domingo (Reyes 1950, p. 195). This small farm later changed owners – one of them was Dona Margarita Fuentes, the spouse of Don Antonio Álvarez, who is said to have founded the community Yaguate in 1818.

160 The rebellious *grifos* from Bahoruco were moved to Buenaventura (Rodríguez Morel 2007).

161 Incháustegui (cited by Rodríguez Demorizi 1974) says that Baní was founded in 1764. In the 1740s, church representatives registered in Baní a population of 525 inhabitants, of which 270 were children and enslaved people. The houses of its inhabitants were said to be two or three leagues from the church; only the house of the priest was near the church. According to the words of one of the founders, José Luis Peguero, the main reason was to facilitate access to the religion. Until then, the inhabitants of the valley Baní (estimated to be 718 people) did not attend any mass due to the remoteness of the small church dedicated to the Virgen de La Regla, as well as because of their poverty, the size of their family or transportation issues (Rodríguez Demorizi 1974).

The history of San Cristóbal is marked by early colonization and the first sugar production along the surrounding rivers.[162] Current San Cristóbal is situated at the fort Buenaventura founded by Miguel Díaz who was married to an indigenous woman named Catalina who showed him gold sources along the western bank of the river Haina. Councilors of Buenaventura (Diego López de Salcedo and Fernando Mesa) were allocated 180 indigenous slaves (Mira Caballos 1997). Around 1517, after the establishment of the fort, sugar mills were built along the Haina, Nigua, and Ocoa riverbanks producing sugar for export. The founding population was composed of African, indigenous and European inhabitants.[163] Since the first half of the 16th century until the end of the 18th century many inhabitants of this region were enslaved and were forced to work at sugar plantations and cattle herds.[164] Also here the limited influence of the official church gave space for non-institutional religious practices.[165] In 1796, the plantation Boca de Nigua inscribed itself into the national history as the site of a famous slave revolt followed by the sanguinary reprisal of the colonial authorities, who feared a revolution like the one taking place in the French part.

At present, the majority (88%) of the population of the municipality Yaguate (42,325 inhabitants in total) lives in the rural area. In this case, no exact number of inhabitants was recorded for the municipal sections. According to Tejeda, the community of Mana counted approximately 2,000 inhabitants in the 1980s.

The Boca de Mana section faces an enormous degree of poverty: 96% of the population was evaluated as poor, and 55% as living in extreme poverty, according to governmental statistics. My own observations during fieldwork make me estimate even higher ranks of extreme poverty for another section called Monte Bonito. As the above-mentioned sections, the villages near the river of Mana face a lack of employment opportunities, which make the rest of the population move to the capital in search for jobs, or rely on governmental subsidies. Many inhabitants of these sections rely on small-scale agriculture (producing coffee, tobacco, tubers as yucca, guáyiga, fruits) and large-scale agriculture (rice and sugar) in the close surroundings of Yaguate.

Few publications have mentioned the ritual use of the cavern La Mancha. Firstly, Tejeda Ortiz (1978) wrote a biography of Bibiana de la Rosa, describing her miracles, prophecies, the places associated with her role as a healer and messianic figure, and

---

162 The history of the Haina region is of interest also because one contributor who provided us with many insights about the importance of the Mana cave is from Haina.

163 In 1538, Diego Caballero, who owned cattle herds and two sugar mills along the river Nigua, founded a village with approximately sixty houses and a church. During this period, the population was composed of Spaniards, indigenous people, and West Africans. Diego Caballero owned two sugar factories, one at the bank of the river Nigua and the other the SepiSepi of Azua.

164 According to the census of Osorio (1606), there were at least 12 sugar mills between Santo Domingo and Azua, along the rivers Haina, Nigua, Ocoa, and Itabo. In the beginning of the 17th century, there were many sugar mills, farms, with their own hermitages, and cemeteries. Nearly one hundred years later (1692) at the river Haina were 10 sugar mills, 33 farms and cattle herds, having a population over one thousand persons, the great majority being black enslaved people (990 persons, only 15 whites and 40 free black) (Carvajal y Rivera 1692). In the first half of the 18th century, there were seven sugar mills, many herds and farms, the great majority of the population being enslaved people: 15 "white", 40 "mulatos", and 995 "black slaves" (Rodríguez Demorizi 1957).

165 Carvajal y Rivera describes also the little interests to spread the Catholic religion among the enslaved people of Haina and Nigua. Although a priest visited this zone by 1692, there was no church, and devotees were unable to pay tithes because of the deaths and robberies. At the end of the 17th century, some families from the Canary Islands settled at Nigua and in Baní (Rodríguez Demorizi 1957).

the celebration of the Virgen Mercedes.[166] López Belando (2011) has carried out archaeological surveys in the area and reports existence of altars of 21 Division in close by caverns. Lastly, Toño Arias Peláez, a visual anthropologist, has conducted long-term fieldwork in the communities surrounding the river Mana, focusing on the religious practices, and at this point is writing a promising thesis on the biography of Mana.

La Jaiba

Different small sections of municipalities in three different provinces -Puerto Plata, Monte Cristi, and Valverde, situated in the Cibao region – were visited during fieldwork. Some of the data presented below are from the small settlement La Jaiba, located in the municipality Villa Isabela in the northwestern part of the province Puerto Plata.

According to the most recent census, La Jaiba had 2,273 inhabitants, of which 67% were evaluated as poor, and 26% as extremely poor. The inhabitants are employed in the public sector, agriculture, small shops, work in larger towns like Imbert or Puerto Plata, or live on remittances from the USA.

As in the case of many other rural settlements, for the history of La Jaiba we have only oral history to rely on. As for the town's origin, the oral history is limited to a few names of founding families. Therefore, the history of the two provinces Puerto Plata and Santiago will be summarized in order to help us understand the broader picture of regional development, because to my knowledge there are no more specific historical data available.

The archaeological examination of Northern Cibao has yielded rich evidence of pre-colonial settlements (Ulloa Hung 2014; Herrera Malatesta 2018). The early colonial history of this region is related to the establishment of the first Spanish towns and fortifications, like La Isabela, Concepción de la Vega, Puerto Plata, Santiago, and small fortifications like Santo Tomás de Jánico, Esperanza, and later Monte Cristi (Hofman et al. 2018; Ulloa Hung & Sonnemann 2017).[167]

La Jaiba is approximately 22 kms from the first European town in the Americas: La Isabela (founded in 1493). Different publications have addressed the history of La Isabela (*e.g.* Chiarelli & Luna Calderón 1987; Deagan & Cruxent 2002). The general consensus is that after the discovery of gold in other regions, early settlers of this town started to move to other places. Around 1498, La Isabela was nearly abandoned. However, it seems that a small part of the population remained, established their herds, engaged in trade with cattle, and hunted wild pigs (Blanco Díaz 2009). La Isabela emerges repeatedly in records as part of a farming area. In 1609, La Isabela had cattle herds and estates producing ginger. In the late 18th century references, a river of La Isabela appears again in a cattle estate of Tomasa from El Castillo (Hernández González 2007). Now, the ruins of the first town are situated in a small community

166 With regard to the cavern of Mana, Tejeda Ortiz (1978) writes about Mr. Reyes de las Rosas, one of Bibiana's associates, active as a healer, was using the cave for his practices and describes this place as a dwelling of indigenous peoples. Knowing their secrets, this associate had its altar at a huge rock, to which the whorshippers were atributing supernatural powers, and he himself used a small piece of it as an amulet.

167 For recent archaeological studies of this region see Ulloa Hung (2014), Ting et al. (2016), Herrera Malatesta (2018), Keegan & Hofman (2017, 2018), Hofman et al. (2018) and forthcoming publications from the ongoing archaeological excavations of the Nexus 1492 project.

called El Castillo. Whether or not the present-day community can be linked to some of the farms or the original town is unclear. The lands around La Jaiba are fertile and used for agriculture but the population has been facing problems of water shortages, which were considered consequences of the large-scale deforestation, linked to large-scale cattle raising.

The existing cultural expressions of inhabitants of La Jaiba should be understood as a part of larger provincial rural history. Within the province where the settlement is situated, different early colonial forts and towns relied on food supplies first produced by the indigenous subjects and later by the population of mixed origins. In the *repartimiento* of 1514, around 1200 indigenous subjects were allocated to Puerto Plata, Santiago, and La Vega.[168] The demographic growth of Puerto Plata during the second half of 16th century was the consequence of an economic boom related to its port, its sugar mills (30-40), and contraband (Blanco Díaz 2009).

Because of the contraband, Osorio's troops forced the inhabitants of the northern region, including those of Puerto Plata, to move to Monte Plata and Bayaguana in 1609, in order to end this illegal trade (Rodriguez Morel 2016b). At the time of that forced removal around 22 farms existed between Santiago, Montecristi and Bayajá.[169] In complaints against the relocations, the majority of the *vecinos* and inhabitants of the northern area were described as *"commoners, mestizos, mulatos and blacks"*, who did not have large houses, or much property to lose. The farms were sustained by their respective resident families, and just one or two enslaved individuals, if they had any at all (Blanco Díaz 2009). Some of the existing farms were relocated closer to Santiago, La Vega, and Cotuí but some of them also stayed (Hernández González 2007).[170] After the beginning of the 17th century there are few historical references to the town Puerto Plata or the settlements in the province of the same name. This lack of information remained until the town's repopulation by people from the Islas Canarias in 1736.

The 18th century demographic increase was stimulated by economic growth, which profited from the free port policy. Among the commodities produced in this region were onions, garlic, tobacco, salted fish, palm and mangle wood (Rodríguez Demorizi 1979). In the 1780s, Puertoplateños were forced to resettle in Santiago and other areas outside of the town, due to severe droughts and lack of medical attention within their town (Hernández González 2007). During the 19th century, Puerto Plata regained its trade town status with the majority of workers focusing on work in the port, caoba exploitation, and cultivation of vegetables, sugar, tobacco and cacao, as well as cattle raising (Moya Pons 2010). During this period, the rural population of Puerto Plata exceeded the inhabitants of the town (17,479 vs. 7,370). Sugar production remained

---

168 For more details on this *repartimiento* see Mira Caballos (1997). The transcript of the original document is to be found in the *Colección de documentos inéditos relativos al descubrimiento, conquista y colonización de las posesiones españolas en América y Oceanía.*

169 For the most recent archaeological study of Monte Christi see Herrera Malatesta 2018; for Bayajá see Sony Jean (forthcoming), and Ulloa Hung & Malatesta (2015).

170 In the Mao region, there were various farms, such as Jaibón, Yaque, or Guayacanes. The farm of Guyacanes and Pontón, owned by Juan Cid, was moved to a location called Payavo, between the towns of Cotuí and Boyá (possible current Payabo at the river Payabo) (Blanco Díaz 2009). Some of the residents, like the owners of farms at Mao, stayed (Blanco Díaz 2009). In the late 18th century, the Tejadas family is said to have owned a farm in Mao, and Tomasa del Castillo had a farm at river of La Isabela (Hernández González 2007).

an important contribution to the local economy until 1930 (Moya Pons 2010).[171] The information about the past economy of this town and the activities of its inhabitants again refers to the rural areas outside of the town.

In general, the provincial histories are based on the histories of the major towns, which are better mapped. In the case of Puerto Plata province, however, the depopulation was accompanied by a silence of the historical records for both the rural areas and the town of Puerto Plata. The town Puerto Plata is quite remote (73 km) from the location of La Jaiba. In fact, Santiago de los Caballeros is not much farther than Puerto Plata (only three km difference). Unlike Puerto Plata, Santiago escaped Osorio's devastation and from 1609 onward it became an economic center of the region in the fertile Cibao valley. Santiago was founded as a small fortification, which was later relocated, repopulated, and which gained town status at its current location.

At the beginning of the 17th century, there were many scattered small communities outside of Santiago, cultivating crops, hunting and trading in cowhides. At the end of the eighteenth century around 26,000 inhabitants belonged to Santiago's jurisdiction (Hernández González 2007). This part of the population is described as poor, living in small villages, dedicated to hunting and raising small numbers of domestic animals, while having little access to the institutional religion (Sánchez Valverde in Hernández González 2007). The agricultural production of this region increased, especially with the boom of the sugar industry in Haiti. In the first half of the 17th century, Santiago already had churches (with eight brotherhoods), a hospital, and around two hundred *vecinos* (Hernández González 2007). From the end of the 17th century to the first half of the eighteenth century, Canarian families moved into the region and contributed to the socio-economic development through their involvement in agriculture (tobacco and livestock) (Hernández González 2007).

In various periods the Santiago population suffered from violent conflicts (1660, 1805, 1822, 1863) and several earthquakes (1775, 1783, 1842), which led to demographic decline.[172] The ethnic composition of Santiago in the first half of the 18th century was highly diverse, including more than three hundred men of arms, the rest being "*mulatos*, free blacks, and *mestizos*" (Hernández González 2007). The lifestyle of farmers in 18th century Cibao was described by a Frenchman, Vincent (Rodríguez Demorizi 1979). Farmers lived in *bohios*, slept in *hamacas*, were self-sufficient, producing everything they needed for alimentation, ate from plates of calabash, and produced their own furniture. With some exceptions, *hateros* in Cibao did not exploit

171 Similarly, the rural population of Mao was around 7,324 while the town had only something over 1,800 inhabitants (Moya Pons 2010). The urban population increased later on with the commercial production of rice for the internal market.

172 Santiago's relative proximity to the French territory led to its being subjected to attacks from there: the town was burned down and surrounding farms were plundered on different occasions. These attacks caused a decline, which in turn stimulated the Canarian immigration.

slave labor to the same extent as the sugar regions in this period. On average one cattle holder would have a maximum of four enslaved laborers.[173]

In the 19th century, Santiago's rural economy was dependent on the cultivation of tobacco and vegetables, as well as on cattle raising, while the town had many craftsmen, tailors working in tanneries, and producers of brick and cigarettes (Moya Pons 2010). In 1904, Santiago had around eleven thousand inhabitants and continued to grow further in the 20th century.[174]

From this brief overview of the local histories it is clear that indigenous predecessors were present in the area where I conducted my fieldwork for much longer than is generally assumed. We must, however, consider these continuities within the general demographic development, wherein the majority of the Dominican ancestry is of non-local origin.

Major tendencies in Cuban ethnogenesis

The early colonial population of Cuba was characterized by huge demographic changes. Besides the well known devastations, Velázquez' landfall and colonization triggered a profound transformation of Cuban demography and spawned unique cultural, spiritual, and social patterns. Like the Dominican history, the Cuban past is punctuated with acts of survival, human suffering, rebellion, and adaptation in the aftermath of the European invasion. After the violent occupation of selected regions, the island was colonized through the establishment of permanent European settlements between the years 1511 and 1515. Even before the first conquest was concluded, Velázquez was already allocating indigenous people to his army. The first inhabitants of the newly established cities were the men of Velázquez with their indigenous captives. The reconstruction of Cuban demographic history faces the same problems as the studies on that process in the neighboring island of Hispaniola. One of the obstacles in comprehending the formation of the Cuban society is our lack of knowledge concerning the colonial history of the indigenous people.

Colonial history of Indigenous Cuban ancestors

As in the case of Hispaniola, the grand narrative argued that the European colonization caused a demographic catastrophe during which the indigenous peoples vanished. Unlike the Dominican case, different studies have revised this traditional vision of indigenous rapid extinction in Cuba. In 1945, Pichardo Moya wrote a pioneering article on indigenous colonial history, in which he argued that historical sources, archaeological evidence and heritage documentation suggest that this disappearance was

173 To illustrate, an owner of one farm at Guayacanes, Melchor de Chaves, is said to have exchanged his tobacco with the French for two persons labeled as Congolese, and another as Bambara (Hernández González 2007). Also Tomasa from El Castillo had one *Creole* from Carolina in North America (Hernández González 2007). In 1776 the Congo group seems to have been quite prominent in this region. Among other groups of enslaved people in this region were also individuals called Congo, Carabali, Bambara, Mandinga, Mina, Senegal, Nago, Cotucolí (Hernández González 2007).

174 For more detailed information about the exponential growth of Santiago from 1800 until now, see the work of Paulino Ramos (2007).

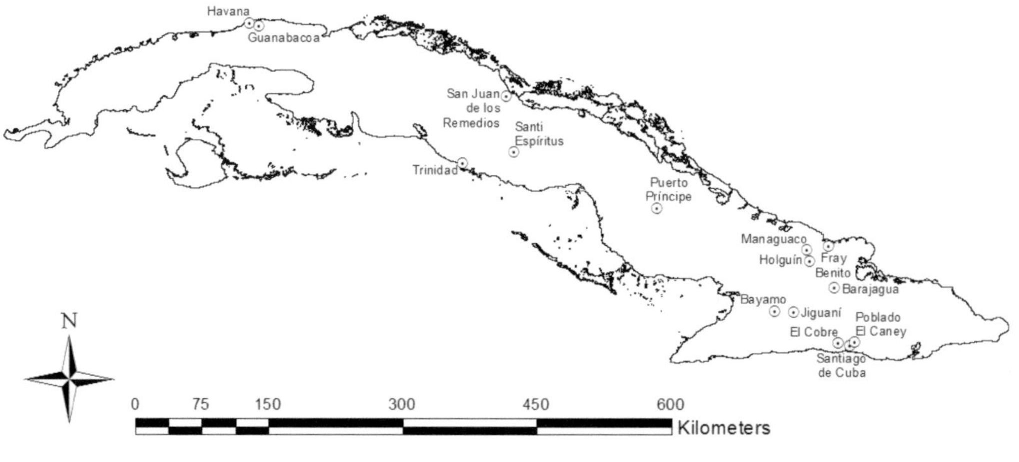

Figure 9 Cuban locations mentioned in this section.

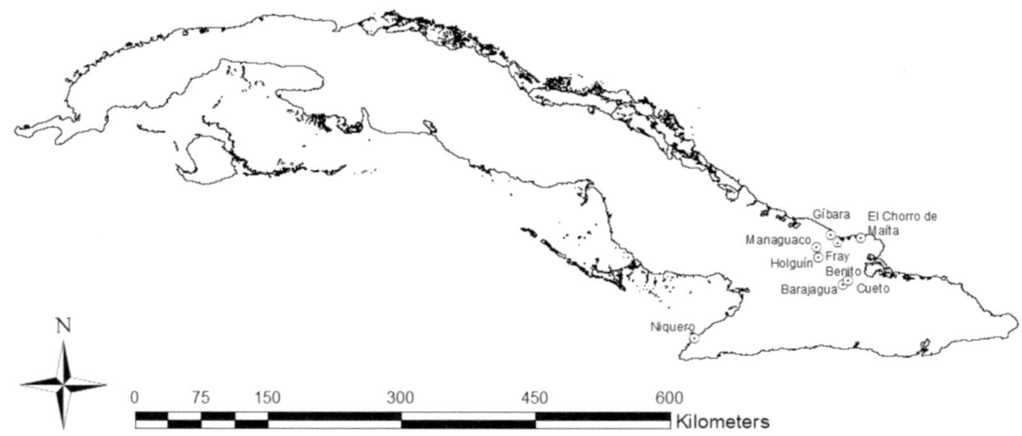

Figure 10 Cuban fieldwork locations.

exaggerated. Similarly, García Castañeda (1949), one of the founders of archaeology in Holguín, was one of the first to discuss the relationship between the indigenous people and the Spanish settlers in eastern Cuba (Valcárcel Rojas 2014). Pichardo Moya's call for more studies on this topic was answered much later when an increasing body of studies from historical, archaeological, and anthropological perspectives nuanced Ortiz′ conclusion about the failed indigenous transculturation (*e.g.* Badura 2013; Barreiro 2006; García Molina 2007; Mira Caballos 2000; Portuondo Zúñiga 2014; Roura Álvarez 2008; Valcárcel Rojas 1997, 2012, 2014, 2016). These studies also suggested that the European colonization led to a complex process of transformations of indigenous life and culture.

As for Eastern Cuba, the investigations by Valcárcel Rojas and his colleagues from the CITMA department have provided new data and perspectives on the indigenous life-ways in the colonial period. Valcárcel's most recent studies (2012 – 2017) expanded the evidence for a wide array of responses of indigenous people to the colonial situation in Cuba. The author suggests, that in spite of the conquest and colonization of Cuba, leading to large-scale destruction, death, and cultural loss, the indigenous people also resisted, took refuge, isolated themselves from the colonialists, or immersed themselves in the colonial society.

As De La Fuente (2009) suggested, it is nearly impossible to establish the extension of this demographic catastrophe. While the quick decline of the indigenous population has been one of the hallmarks in the historiography, the size of the Spanish population in the same period seems to have been even smaller. Expeditions for riches in New Spain, Peru, and other regions of Tierra Firme provoked a decline of the indigenous population and destabilized the early Spanish strata. In 1519, about one to three thousand Spaniards were living in Cuba (De la Fuente 2009; Guanche 2011). Before the Spanish governor Velázquez died in 1524, many early colonial towns became depopulated (Portuondo Zúñiga 2012a). The estimates of urban populations are sometimes likely to be downsized intentionally as these were done in a period when local authorities sought to maintain the population on the island. The first two decades after the conquest, the indigenous inhabitants were more numerous than the colonizers (in 1520 about 18,700; in 1532 about 5000). Around 1544, registers speak of only 750 persons of Spanish origin, the majority of which were men living in the new established towns with indigenous subjects.

Considering the indigenous influence in the Cuban genetical makeup it is indicative that in the context of the male predominance of the colonizers, one year after the European invasion in Hispaniola, the first child of a Spaniard and an indigenous woman was born.[175] Still in 1534, inhabitants of San Salvador, Puerto Principe, and Sancti Spiritus were said to have frequent sexual relations with *naborias*, natives (*naturales*) from the island and enslaved people (Portuondo Zúñiga 2012a).[176] One of the observers, Manuel de Rojas, complained about this and argued that the fact that Spanish and "*mestizos*" married indigenous women lead to the indigenous "disappearance". According to de Rojas, to avoid this disappearance, indigenous women from Florida should be sent to the island. De Rojas' petition was repeated word for word by Bishop Diego Sarmiento twenty-two years later, using the exact same arguments for bringing indigenous women from Florida (Portuondo 2012a). A prominent Cuban historian, Portuondo Zúñiga, agreed that one explanation of the indigenous "disappearance" is the process of "*mestizaje*" (2012b). This disappearance refers to groups that are distinguished by visible aspects such as skin color and hair type. Therefore, these accounts then speak about demographic loss of population, which in the public display

175 The Spanish conquest and colonization were executed primarily by Spanish men. Iberian women were incorporated much later into the colonial endeavor. Similarly, later transatlantic human cargoes mainly consisted of male adolescents, not of families (with the exception of Angolans, see Guanche 2011). The percentage of women arriving from the Hispanic peninsula to Cuba increased especially in the 19th and 20th centuries, but even then it never exceeded 30% of the total Iberian migration (Guanche 2011). The gender balance was recuperated later through the demographic growth.

176 There are numerous accounts of how colonizers used sexual abuse and gender violence as weapons (Mira Caballos 2000). The sexual conquest of indigenous women, and later of African women, together with less violent encounters in the colonial society created a new class of people whose social status contested the colonial categories of colonizer and colonized.

and outsider's evaluation would imply loss of linguistic skills, continuity of beliefs, and other cultural traits.

This "disappearance" should however be placed within the context of imposition of colonial power through the introduction of the colonizer's genes, language, religion, and culture, within a society in which all non-European traits became a cause of stigma and a justification of exploitation. In contrast to Ortiz' idea of failed transculturation the invisibility of certain physical and cultural markers could be explained by their integration into the new genetic and cultural reality.

The colonization profoundly affected the indigenous life-ways. After birth many people were baptized, received Catholic names, spoke Spanish, and dressed in Spanish clothes (Valcárcel Rojas 2012, 2016). For some of these changes there is documentary evidence, for example during the *repartimiento* of 1527. Catholic names prevail among the mentioned individuals, sometimes in combination with non-Catholic names like Bartolomé Zemcubadahaguano, Ximón Çococamayaciniguaya, or Beatrizica, who is now called Constanza Puacayma (AGI, Justicia 52, N. 11 in Mira Caballos 1997a).

The cultural changes did not restrict themselves to renaming, but extended to the whole spectrum of social positions and daily occupations. Indigenous people occupied different positions in society. There have been various cases of indigenous men that had a quite high social position. One of these was Miguel Velázquez, of indo-hispano ancestry, who was canon and musician in the cathedral of Santiago de Cuba around 1544 (Portuondo 2012a).[177] During the same period (1531), indigenous enslaved persons owned by Miguel Ramírez, bishop of Santiago de Cuba (1530-1534), constructed the Franciscan convent and church in Santiago (Mira Caballos 1997a). Some of the friars of the Franciscan convent instructed indigenous children in the Catholic beliefs (Portuondo 2012a). Similar to the early and later colonial history, Santiago church officials seem to have had servants of indigenous origin as late as 1695.[178] In addition, indigenous descendants worked as servants, military troops, carpenters, potters, agriculturalists, watchmen on the coasts, constructors of the main roads (*caminos reales*), and carried out paid labor in sugar mills (Valcárcel Rojas 2016).[179]

Some individual and small communities such as Macurige withdrew from permanent contact with the Spaniards and their history remains untold (Valcárcel Rojas 2016). During the initial phase of colonization some independent groups attacked Spanish farms and settlements (*e.g.* Baracoa 1538 and a series of insurrections in 1524-1550). One of the Spanish complaints addressed the attacks of indigenous Maroons that burned ranches, killed servants and other "tamed Indian" servants. The

177 But also see: AGI/10.42.3.300//CONTRATACION,5506,N.1,R.3 1763, Expediente de información y licencia de pasajero a Indias de Juan Basilio Rodríguez, ministro provincial de Santa Elena de La Florida, fraile franciscano, con Juan de Dios Rodríguez, franciscano, donado, mestizo, natural de Cuba, a Florida.

178 AGI/10.42.3.249//CONTRATACION,5456,N.3,R.40. Expediente de información y licencia de pasajero a indias del doctor Andrés de Olmos, racionero de la catedral de Santiago de Cuba, con su criado mestizo Tomás de Olmos, a Cuba.

179 During the attack of Havana by Jacques de Sores, indigenous, African and Spanish people fought together, the latter being a minority. The fear of depopulation, reinforced by attacks, gave the colonizer space to negotiate the implementation of the New Laws, which could be postponed up to 1553. See also 1756 AGI/27.29//MP-VARIOS,5.

social organization and sense of identity of these Maroons may have been based on the still continuous practice of *areítos* (Portuondo Zúñiga 2012a, p. 55).[180]

Thus the colonial landfall provoked a large-scale internal movement of people, which forced indigenous ancestors to enter into contact with other people of local and non-local origin. At first, these movements of people were related to the initial phase of the conquest, when people were searching refuge in the areas that were remote from the Spanish occupation. When Velázquez forcibly divided indigenous ancestors (through the *repartimiento*) he brought together inhabitants from different villages and even provinces, several of whom spoke different languages.[181] In the 1530s, Spaniards from Bayamo, Baracoa, Puerto Principe and Habana were allotted persons who belonged to at least 75 indigenous settlements.[182]

These movements continued with the establishment of indigenous towns after the *encomienda* period, such as Guanabacoa (1555) or Caney (Badura 2013). The foundation of settlements such as Guanabacoa seems to have been stimulated by the fact that indigenous people already inhabited this place in 1525 (Roura Alvarez 2011). Economic developments and the establishment of new settlements further motivated indigenous intra-island and inter-island migration in the 17th and 18th centuries. Concretely, in the 18th century indigenous people from Jiguaní and Bayamo moved to Camagüey, and in the 18th and 19th centuries indigenous people from Bayamo, Jiguaní, El Caney, and Baracoa moved to Holguín, from Caney to Tiguabos and Yateras, and from Bayamo to Jiguaní (Valcárcel Rojas 2016).[183] Moreover, these population shifts did not remain within the boundaries of the island. The Spanish conquest implied large-scale displacement of people. The invasion of the mainland was carried out on the shoulders of the indigenous people from Cuba and Hispaniola, who were used as logistic help. Although it is not clear how many indigenous people were displaced in this way from Cuba, around three thousands of them were transported from Hispaniola to Tierra Firme in the 16th century (Mira Caballos 1997; for Cuba see further Morales Patiño 1945). The Spanish colonial enterprise on the mainland implied in turn an influx of local inhabitants from there to the Caribbean.

Non-local indigenous peoples in Cuban history

After the colonization of the mainland, indigenous peoples from the continental Americas reinforced the plurality of indigenous cultures in the Caribbean, also in Cuba. As earlier suggested, the interregional links with other islands and with the mainland were already established prior to the European conquest. The conquistador Bernal Díaz del Castillo (1844: Ch.8 [1568]) gives an interesting eye-witness account of how during the expedition of Grijalva from Cuba to Mesoamerica (1518) the Spaniards

180 The indigenous descendants from Caney and cobreros attacked Santiago and put into jail governor Villalobos 1692. During attacks of Britain militias composed of the people carrying the following colonial categories: *"mulatos, negros libres, esclavos and indios"* in 1740-41 (Portuondo 2012a).

181 Real Cedúla a Gonzalo Guzmán, 1529, published by Mira Caballos (1997).

182 Some of these settlements are: Gueynaya, Guanacobi, Guanarabi, Tinama closeby to Bayamo, Mayci, Mayaguano, Guanyguanyco, Banibacoa, Guamanicao, Barajagua.

183 As Valcárcel suggests, these movements may be explained by a search for ways to improve wellbeing or by existing land conflicts, and in some cases they may have been motivated by relationships between families, friends, and by solidarity among the people (ethnicity) concerned. Such internal migrations were likely accelerated due to the demographic growth and changes in economic developments.

encountered on the island of Cozumel (in front of the Yucatan coast) an indigenous woman from Jamaica, who had got there two years before by accident (the large canoe with which she and ten other indigenous persons had set out to go fishing, had been driven by the currents to the shore of Cozumel). The indigenous language of Jamaica she spoke was the same as that of Cuba, so that several Spaniards, including Bernal Díaz himself, could communicate with her. She had also learned the local (Maya) language and could communicate with the native people of Cozumel. It is likely that this was not a unique incident but that such casual (but without doubt significant) encounters and communications between the indigenous peoples of the Caribbean and Mesoamerica did occur more often in the pre-colonial period.

The interregional movements of Caribbean indigenous inhabitants evoked by the Spanish colonization can be considered another motor of enhancing the cultural diversity of the indigenous segments of local societies. Furthermore there were the raids and enslaving voyages of the Kalinagos and indigenous peoples from the Circum-Caribbean.

Yaremko (2016) presents the dynamics of the indigenous movements from the American continent under various conditions from the 16th century through the 19th century. During the colonial period thousands of peoples including Yucatec Mayas, Chichimecas, Nahuas, Calusas, Timucuas, Creeks, Seminoles, Apaches, and Pueblo further diversified Cuban cultural heritage. Yucatecos and Panucos were shipped to Guanabacoa close to Havana and Baracoa since the first half of the 16th century. Archaeological evidence confirms Maya presence in rural Eastern Cuban in the first half of the 16th century (Valcárcel Rojas 2012). In the first half of the nineteenth century some indigenous families from the Florida Keys and others from the Yucatan peninsula were brought to the Cienfuegos area (Zapata 2011; see also the Census of 1845 and 1861).[184] Later ethnographic studies affirm that some of these forced migrants were inserted in small rural settlements like Madruga in Mayabeque, Los Palos, Nueva Paz, Sabana, Cubacanacán, and Hanábana Quemada. Yaremko (2016) suggests that in the location of Hanábana Quemada there is a case of a man of Arawakan ancestry who married to a women of Yucatec Maya origin.

African ancestors in Cuban ethnogenesis

As long as the Spaniards could exploit the indigenous workforce, the transatlantic human trafficking was restricted. In 1526, it was prohibited to put indigenous people to work in mines. This abolition lead to many complaints of the Spaniards, who argued that the mines on the surface were not physically demanding for indigenous laborers (Mira Caballos 1997). The same year, the king (Charles V) was convinced by those arguments and authorized that indigenous people might be put to work in the mines again. In 1528 the Spaniards started to exploit the copper mines of Santiago. Only one year later, smallpox epidemics caused the death of thousands of indigenous people. Like in the Dominican cases, the quick decline in population was used as an argument for bringing peoples from Guinea to Santiago de Cuba (De la Fuente 2009). The

184 In 1743 Governor Juan Francisco de Güemes y Horcasitas in his letter to the King about the instruction of the indigenous peoples of Los Cayos at Florida writes that they were fleeing because they were afraid to be sent to the Bay of Jagua (Yaremko 2016).

extent of this decline might have been exaggerated in order to convince the Crown to send more enslaved Africans. The replacement of indigenous forced labor by African ones was much more profitable, as the taxes on the gains made by using African labor were half of those on gains made by using indigenous labor (Mira Caballos 1997). In addition, the exploitation of these enslaved men was not restricted by the Burgos Laws nor complicated by obligations of providing religious instruction.

In 1532, another appeal was issued to send new enslaved peoples from Africa. This appeal explains that it was important to bring in this workforce before indigenous peoples declined further, as Spanish survival depended on forced labor. Without these laborers the colonizers were forced to leave and exploit the peoples of Peru. In 1535, Santiago de Cuba officially estimated that there were around one thousand enslaved people originating from Africa. This African labor was employed in the construction of urban centers, mines, and agricultural fields. Some of such petitions, like that of Gonzalo Guzman (1535), asked to receive more enslaved peoples by pointing to the inequality in the allocation of indigenous laborers. Guzmán claimed that indigenous people should not be allowed to have freedom because it was neither useful for them nor for the colonizers.[185] Four years later, the same person asked to bring African enslaved peoples, because, as he explained, *"they (indigenous people) are few to serve but many to rise and damage".* Around the same period, permission was asked to bring forced labor to help develop sugar mills (Fernando de Castro 1534; Ortiz 1947). After the New Laws, the *encomenderos* from whom the indigenous enslaved individuals were taken away, applied again for permissions to bring Africans. As Fernando Ortiz (1947) suggests, *"there was no end to the requests: governors, bishops, monks, municipalities, landowners, and merchants asked for slaves and more slaves. And this went on for over three centuries"* (1947, p. 280).

The newly emerging population of people born on the island (*Creoles*) should be seen in the context of general demographic developments. De la Fuente (2007a) suggests that the Cuban free population (*vecinos*) grew according to the following estimates: 1,100 in 1608, 6,000 in 1689, and 12,000 around 1755.[186] According to the account of bishop Juan de las Cabezas Altamirano in 1604 the Oriente region had around 1800 people of African origin (Portuondo 2012a). This is considerable less than the 6,000 estimated for Havana alone in the same period (De la Fuente 2007a). Both numbers suggest that by the beginning of the 17th century the process of transculturation continued and incorporated large numbers of Cuban ancestors of African origin.[187] The overview of data relevant for Cuban demographic history since 1750s until 2012 is presented in Table 2.

185 Gonzalo de Guzmán sobre la condición de los indios y su sustitución por africanos (1535).

186 The differences in the estimates of De La Fuente (2007) and Engerman and Higman (1997) are considerable if we keep taking into account that the population size was five times the number of the *vecinos*. According to SVD only around three hundred enslaved subsaharans were brought to Cuba in the 17th century. This obviously does not include the illicit trade, which was prominent in this period.

187 If we take into account that the size of the free population was five times the number of the *vecinos*.

	1750s	1774	1792	1817	1827	1830s	1841	1880s	2012
Total	170,000	171,620	273,979	553,033	704,487	775,695	1,007,624	1,494,966	11,167,325
White (%)	69	56'2	48'8	43'4	44'2	44	41'5	66	64
Free of color (%)	14	18	20'4	20'6	15'1	15	15'2	18^{A}	(36)
Enslaved (%)	25	25'8	30'8	36	40'7	41	43'3	13	

Table 2 Demographic development in Cuba in the last 250 years. Based on Engerman and Higman (1997) and the census of 2012. The estimate of the Cuban population between 1774 and 1841 is based on Naranjo Orovio (2007). ^{A} *Plus 3% Asians.*

	1750s		1830s	
	Cuba	**Hispaniola**	**Cuba**	**Hispaniola**
Total	170,000	70,625	775,695	
White (%)	69	44	44	42
Free of color(%)	14	44	15	42
Enslaved (%)	25	13	41	16

Table 3 Comparison Cuba and Hispaniola in the 18th and 19th centuries.

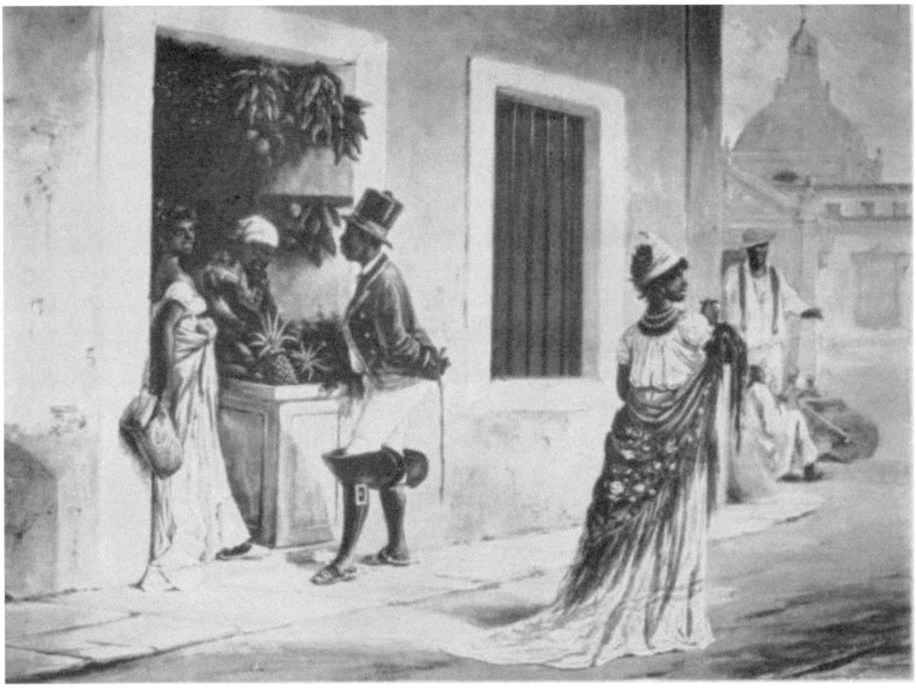

Figure 11 Scenes from Havana, end of the 19th century by Landaluze in Bachiller y Morales (1881).

In total, at least 778,541 persons came from Africa to Cuba (SVD 2017).[188] The horrors of the slave trade are not easy to be quantified, as this has had an enormous negative impact on many societies, with consequences even today. Large-scale slave trade began in the 16th century with the Portuguese traders. Gómez Reynel received a

188 Based on official registers, it has been estimated that at least 111,000 persons, who were embarked with the destination Cuba, passed away on their journey (SVD 2017).

royal decree to bring every year approximately 4,500 enslaved men to Cuba (Rawley et al. 2005). The peak of the slave trade is related to the expansion of the sugar industry between 1790 and 1860. In the 18th century there were approximately 68,000 enslaved persons, and in the 19th century disembarked around 710, 000 enslaved people in Cuba (SVD 2017). According to Engerman and Higman (1997), between 1815-1819 and 1835-1839 more than 1,137,300 enslaved individuals was seized in various regions of West Africa and brought to Cuba. The sugar and coffee boom in Cuba has lead also to considerably differences between Cuban and Dominican demographic histories (see Table 3).

In total, there has been also much more African captives brought to Cuba then to Spanish speaking Hispaniola. The West-Central African influxes have been constantly renewed, with new ships coming to the Cuban harbors. One of likely factors in differences in the demographic development in Cuba and the Dominican Republic is the fact that the slavery in Cuba was abolished in 1886, which was 64 years later than in Hispaniola and 93 years after the revolution in Haiti. This is an important factor for the preservation of cultural traits, oral history, and knowledge related to slavery. One of the breathtaking testimonies of the late Cuban slave period is Esteban Montejo's description of his life in Barrancones, and later his flight and survival in the Cuban mountains (Barnet 1966).

The heterogeneity of the Cuban ancestors of African origin

Similar to what happened in Dominican history, the forced African migration to Cuba was marked by great heterogeneity. According to Guanche (2011), based on parochial books, the majority of the enslaved people that were brought to Cuba throughout the colonial history belonged to the Niger-Congo language family.[189] Their presence in ecclesiastical statistics may be due to the early conversion of this region to the Catholic faith. Another important multi-ethnic group called Lucumí grew especially between the second half of the eighteenth century to the first half of the 19th century (Guanche 2011).[190] From the present-day Benin area (the old kingdom of Dahomey) came Ararás, while present-day Carabal on the Nigerian coast was the homeland of the so-called Carabalís. This hyper-diversity was also related to a high percentage of exogamy. However, parochial books from Pinar del Río (1822-1870) show also some cases of couples married within their own ethnic group (see Guanche 2011).

As the popularity and composition of the Cuban brotherhoods indicate, transculturation went beyond genetic exchanges. In spite of being considerably fragmented by the process of colonization, the colonized shared religious ideas and practices around established models of "colonizer institution", which were consequently reinterpreted in a creative manner. As the richness of the Cuban religious practices indicates, also

189 According to Guanche, the Congo included different groups from those living across the region below the Congo river up to the south of Angola. These included Banda, Boma (probably from the surroundings of the city Boma, not the ethnic group Boma), Bubi, Kamba, Kongo, Kuba, Mbala, Mbamba, Mbundu, Ndamba, Orimbundu, Songe, Sundi, Yaka (Guanche 2011).

190 In the Lucumí group Guanche included Yoruba, Bariba, Bini, Bolo, Chamba, Gbari, Hausá, Mosi, and Nupe. Others have argued that among the Lucumí were also Yorúbá, Nago, Arará, Ajá, Fon, Mahi, Ewé. According to Guanche's description the Arará coincide with the present-day Ewe and Fon-Gbe people from Benin (former Dahomey).

Period/ Region	Senegambia &off-shore Atlantic	Sierra Leone	Windward Coast	Gold Coast	Bight of Benin	Bight of Biafra	West Central Africa	South-east Africa	Totals
1601-1700	0	0	0	0	336	0	0	0	336
1701-1800	2702	10282	713	19817	5241	15241	10007	4030	68033
1801-1900	18453	79219	12236	16727	106161	173925	233530	69921	710172
Totals	21155	89501	12949	36544	111402	189502	243537	73951	778541
% of Total	2,72%	11,50%	1,66%	4,69%	14,31%	24,34%	31,28%	9,50%	

Table 4 Overview of regions prominent in Transatlantic Slave Trade Cuba 1601-1900. Retrieved from from slavevoyages.org, accessed on 1 August 2017.

Cuban ancestors of West African origin managed to maintain many of their own traditions and worldviews.

Distinctive character of the demographic history of the eastern Cuba

Various economic specializations within specific regions have contributed to the formation of distinctive regional demographic characteristics. When Havana started to gain significance as a port, the 16th century economy of the Eastern Cuba (Oriente) started to shift towards the construction of estates with cattle ranches relying upon indigenous and African labor.

As earlier suggested, the population of the first colonial settlements in Eastern Cuba was of small size and there were many mixed marriages. The posterior composition of the Eastern Cuban towns is displayed in the Table 5.

First displayed accounts from 1570 are from Bishop Del Castillo who registered inhabitants with the status of vecino and indigenous persons who were married in some of the towns in the Eastern Cuba (Portuondo 2012a). Accordingly, Bayamo was the major town, considered to be the best off economically, profiting from farms in the surrounding area. In addition, the richness of the Bayamo was closely related also to contraband (Portuondo 2012a).

Another important document that gives us insights into the early 17th century composition of Cuban society is the account of the visit of Bishop Cabezas (1608). Bayamo continued to be the biggest town, followed by Santiago de Cuba, El Cobre, which gained clearly in economic importance, Puerto Principe and Baracoa, which appears as a predominantly indigenous town (Portuondo 2012a). The composition of these towns is of multiple origins including still communities of indigenous descedants.

In his later description (1608) Cabeza reveals the criteria of the Spanish definition of indigenous population: for Cabezas some villages could not be called indigenous because they had been "hispanized". Most likely, this notion was also applied to hispanized indigenous inhabitants of Baracoa. The indigenous segment of society was definitely changing in its culture and ancestral heritage. The indigenous descendants lived in a society of strong Spanish influences but of African ancestors and an influx of indigenous peoples of non-local origins. According to Cabezas, part of the indigenous population localized

Period	1570[A]			1604[B]		1620[C]				1774[D]			1861[E]		
Place	*Inhabitants*[F]	Married *Indians*	*Indians*	*Blacks*	*Whites*	*Inhabitants*	*Souls*[G]	*Indians*	Persons	*Whites*	*Free of Color*	Enslaved	*White*	*Free of color*	Enslaved
Baracoa	8	17	100			20	30		350	1001(45%)	1001(45%)	220 (10%)	4342	4308	2708
Santiago	32	20 Caneyes	77	221	327	65	250	12	313	6525 (36%)	6084 (33%)	5765 (31%)	25406	35295	34500
Caneyes		20							294						
Puerto Principe	25	40	150	600	750	150	300	6	2539						
Bayamo	70	80	250	1000	1250	250	1500		4180	5995 (48%)	4023 (32%)	2430 (20%)	12081	10803	2708
Holguin jur.										1606	547	287			

Table 5 Selected census of the Cuban East demographic history.The information in this table is from various historical documents as published by Portuondo Zúñiga (2012a,b,c).
[A]Visit of the Bishop Juan del Castillo through the island of Cuba, 1570 in Portuondo Zúñiga (2012b). [B] The census directed by Bishop Juan de las Cabezas Altamirano, Wright and Macías Dominguez summarized by Portuondo Zúñiga (2012a). [C] Relación del obispo fray Alonso Enríquez de Armendáriz, 1620 in Portuondo Zúñiga (2012b). [D] Ramón de la Sagra (1838) cited in (2012a). [E] Noticias estadísticas de la isla de Cuba en 1862, as published by Portuondo Zúñiga (2012a). [F] Vecinos is generally to be translated as inhabitants. See earlier explanation of the vecino. [G] This count included together the following categories: Spanish, Blacks, Indians, and Mulatos.

at peripheries of Bayamo and Puerto Principe seems to have been brought in from New Spain.

Bishop Alonso Enríquez de Armendáriz registered more details of the composition of these towns in 1620 (Portuondo Zúñiga 2012a). Bayamo maintained its primacy with a population. The Bayamo town was criticized for not being devoted enough to the Catholic religion. Like Bayamo's Santiago's inhabitants (including those closeby copper mines) were of including colonizers and colonized (*i.e.* indigenous people, of African ancestry and people of mixed origin). This bishop furthermore argued that the individuals of combined indigenous and Spanish ancestry were "not truly indigenous" and were to be treated and instructed in the same way as the Spanish population. For example, indigenous inhabitants of Bayamo were said to be so mixed that it was difficult to distinguish between the different groups, and in Santiago they were assimilated with Spanish so that it was not necessary to instruct them separately in the religious doctrine. Again, we see here how Spanish authorities saw the imposed acculturation – or at least the public exercise of Spanish religion and customs – as incompatible with the continuation of indigenous traditions.

The 17th century economy of Cuba was dominated by large estates with cattle and mines. In Santiago there were sugar mills and many farms with cattle; in Bayamo the greater emphasis was on legal and illegal trade with sugar, tobacco, and cattle (especially cowhides). The demand for copper and cattle from Jamaica and Saint Dominque and an increase of the plantation production increased the contraband. The peace treaty of Rijswijk (1679) had a positive impact on the economy of Eastern Cuba as it reduced piracy. With the English occupation of Jamaica, the local Spanish families, freedmen of color, and enslaved people were forced to move to Bayamo, Santiago and Trinidad (Portuondo 2012a). The fortification of San Pedro de la Roca was built in Santiago and sugar plantations relied also on an immense amount of slave labor in Santiago. In contrast to the sugar industry and the mines, the cattle estates relied upon the labor of only a few enslaved men. In this context, the family members of the owners of small farms participated in carrying out the work.

The 18th century was a period of progressive demographic development also in Eastern Cuba. In comparison to the populational growth of Habana in the same period (1774) the amount of the enslaved population in the Western jurisdiction was three times larger than in the Eastern Departement. The jurisdiction of Santiago focused on growing coffee, on sugar plantations, and copper mines and had more enslaved black laborers than Holguin, Jiguaní, and Bayamo, where the free populations (of Hispanic or mixed origin) worked on farms and tobacco fields. In fact, the North East has maintained the farms since the second half of the 16th century up to the 18th century.

Because of the Haitian revolution, thousands of people of different social statuses fled to Cuba in the years 1791-1805 (Portuondo 2012a). Owners of sugar and coffee plantations contributed to the transition towards monocrop cultivation with extensive exploitation of enslaved labor in Eastern Cuba. This process was also accompanied by a move to populate the interior of the island and to construct railways, which led to the foundation of new settlements and to support for the infrastructure of the sugar industry (Portuondo 2012a). The sugar revolution and the associated influx of Africans in the years 1792-1846 changed the general composition of the Cuba population, as people of Afro-European ancestry became more numerous than those of Hispanic origin. The new character of the population was further modified by official policies in the first part of the 19th century when royal decrees stimulated an influx of "white" migrants to the island.

The increase of the plantations also led to the growth of urban centers. Therefore, enslaved people were concentrated in the city and sugar mills. The census of 1861 shows clear differences between populations in relation to their economies (see the following table). This census is also one of the few that specify what is meant by the category "white". In this census whites are defined as "whites, Asians, Mexicans, Yucatecos". The growth of the white population in rural areas was stimulated by the official policies to "whiten" the island, establishing new settlements in regions that until that time had been depopulated, in order to create services for the sugar plantations. The war of ten years and the abolition of slavery in 1886 stimulated the internal migration.

A brief overview of demographic background of selected Cuban sites

Within these regional demographic developments particular histories of localities should be considered as well. The following pages discuss briefly some of the known aspect of the history of locations where I did my fieldwork (the data which will be presented in Part II). Again the emphasis is on the information about the indigenous inhabitants during the colonial time.

Jiguaní

Jiguaní is one of the municipalities in the province Granma, situated approximately 25 km from Bayamo, one of the towns founded by Velázquez in 1515. Together with Caney and Guanabacoa, Jiguaní was one of the officially founded villages of indigenous descendants in Eastern Cuba. Various archaeological sites have been registered in the surrounding areas of Jiguaní. In spite of the archaeological sites' great informative potential regarding the transformation of indigenous cultures after the European conquest, systematic excavations have not yet been carried out at these sites.[191]

The first historical references to the region of Jiguaní date from 1535. In that year, Manuel de Rojas mentions that close to Bayamo a village was to be founded where indigenous peoples would be located in order to experiment whether they can live in freedom. Whether this settlement has any link with the later village of Jiguaní is unclear, however. About one hundred and fifty years later, General Pardon (1684) identified communities of indigenous descendants in the surrounding areas of Bayamo.[192] These settlements enter the registers because of disputes among the herd owners in these locations. Miguel Rodríguez, son of a Spanish man and an indigenous woman of Bayamese origin, owner of one of the herds in Jiguaní Arriba, disputed with Géronimo Palacín, owner of Jiguaní Abajo, about land rights. Miguel Rodríguez opposed Palacin's intention to sell the herd in Jiguaní Abajo because he claimed this land was granted to indigenous people, it was common property, inalienable, and therefore its sale was against the law (Frómeta Suárez 2003). Their dispute informs us about successful integration of indigenous descendants into colonial society preserving their own cultural concepts.

Soon after, in 1701, Miguel Rodríguez succeeded in founding Villa San Pablo de Jiguaní, which was populated by indigenous descendants that had suffered mistreatment by the Spaniards (SEH 1847).[193] The town is named after the river Jiguaní; its Patron Saint, San Pablo, was renowned as the Christian symbol of conversion. In 1703 Jiguaniceros were granted a substantial part of land. The construction of the church (1720) and the municipality building (1737) also display the wealth of the local inhabitants. The first priest was Andrés de Jerez, who baptized in the church since 1739 (SEH 1847).

Over one hundred years later (1847), the population of Jiguaní was estimated as approximately 2,000 people, and the total of its jurisdiction exceeded 10,000 people (SEH 1847). The majority of its urban population was identified as "white" (1340), with 275 "free brown (*pardos*)", 25 "brown slaves", 90 "freed black", and 212 "black slaves" (SEH 1847). The number of the indigenous descendants in the jurisdiction is difficult to estimate. If there were indigenous descendants they seem to have been integrated into of these categories. Valcárcel has confirmed in his study (2017) the bias of the official censuses and has argued that this bias was motivated by the formation of the sugar industry and commercial agriculture. Although the baptismal records have not been preserved, at least in Bayamo, the church kept using a separate registeration for indigenous people until 1803 (Yero Masdeu 2016). In the censuses of 1778 and 1814, the indigenous descendants of Jiguaní, Caney, and Tiguabos were catego-

---

191 Among the registered sites are La Yaya, Dos Ríos, La Pelua, Jiguaní Abajo, Jiguaní Arriba, El Fuerte, El Huerto, Calabazar, El Faldón, Las Cabezas, La Rinconada, and Cuatro Caminos. Some of the materials together with the map of the sites are displayed in the Jiguaní Museum.

192 Among these were location Santa Ana, Guanarubí, Jiguaní Arriba, Los Quemados and Sao Cautillo.

193 Rodríguez executed this together with his brothers Domingo and Antonio and with the help of other countrymen, including a foreigner: José Sanchez from Mexico (SEAP 1847).

rized as "whites" and "*mulatos*" in order to diminish their right as indigenous people (Portuondo 2012b; Valcárcel Rojas forthcoming).

The 19th century economy of Jiguaní and places in its jurisdiction was based on agriculture, cultivation of tabacco (important for the national market), corn, yucca, plantain, rice, but also on manufacturing tiles, brick, hats of *yarey*, and wax. The census of 1847 shows that the tradition of weaving was alive. Finally, according to this census the Jiguaniceros cured themselves on large scale with green medicine. In 1824 Jiguaní lost its rights and privileges as an indigenous village. At the onset of the Great War a fort was built (Frómeta Suárez 2003).

According to the most recent census (2012) Jiguaní had 60, 573 inhabitants, of which 45% lived in the rural area outside of the town.[194] This census documents that 46% of the population was "white", while 51% belonged in the category "*mestizo* or *mulato*", and 3% were "black".[195] The present-day economy relies on the production of marble, tobacco, poultry, and asphalt. There are plans for the promotion of tourism. Consciousness about the indigenous past is very much alive.[196] The local museum, library, *casa de la cultura*, radio, publications, different schools, all disseminate the knowledge about Jiguaní's indigenous past. Hugo Armas, the historian of the town, could establish a genealogical link between certain families and indigenous ancestors: for example the Anayas family can be linked to the cacique Anaya mentioned by Manuel de Rojas.[197]

Barajagua

Barajagua is small settlement, situated in the Holguín province that holds a great importance for the national history because of being one of the sites displaying a contact of material Spanish and indigenous expressions and because of its link to the appearance of the Virgin of Charity, the Patron Saint of Cuba in 1612.

Barajagua (Bacaxagua) is one of the first regions in which Velázquez had contact with indigenous people in 1513 (Portuondo 2012a). In the first half of the 16th century (1547) indigenous people were raising pigs in one of the estates of Juan Escribano (Mira Caballos 1997). Also, later in the 16th century some of the resistant indigenous troops were residing in the Barajagua province (Mira Caballos 1997). The first settlements in Barajagua supplied the royal copper mines next to Santiago (founded in the 1530s) with crops, meat, and salt (Peña Obregón et al. 2012). The archaeological excavations of sites in the same location confirmed pre-colonial human occupation of these sites, which seems to have continued up to the first half of the 16th century (Valcárcel Rojas 1997). The human presence in the colonial period can be related to the estates with cows that appeared in 1598 (Valcárcel et al. 2014; Peña Obregón et al. 2012).

---

194 Población de Cuba. Retrieved from http://www.one.cu/EstadisticaPoblacion/EstadisticaPoblacion.asp. [accessed on 18 May 2017].

195 Retrieved from http://www.one.cu/publicaciones/cepde/cpv2012/20131107resumenadelantado/Tablas/4.pdf. [accessed on 18 May 2017].

196 But also proud for its role in the independence war and for being a place where José Martí has died. This event is commemorated in the museum by a vessel with earth at display with the following description: The Earth of Dos Ríos, the sacred place of the nation where General José Martí Pérez has fallen.

197 In 1535, Rojas informs us that one cacique called Anaya, was removed with his wife and allocated to one of the *vecinos* of Bayamo. A la Emperatriz Manuel Rojas Santiago 1535 (in De La Sagra 1861).

During the early colonial period, Barajagua maintained itself as a farming region, and continued to do so in the following centuries. This small settlement entered national history with the Marian manifestation during the beginnings of the 17th century. An account by Juan Moreno (1687) described how the Virgin of Charity manifested herself at the Nipe Bay to three children, two of indigenous descent and another of West African origin. After the discovery, these boys went to announce the miracle in the *hato* Barajagua where also the first hermitage was built (Valcárcel et al. 2014). As in the case of Bayamo, the 17th century economy of this region profited from the proximity to the Bay of Nipe, securing a safe harbor for contraband in meat, cowhides, candles, soap, and salt (Valcárcel et al. 2014).

Managuaco

While Managuaco is distant from Barajagua (approx. 60 km), both settlements have some similarities in their importance for the regional religious history. Managuaco is also a small rural settlement in the Holguín province, where the first Catholic hermitage was built in 1692.

The inhabitants of Managuaco engaged in small-scale farming and cattle raising since the end of the 17th through the 19th century (Rodríguez Bruzón 2015). Animal husbandry (especially pigs, horses, and cows) and the cultivation of crops (most likely yucca, corn, plantains, sugarcane, coco, tobacco) appear to have been the major sources of income throughout recent centuries (Rodríguez Bruzón 2015).

The scarce information about the history of Managuaco and Barajagua guides us to see their development as a part of the provincial history. In the present-day Holguín province there are multiple lines of evidence confirming the integration of the indigenous population within the urban and rural societies. Vega Suñol's study (2014) of parochial books from the church of San Isidro provides data that show that indigenous descendants were part of the 18th century population of Holguín province. More specifically, that study suggests that in the years 1713-1819 there were at least 274 indigenous baptisms, of which the majority were of persons who descended from two indigenous parents (173), or at least from an indigenous mother (96), but in some cases (6) from one parent of African ancestry (Vega Suñol 2014). The last baptism of an indigenous child was registered in 1860 in the church of San José de Holguín (Vega Suñol 2014). These findings are confirmed by Novoa Betancourt's analysis (2014) of the rural census from 1775 wherein 7,5% (137) of the total of 1,830 inhabitants were registered as indigenous people. Some of these were foremen, owners of estates in Ejido, but the majority were laborers. The excavations of the first colonial buildings in Holguín where ceramics of indigenous traditions were found confirm that some of indigenous pottery skills were existent between the 17th till the 19th century in this urban section (Jardines Macías et al. 2014).

The indigenous people were present also throughout the colonial period in different rural settlements in the Holguín province. Early in the 1550s, Castañeda (1949) addressed the transculturation mechanisms within these spaces. Drawing on material evidence from sites at Barajagua, Banes, El Yayal and El Pesquero, Castañeda argued that the first two were contact sites, while the latter two were long-term occupations, showing intensive relationships between the Indigenous people and the Spaniards (Valcárcel Rojas 2014). Local investigations have registered more sites where materials

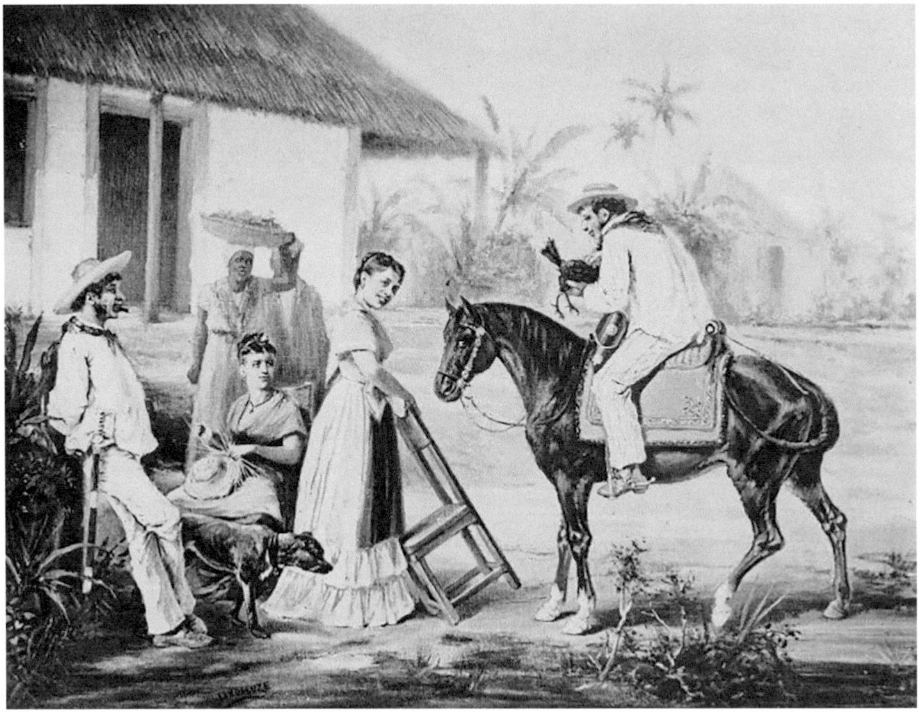

Figure 12 Scenes from the Cuban rural area at the end of the 19th century by Landaluze in Bachiller y Morales (1881).

of European and indigenous traditions were encountered together.[198] Of these sites, Chorro de Maíta exposed complex place formations, where the local and non-local indigenous individuals coexisted (individuals from Cuba, other Caribbean islands, and Mesoamerica), with some people of West African and mixed origins (Afro-hispanic, Indo-hispanic) (Valcárcel Rojas 2012). The analysis of the data from Chorro de Maíta also suggests influences of the Catholic faith in indigenous mortuary treatment, causing the modification of some of the indigenous cultural traditions. A particular case, exemplifying both continuity and change of indigenous culture, is a child's burial. The forehead of this child (age 3-5) was modified in conformity with a pre-colonial tradition, but several grave goods, such as a brass tube and coral beads along with a jet bead, indicate colonial influences. The jet stone is one of the Moorish influences in Catholic religion, and is currently used in the Caribbean as well as the Iberian Peninsula for protection against the evil eye.

In both Barajagua and Managuaco, the awareness of a link with the local indigenous past has been reinforced by recent archaeological research conducted by Valcárcel and his colleagues from the CITMA Holguín. In the case of Barajagua, this identification is further developed through the historical knowledge about the manifestation of the Virgin. In Managuaco the connection to indigenous ancestors has been developed

198 Among these sites are: Alcalá, El Porvenir, Los Buchillones, Potrero del Mango, Maniabón, Loma de Baní, Loma de los Mates, La Siguaraya, La Guanaja, María Luisa, El Jobo, and El Chorro de Maíta (for more details see Novoa Betancourt 2015 and Valcárcel Rojas 1997).

through *Espiritismo del Cordón*. One of the *Espiritismo* believers has attributed his spiritual link with the indigenous ancestors to a possible genealogical descent. This would not be unique in the region as according to the oral tradition of the Zaldívar family from Fray Benito they are indigenous descendants as well; and other members of the community share this conviction.

Revising the indigenous component in demographic histories

Understanding the indigenous contributions to the present-day medicinal culture is conditioned by knowledge of demographic history, including that of relations among different population groups. This chapter highlighted some major tendencies of the development of the indigenous component within the demography of Hispaniola and Cuba. The earliest, more or less accurate documentary information on the size of the indigenous population in Hispaniola comes from 22 years after the first colonial encounter in Hispaniola and from the same time in the early colonial history of Cuba. Although the vast majority of the 26.000 people was located in mining towns, a substantial number was also sent to towns with agricultural and trade based economies.[199] Only four years later, before the friars were able to reallocate the indigenous people into new villages, their number officially dropped to four thousand. Some of these survivors were distributed to indigenous villages which were established in 1519.[200] While some of the names could suggest that these where located in the vicinity of towns that have the same names today (Yaquimo, La Sabana, Santo Tomás de Jánico, Verapaz, San Juan, Báni), their exact location as well as the later history and the biographies of their inhabitants, are unclear.[201]

After the *encomienda* was dismantled, indigenous people were settled in the regions of the cape of San Nicolás, Tiburón, the province of Ciguayos, and Samaná. In the second half of the 16th century, indigenous persons were residing in Boyá, La Mona, Sabana, Santo Domingo, La Yaguana, Yaquimo, and settlements nearby La Vega, Buenaventura and Santa Cruz de Acayagua.[202] The 17th century resources briefly mention indigenous descendants in Azua, Boyá, Cibao, Yaguana, Tortuga, and on the bank of the river Yguamo. At the end of the 18th century, inhabitants of Bánica and Boyá are acknowledged as indigenous descendants. While in this period more people self-identified as such, their identity was doubted because, according to one author (Moreau de Saint-Méry 1796), it could not be proven historically. Some people of mixed ancestry (indigenous, African, and European) were registered by other sources in Santiago. By the end of the 19th century the inhabitants of Boyá are described as having mixed racial composition including phenotypic traits that are considered to be typical for the indigenous peoples of the Americas.

---

199 These were Azúa, Buenaventura, Bonao, Lares de Guahaba, Puerto Plata, Puerto Real, San Juan de Maguana, Vega, La Sabana, Santo Domingo, Salvación de Higüey, Santiago, La Verapaz, and Yáquimo.

200 The seventeen indigenous villages that were earlier mentioned by Mira Caballos (1997).

201 Whether San Juan de Ortega and one of the first villages San Juan de Maguana or San Juan Bautista, were among the villages established by the Hieronymites is unclear. While Mira Caballos (2007) locates some of the villages such as Santiago and La Mejorada, in the vicinity of the earlier Spanish settlements carrying the same name, both San Juan Bautista and San Juan de Ortega are located quite far from San Juan de Maguana.

202 At present there is a small village Dicayagua next to the Jánico, near to San Tomé de Jánico, one of the first forsts established by Spaniards in this region.

Cuba's demographic development is marked by similar long-term continuities of people of indigenous origin in both urban and rural locations. The small size of the indigenous people present in the major towns in the second half of 16th century and the first half of the 17th century have to be considered within the context of the overall small size of the population at large. The focus on the regional and local history brings to light significant differences not only in the economic but also in the demographic history. Colonial authorities registered indigenous people and in the later period their descendants in the following Cuban settlements: Bayamo, Baracoa, Puerto Principe, Sabana/Los Remedios, Sancti Espiritus, Habana, Guanabacoa, Caney, and Macurige. With the exception of San Juan de Remedios, all these settlements maintained indigenous population or its descendants in the 17th century. Camagüey, Caney, Guanabacoa, Jiguaní and Holguín had populations of indigenous origins throughout the 18th century, and Holguin until the beginning of 19th century. As the histories of Boyá, Jiguaní, Caney or Guanabacoa illustrate, indigenous people lived in settlements that were not isolated but rather close to important economic centers.

On both islands, demography was profoundly shaped by the decline of indigenous people, the Transatlantic Slave Trade, the series of immigration waves (including Canarian and Caribbean immigration), emigrations (16th century till present), epidemics, population movements after the Peace Treaty of Basel in 1795, series of foreign occupations, together with other particular local historical events like the evacuation of the North, the profound economic changes (production of monocultures, industrialization), agrarian reforms, and technological changes.

Based on this overview of historical references to the indigenous people of Hispaniola and Cuba, we conclude that the hypothesis of the failed indigenous transculturation needs to be revised. The indigenous population lies at the foundation of the early colonial Creole societies on both islands. It is also worthwhile to emphasize that the indigenous population was composed of people of local and non-local origin, and that the labels defining their identities were imposed by the colonial regimes and likely ignore self-identification with their own ancestors and heritage. The colonial emphasis on race should not blind us for the multiple ways in which indigenous descendants were able to maintain distinct ethnic identities, medicinal cultures and cultural transfer.

The consideration of the indigenous influences in the transculturation process does not deny that the number of people of indigenous descent was always relatively small when compared to the immigrant population in each of the particular historical trajectories of the discussed settlements and regions. The regional and local histories complement and nuance the general developments defined earlier for Cuba as the counterpoint between the sugar/African ancestors and tobacco/European ancestors. This development creates a historical context from which the present healing traditions emerges.

The colonization and the transculturation made large part of the strata of the population including indigenous descendants invisible in the historical records. The poem of Morales (2001), drawing our attention to the indigenous women of low social status, cited at the beginning of this chapter, reminds us how little is known about the commoners and marginalized strata of the population. The demographic overview clearly shows that neither *caciques* nor *conquistadores*, but the commoners of plural origins were the forefathers of the majority of the present population.

Part 2

CONTEMPORARY TRADITIONS

6

Qualities of the landscape in daily life

The previous chapters guided the reader on a journey towards the understanding of how the current memory of the indigenous past has been constructed through institutional means of remembering such as written history. The memory of the indigenous past emerges from the colonial institutional domain but also from the public production of knowledge. The second part of this dissertation addresses the cultural memory of a wider public and provides some insights about how the past is reenacted in more or less conscious ways in the domain of ecological knowledge as applied in daily life, particularly in the case of an illness, when healing performances are necessary.

Chapter 6 concerns the ecological knowledge that has been transferred in foodways, crafts, house building, and agricultural activities, including a broader spectrum of associated cultural practices. After presenting the main character of healing landscapes in the Dominican Republic and Cuba, Chapter 7 will introduce us to the popular concepts of illness, the role of healers, their working settings and their ways of collecting and using medicinal plants. The subsequent Chapters 8 and 9 will elaborate on particular caverns and water sources as healing and ceremonial places. Various examples will be presented to illustrate connections between different landscape elements and to provide us with insights into the more or less conscious ways of remembering, creating a link between contemporary and previous generations.

All data presented in this part, if not referenced otherwise, come from my ethnographic fieldwork conducted between 2013 and 2016 in the Dominican Republic and Cuba. Those data that are not referenced directly as particular interviews originate from various interviews at different locations or fieldnotes. For the locations where the data have been collected see Figs. 7 and 10.

When approaching the healing landscape in a holistic manner, we find that individual wellbeing and health are connected to communal wellbeing, wherein daily activities transform flora into alimentation and natural resources into materials for living and crafts.[203] The rich botanical knowledge is a tenet of agricultural life and culture. The awareness of the intimate human/nature interdependency is expressed in people's own spirituality, which is here illustrated by prayers for rainfall and offerings to earth.

203 For another work on the close of wellbeing, environment and heritage see the dissertation of Stancioff (2018).

This chapter concludes with a short reflection about how the environmental knowledge displayed in the first part carries the cultural memory of the indigenous past and about whether this includes also continuities of indigenous worldviews and knowledge. The outcomes of this analysis will be further discussed in Chapter 10.

Flora as a source of alimentation

The knowledge of local flora is materialized in cultivation, preparation and consumption of crops. This knowledge, however, does not only develop from daily interaction with the local environment but also from other regions and time contexts. Local menus are testimonies of the cultural history of the region, marked by a long process of immigration to the islands. As a result, the Cuban (C) and Dominican (D) culinary tapestry includes dishes and crops of local and non-local origins. As Ortiz's (1995) metaphor of *ajiaco* showed, typical Cuban dishes are often a combination of ingredients from different origins. Similarly, the Dominican traditional dish *sancocho* combines local and nonlocal ingredients. In both study areas, native crops like yucca, corn, *boniato* but also exotic crops like plantain, yams, and rice, become naturalized as an inherent part of the local diet. In the meantime, exotic crops like rice, first introduced during the second voyage of Columbus, were cultivated in rather small amounts until the end of the 19th century, when they spread nation-wide. The rice is then combined with native beans into the popular dish *moro* (C: *moro cristiano* using rice and black beans, *congrí* using red beans, local variants of beans first described by Fernández de Oviedo (2002 [1535]) or is seasoned with *bija* (*Bixa Orellana*) thereby obtaining a local flavor. Like rice also plantains (*Musa paradiasaca)*, guineos (*Musa sapientum*), and yams, a common source of food on Portuguese ships, were introduced to the Caribbean during the early colonial period and are components of other popular dishes: Dominican *mangú* (also *mofongo*), and Cuban *fufu* (mashed green plantains with yucca).

Native plant species like yucca, corn, and guáyiga are used today for a wide range of recipes and traditional utensils with their own specific vocabularies. A variety of dishes is prepared from yucca. The sweet type is used to make *chulitos, roketas, conconetas*, bread, *panecico*, and *hojaldra* in the Dominican Republic, while the same crop is used to prepare *buñuelo, masamora, matahambre, ñape, panocha,* on the neighboring island. The starch from yucca mixed with milk (D: called *natilla*) was used also for alimentation of babies or mixed with eggs and milk into another dish called *cusubé* in Cuba. Without any doubt, the most popular dish prepared from yucca (both sweet and bitter) is until now cassava bread. The recipe for cassava is as follows: after the yucca root is scraped (without removing the starch/*sagú* layer, which is vital in holding the dough together), the roots will be grated on a tin grater to be later stuffed into a special type of woven container (Dominican term: *macuto, capacho;* Cuban term: *catauro/júkaro/sibucán*), a guano, yute or henequen bag, which is placed into a press (lying in horizontal position) to extract the juice. The remaining dough (D: *catibía*, C: *naiboa*[204]) is later deposited in a vessel (D: *canoa* from yagua[205]) to be spread on a *circular metal griddle (D: burén),* which stands on U-form walls made of stones and

204 The word naiboa is also used in Dominican location Bánica.

205 Yagua is a fibrous tissue from the upper part of a specific palm.

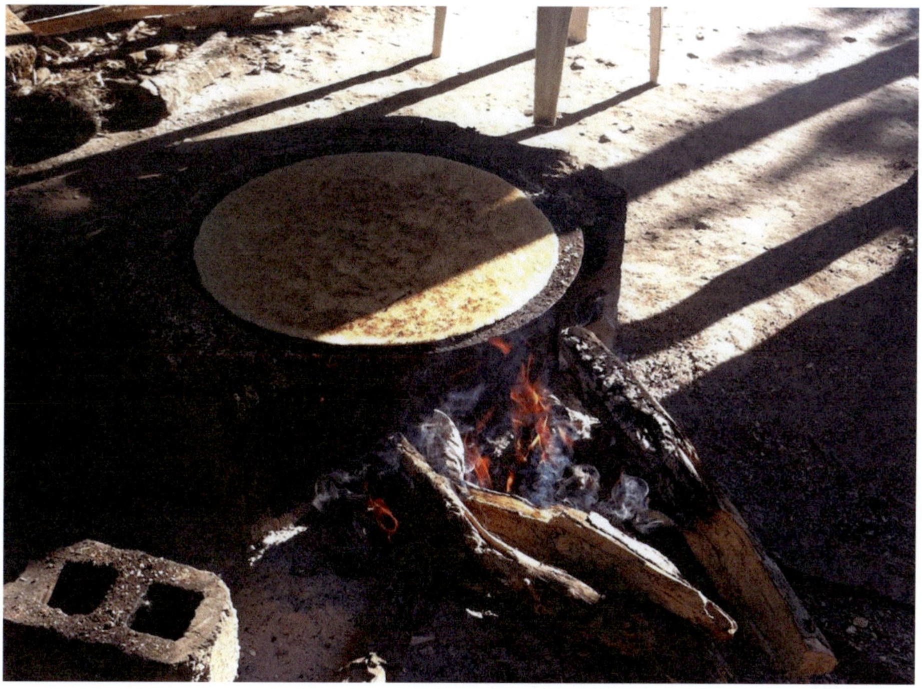

Figure 13 Cassava being baked in Mamey, Dominican Republic.

clay (C: *cocoa* mixed with *apartillo* herb). The round shape of the bread is achieved by using a wooden circular frame (C: *aríto*), on which the dough is placed from a sifter (woven from *guano*). When the cassava bread is dry, it is flavored with peanuts, garlic, and other ingredients.

Another native plant widely used in a great variety of Dominican dishes is corn. From corn are prepared *arepas, arepetes, boyos, bucheperico, chaka, empanadas, guabara* (corn milk), *guanibos, guánimos, gofio, majaretes, tortas, chenchen*, corn wine and corn is added to a chocolate beverage. Cuban corn dishes include *boyo*, corn flour with milk, *frituras, pinol, pan de maíz revuelto*, and *tamales*. The corn silk is used in Dominican for infections in general, and added to herb decoction called *botellas*, literally bottles. Corn, as well as fruits like *chinola*, tamarind, or herbs as *mabí/prú* (a naturally fermented beverage from *behuco del indio*) are used in some locations also to make wine and light fermented bevarege called prú or mabí.

Besides the vocabularies and skills related to the preparation of cassava bread, there are multiple references to crops also in metaphors, songs, poetry, riddles, and proverbs. One of the common Dominican expressions is "*guayar la yucca*", meaning to work intensively and exhaustively. Such traditional expressions inform us about the importance of these crops. Another example is a song about the counterpoint between yucca and corn. These two crops had a dispute about who governs the country; both crops name different dishes having themselves as main ingredients. A fragment goes as follows: "*Say the yucca I am the one who governs the country, and the corn responds I am the governor, says the grater ruku ruku I have not got so many teeth or tooth to grind the flour, and the parents of the family say where is the poor person?"*[206]

Traditional ecological knowledge in Dominican housing areas

For a long period, the wellbeing in agricultural settings has relied upon ecological knowledge, which is reflected in specific skills, including house construction, house furnishing, and the creation of equipment for economic activities. Ironically, this type of material culture is nowadays associated with poverty. Consequently, the change in lifestyle and upward social mobility towards a higher social class result also often in gradually loss of the knowledge accross generations.

Different tree species, for example, were used for building houses. Although the selection of wood varied according to its availability, specific species were preferred because of their durability, water resistance, and flexibility. For house poles roble is considered to be the best wood (different species, *i.e. Catalpa longissima, Tabebuia spp.*).[207] Depending on the type of the house, walls can be made of palm boards (from palm trunk), yaguas (palms called after fibrous tissue from the before mentioned palm tree) or *tejamaní*. The latter are woven from small tree branches, which are later filled out with a manure or clay (C: *cocoa*) mixed with *pangola* (*Digitaria spp.*) or *jiribílla* herb (*Dichanthium caricosum* (L.).[208] The roofs have been often thatched with *yagua/guano* (Coccothrina spp.)/*cana* (Sabal spp.), which would be spiked to radial rafters and beams or tied with *bejuco vieja* (*Hiprocatea volubilis L.*, but also different *lianas*) or *yarey* (*Copernicia spp.*) to the palm stalk.[209] The thatched roofs are said to be cooler in the summer and safer during the storms compared to zinc roofs.[210]

Currently, houses are often furnished with furniture from mahogany, *roble, pino, caoba*, often embellished with weavings from *cana/guano*. The hammocks, now rather used for the afternoon break are woven from *cabuya* (*Furcraea hexapétala*). In the Monte Plata region, some people were sleeping in the past on small carpets from *cana, cabuya*, banana leaves or *huncos* (*Cyperus ligularis* L.). At night, houses are lit by lamps decorated with cotton fiber and embellished with seeds of peonía (*Abrus precatorius* L.). When necessary, the mosquitos are repelled by burning *copey* resin (*Clussia rosea*). When leaving the main house, a visitor might pass under the blessed bread, palm leaves, or *sábila* (*Aloe vera*) hung with a red scarf at the main entrance for protection of the house.[211]

---

206 *The Spanish original is: "Dice la yuca yo soy la que gobierna el país y allí responde el maíz yo soy el gobernador, dice el guayo ruku ruku no tengo tantos dientes ni muela para moler la harina, y dicen los padres de la familia la prangana dónde está metida."* Some of the additional crops such as the yucca, or malanga have double meanings, which sometimes also figure in oral poetry.

207 Fieldnotes taken in conversation with the González family and several other inhabitants of Loma Atravesada.

208 The identification of the flora was based on Acevedo-Rodríguez & Strong (2012). The information on the Cuban flora was crosschecked with the publication of Roig y Mesa (1974).

209 Palma, one of the varieties most popular for walls, but other species of palm called guano, yarey, and cana are also popular.

210 For different traditional house structures see the appendix.

211 As the commemoration of Jesus' entry into Jerusalem, palm leaves are blessed and given to the faithful on Domingo de Ramos (Palm Sunday).

The kitchen is typically a separate building so that the main house remains free of smoke from the fireplace/*fogón* (made of white clay and fine herb). On the *baracoa*[212] (an additional table or repository made of branches and situated above the fireplace) may be found plates, spoons, made from the *higüero* (*Crescentia cujete* L.), sieves (jíbes), vessels for sorting grains (la yo), both woven from *guano*. In the Cuban settlement Los Zaldívares, next to the Cuban town Fray Benito, a visitor might encounter also *achiotera* (sieves made of small calabash) and *arítos*, which are circular in form for preparing cassava and made of *bejuco vieja* or *bejuco manteca*.

Rice accompanying the dish might be somewhere peeled in a wooden mortar called *pilón* (of *caoba*) in Cuba, made of *guyacan* or *cagueyran,* using one, two or three pestles. Coffee beans ground in the pilón, have been sometimes served in small vessels made of *higueritos* (*Crescentia linearifolia).* When drinking his coffee the visitor of a Dominican household might see in the kitchen a large ceramic jar for water that is kept clean by adding carbon; roots of *bejuco caro* (*Vitis vitiginea L.*) are also used to keep the water fresh. A thunderstone lying on the bottom of the jar to keep the water fresh and protect the house from lightening can also be found in some households. In Bánica and Boyá, water was extracted by a ladle made of *higueritos*. The earthen kitchen floor is kept clean with cocoa clay and a broom made from *guano* or swab made from *cabuya.*

Frequently, one of the living areas has an outdoor seating space covered with a roof made from *guano/yarey* or under a tree providing shade on a yard. Basketry, woven from *guano*, can be also easily found at house yards. *Guano* and *cana* are the main materials for the traditional weaving of baskets, bags, hats, or sandals. There are different types of baskets (D: *macutos, cerónes*) with more and less elaborative decoration depending on their function. For example, Dominican *macutos* are without much decoration because they are used for collection of coffee and cacao beans.[213] *Yarey* is frequently used material in Cuban basketry. Another plant used for basketry is *guaniquiqui* (*Trichostigma octandrum).* There are different baskets of more and less elaborative designs. Furthermore, there are crafted: thread of cotton, saddles for donkeys, jibes, or ropes (*henequen), majagua* that is the inner part from *jaguey, guacima tree*). Grandfathers sometimes give children playing in the yard a woven toy (*coge el dedo*, C: *jubo*, called after a type of snake).[214]

Different plants are used for personal hygiene, like soap (made from *cuaba, muñeco/musuy*), Luffa sponges and toothbrushes (from *limpia diente, caimito*). In the past, before the introduction of running water in the villages, women carried clothes in *bateas* (vessels from *almacigo, cedro, roble, jiga* or *caoba*) to the river and washed them with *magey, guayacán, palo amargo, palo piojo* and *quiebrahacha*.[215] The clothes were also stiffened with starch from yucca or corn. *Tuna de España* was used to give more shine to clothes.[216]

---

212 In Monte Plata *baracoa* is the name for a special type of table that functions as a structure for drying the meat.

213 For more on the Cuban basketry work see Moreno (1998).

214 This particular item is also produced among the Kalinagos of Dominica (see Appendix, Table 9).

215 Many Dominican households don't have direct access to drinkable water and have to bring it from the rivers. The consumption of water in this ways carries obvious health risks.

216 Besides offering important construction material, wood may also be used as fuel for the kitchen (different preferences, for lightning for example cuaba), for tint (campeche, manglares, caoba), and of course for being ornamental, or to control erosion and deforestation.

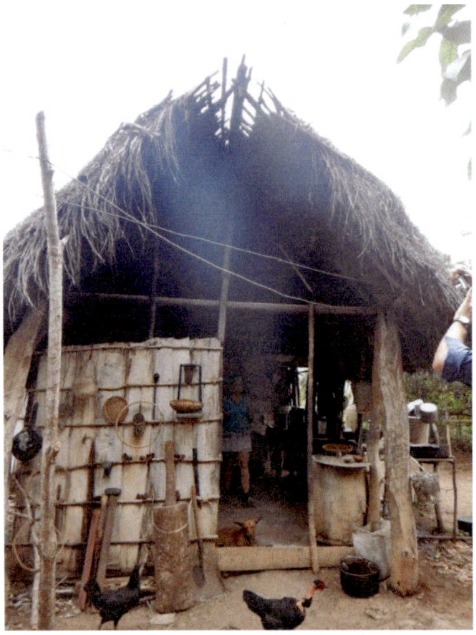

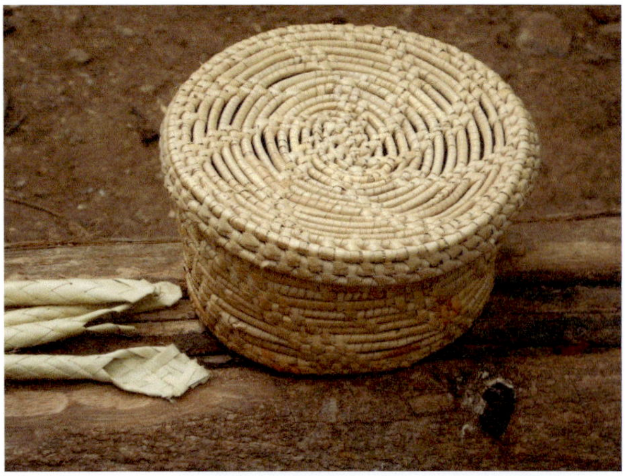

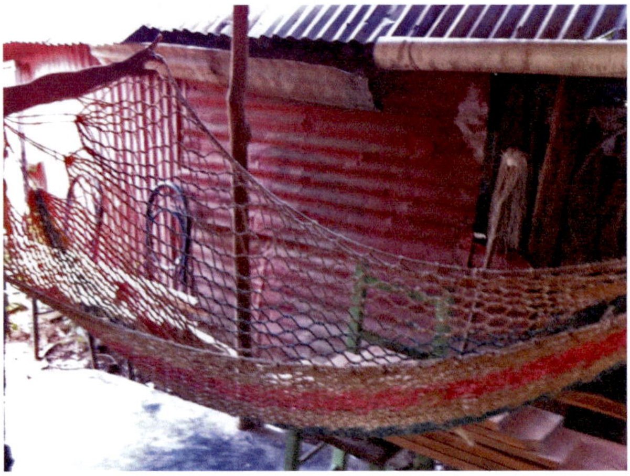

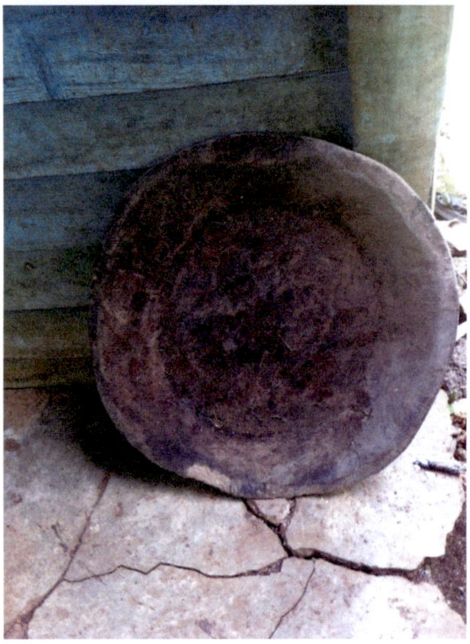

Figure 14 A kitchen in Fray Benito, Cuba (upper row, left).

Figure 15 A basket from Fray Benito, Cuba (upper row, right).

Figure 16 A hammock from Padre de las Casas, close to Bánica, Domincan Republic (lower row, left).

Figure 17 A batea from Boyá, Dominican Republic (lower row, right).

The collective botanical knowledge in agricultural setting

The wellbeing of the people depends on agriculture as a major source of economic activities: often entire communities cultivate individual *conucos* (fields) for self-consumption, while the production of cash crops such as tobacco is a main source of income.[217] The cultural history and interviews in the visited regions yield that tobacco has been an im-

217 At the small-scale fields different crops can be found: tubers (batata, ñame, papa, yucca, yautía), cereals (rice, corn), oleaginous (maní, coco), vegetables, fruits (plantain, guineo, piña, mango, citrics, avocado).

portant cash crop contributing to local economies in different locations in the Dominican Republic and Cuba (see the previous chapter). The example of tobacco illustrates how the traditional ecological knowledge is displayed in a whole set of cultural practices.

Some communities that have sold tobacco as an income source also appreciate tobacco's medicinal properties and spiritual character. Tobacco juice has an emetic effect, used for indigestion, food poisoning, and stomach aches. Tobacco leaves are placed on the forehead to help overcome headaches. During the consultation with a healer, tobacco smoke is the medium for making divine entities descend onto the head of the healer. Tobacco smoke also induces transformations during which a *lwa* (deified being) incarnates into the body of a healer to provide advice and remedies for the patient. The same plant is also a favorite offering for different 'divisions' in Dominican 21 Division, including the water division of indigenous ancestors, Belies, *Ogunes*, or *Petroses*.[218]

The cultivation of the tobacco is also indicative of the cultural diffusion of botanical knowledge and associated traditions, and of how communities are constructed through shared experiences and practices. One tradition, related to the cultivation of tobacco (and other crops), is known as a *junta*. The *junta*, or *combité* (gathering, from Spanish *convite*), was a form of voluntary cooperation between neighbors and family members to help each other with the work on the *conuco* (field), or with other types of collective work like building a house or road. One of the Dominican contributors, Mr. Álvarez from Loma Atravesada remembered how he was harvesting tobacco in a *junta* in the past: people were called together in the first agricultural phase for clearing the fields as well as in the last phase for the collection of the harvest.[219] The collective activities included clearing a new patch of land in order to make a *conuco,* using the slash and burn tradition, felling trees, and sewing plants. The whole community (inhabitants of the village) participated in collecting tobacco: a group exceeding over one hundred people collectively worked on the field.[220] The group sang, ate, and drank together; the refreshments were typically prepared by the family of the owner of the land. The person who received this help from the community would in return give support to the other

218 Indigenous ancestors are part of the Indian Division, which is one of other categories of *lwas* including belies, ogunes, petroses in Dominican Vúdu. Belíe Belcán/San Miguel is the master of the belies. Belíe Belcán is the popular patron of the Dominican healers and is fighting against injustice and black magic. Petroses are earth *lwas*, controlling the world of deaths like the Barón del cementerio, or controlling men as Santa Marta la Dominadora. The master of the division of ogunes is Ogún Balendjo/San Santiago, who is a symbol of a fight. For more details on these *characters* in the Dominican 21 Division see the study of Tejeda Ortiz (2013), which also explains the differences between Haitian Vodou and Dominican 21 Division.

219 In spite of the official prohibitions, the old vegetation (old grass, bush, hollow trees) but sometimes also parts of forests are frequently cleared and burned in order to establish a new field for cultivation. Sometimes, the wood would be used for charcoal (e.g. invasive species such as cambron/bayahonda/ *Prosopis juliflora (Sw.)*) or for fences, but often just burnt. In general, people are aware that these activities are illegal. In their campaign against deforestation, the governmental representatives have referred to this custom as 'slash and burn', which according to them is an aboriginal custom. However, the unsustainable burning of the vegetation and indiscriminate cutting down of the forest have antecedents in colonial history, especially in regions that in the past profited from cattle raising, timber extraction, sugar industry and exploitation of charcoal.

220 Mr. Álvarez from Loma Atravesada explained: *"De antes usted hacia una cosecha grande de cien cerrones de tabaco y no gastaba más que la comida, porque del lugar entero venían y recogían tabacco, y si hacia una junta con hacha para tumbar un conuco, se le juntaban hasta cien personas pero ahora no si usted hace la junta usted va y su mujer para cocinar pero ya no más nadie. Ya el amor va cayendo, ya el amor murió."*

community members when they needed it. Mr. Álvarez perceived this system as a way of increasing social solidarity.

According to testimonies of different contributors, the *juntas* varied in size. Sometimes people would not only receive a meal, but if the harvest was very successful, a feast would be organized or the invited workers would be rewarded with a small portion of the harvest. Dominican and Cuban *juntas* seem to be preserved now only in memory.

Junta was a matter of manual work.[221] The cultivation of fields (of any type) was frequently accompanied by music. Tools such as axes, hoes, and pestles were used as musical instruments whose beats were integral parts of a song. A leading singer/worker at the head of the group was followed by the rest of the group, repeating only the refrain, which often consisted of improvised words. The rhythm of the music indicated the pace of work. The lyrics of the oral poetry were often improvised but common themes included labor, love and some of them were called after the tool used for the work (*e.g.* hoe or axe). Mr. Alvarez from Chacuey sang a song for an axe, wherein strikes of ax were incorporated into the melody and functioned as well as a technique to help the group of workers synchronize their work.[222] Songs also accompanied other daily activities such as washing, weaving, grinding (*e.g.* coffee, cacao), or nightly gatherings. Topics of these songs include love, refusal, disaffection, social critiques, or counterpoints between the singers.[223]

Another tradition related to the cultivation of tobacco (and other crops) was the regulation of plant cultivation according to the lunar calendar. The lunar cycle is not only important for the cultivation of tobacco but is also considered for planning different agricultural activities. Julián de La Rosa from Boca de Mana explained that the moon *"is related to all living beings"*. The new moon is associated with infertility and during this period it has to be respected and the harvest is not collected. Instead, weeding is planned. Similarly, during the new moon, wood is considered to be more fragile and more likely to be attacked by *comején* (termites) and therefore not used for the construction of houses or other structures.[224] The full moon is a period favorable for sowing and for collecting some medicinal plants.[225]

---

221 Some Dominican respondents suggested that there was also a gender specific task specialization in the fields. Mr. Gómez from Bánica described this division of tasks. For example, in the period of maní men tore the plants, and made packages of it, while women beat it and collected the harvest. The beans were collected by men, after it was beaten and women sort it out. In other regions, the women would come to do minor tasks like weeding, or come to cook.

222 These refrain of this song for the axe was: "*Wo wo wo caramba wo wo oigame mi hermano wo wo yo los invitaba wo wo paque piquemos con mi hermano*".

223 One of the décimas mentioned in both regions of the study was the following: *"El carpintero cenizo se le murió su mujer, Y era tanto su querer que de madera la hizo, La metió en un paraíso y ella cuernos le pegó, Y por eso digo yo que ni de palo la mujer es buena.* The reference to carpenter (both person and bird), who has made from the wood his wife resembles Pané's reference to the origin of women, who are said to have been carved from a tree by a carpenter bird. However, the current main message of this song is rather about female ingratitude in general.

224 According to *Diccionario de la lengua española* (*DLE*): comején from the Arawakan *comixén.*

225 More oral poetry includes the theme of the moon. Mr. Alvarez from Loma Atravesada cited the poem: *"El sol le dijo a la luna que se fuera recoger que sola de la noche no anda ninguna mujer, y la luna le contesta con toditos su primores que es mejor andar de noche y no al día con el sol."* The storyline of ...

Present-day agricultural activities are guided by the lunar calendar, which is integrated in the European liturgical calendar that is used to organize Caribbean patronal celebrations and other ritual activities. The official Catholic liturgical calendar marks the time for celebrating Catholic Saints but also other associated divine beings and spiritual entities. The divine beings have powers to influence the wellbeing of communities by means of their influence on harvesting, and on the breeding of animals. Processions in time of droughts, insect plagues, hurricanes, as well as periodical celebrations of patronal Saints often aim at communal wellbeing. Boyá has one of the patronal celebrations that illustrate the divine influence on the harvest. This particular case demonstrates that sometimes the patronal celebrations are interwoven with the memory of the indigenous past.

Prayers for rainfall in Boyá

Since the second half of the seventeenth century inhabitants Boyá cherished their patronal Virgen of the Holy Waters. Like other patronal Saints, this Virgin looks after the (spritual) wellbeing of inhabitants of Boyá and her devotees from surrounding settlements. Among the miracles that this Virgin has performed is due to her power to regulate the rain. This happens periodically at the occasion of her patronal celebration on the 15th of August. Before describing this celebration and the meaning of the Virgin for inhabitants of Boyá, let me briefly summarize oral history about her appearance.

According to oral tradition, the Virgen de las Aguas Santas appeared in an orange tree to a group of hunters (of lost cattle) in the early 16th century. The miracle led to the establishment of the church, which is said to have been built by Spaniards and indigenous people. Some argue that the miraculous appearance of the Virgin was followed by another miracle, which made the church appear overnight.[226]

The Saint's day mass is preceded by nine days of mass. The celebration culminates on the last day with the arrival of devotees from nearby and from more remote areas, like the brotherhood of Jezus from Bayaguana. After Mass is celebrated and children are collectively baptized the respected members of the congregation carry the Virgin on their shoulders out of the church to conduct the procession through the whole village along with the rhythm of drums and *güiras*.

According to devotees, the procession is ended by the rain sent by the Virgin.

The Virgen regulates rain: she sends rain as a blessing during droughts and protects devotees during hurricanes. When people from a neighboring settlement (now nearly abandoned) were troubled by severe rains, which caused floods and isolated them from the outside world, they prayed for the help of the Virgen de las Aguas Santas and made

...another narrative about the moon tells that one day Moon and Sun had a fight during which the moon took the eye from the sun and that is why no one of them has two eyes. There were more beliefs related to the moon. One of them is that Moon has cold, which is especially dangerous for pregnant women because it can hurt a baby or leave a "lunar", birthmark on their skin.

226 The miraculous character of the Virgin's shrine is perceived in various signs today. These include the beehive in the church, a part of the orange tree trunk, presumably from the orange tree in which the Virgin appeared, hidden behind the altar, and the watermarks left on the walls of the church after the rain, all together reinforcing the extraordinary powerful character of this place and its patron.

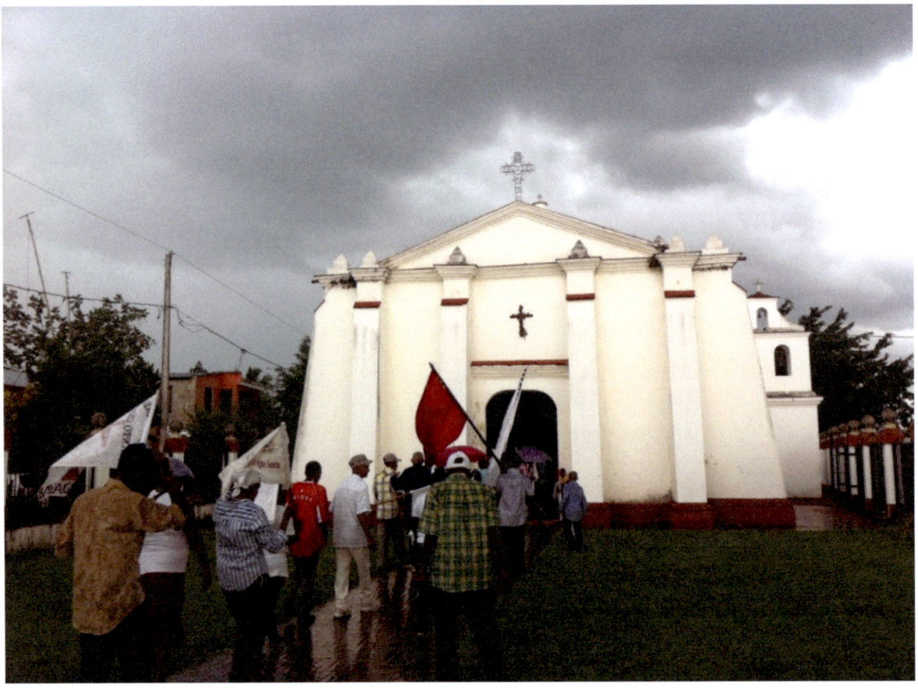

Figure 18 The Celebration of the Virgin of the Holy Waters in Boyá, Dominican Republic.

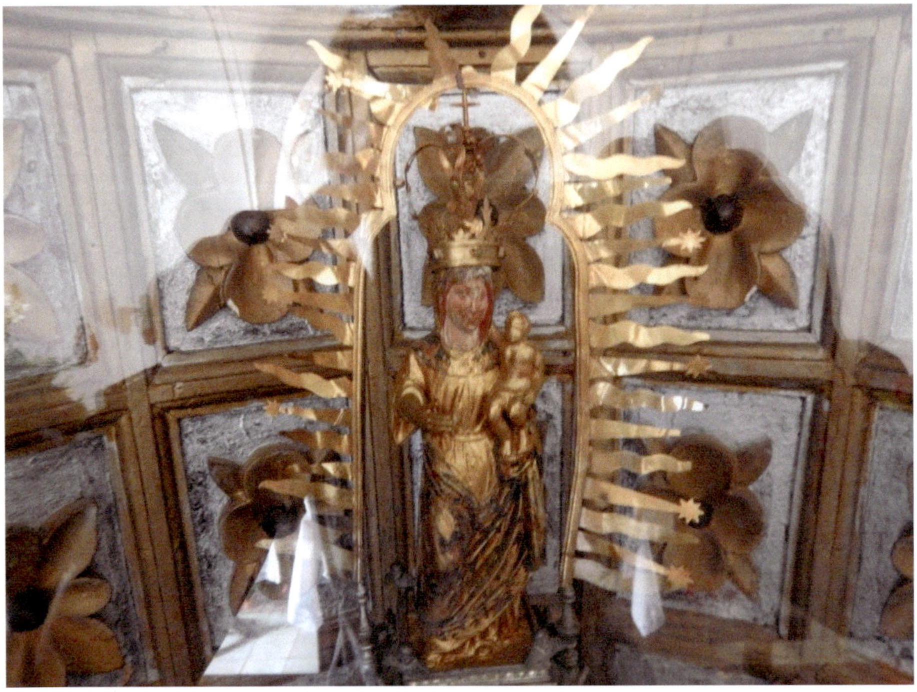

Figure 19 The Virgin of The Holy Waters in Boyá, Dominican Republic.

a vow, which resulted in the commitment to bring her a calf as an offering every year. The offerings were brought for many years until the settlement was depopulated.

The link between the Virgin and water symbolism is also expressed in a song dedicated to her. During the procession, devotees sing: *"The indigenous lady comes, the indigenous lady goes, the indigenous lady lives under the water."* As in the case of other liturgical hymns, this song is sung by the whole crowd of devotees walking in the procession, publicly displaying their faith. The lyrics of this plena (special musical genre) are similar to those of a text recited during the Saint John celebration in the cave in Mancha (see chapter 9).[227] The same hymn is sung once more when the procession is completed. After singing the official hymn some of the Boyá devotees stay and sing the hymn addressing the Virgin as "indigenous lady".

The explanation for this song was given by Mrs. María Mejía, the main singer during the procession. According to her, she and the other participants in the procession sing this song *"because the Virgin is Indian,"* and she adds: *"as the church has appeared there, and was built by the Spaniards and the Indians, we have this song (*repeats the lyrics*), and because Indians live under the water".* Her sister, Dorotea Mejía, adds: *"She (*could be referring to either the Virgin or the Indian woman*) lives under the water and when she submerges, she returns under the water. Because she was not on the earth, she was living under the water, when she is raised to sing she sang and returned and submerged again, because they had a house under the water. Because there was a mine that the old people were saying that could never be demolished and in the period of Trujillo they made a road there and they destroyed it."*[228] To clarify, in Boyá the river and especially deep water-pools are considered dwellings of indigenous ancestors, and are potentially dangerous places, being symbolic for both life and afterlife. Indigenous ancestors are also sometimes observed at archaeological places or places related to their history. As the next chapter on healing as a subaquatic journey to ancestors will explain, the underwater world and afterlife are returning topics in the Dominican belief systems.

The celebration of the Virgin of Boyá is an event that reinforces the relationships between the Virgin and the community. The community publicly displays its devotion through attendance and through fulfilling its vows. The patronal celebration in Boyá fits into the broader acceptance of devotees in agricultural settings praying for a successful harvest and rain during mass. If problems affecting the harvest persist, petitionary processions are organized with patronal Saints, during which the Saints' images are carried on the shoulders and hymns are sung. San Isidro, as the protector of the farmers, the Virgin Mary or the Holy Cross are often invoked in matters of agricultural wellbeing. San Isidro was celebrated also in Boyá. Celebrations for San Isidro

227 This song is not the official hymn. The latter was composed by a nun called Maria Bautista who came to the village in 1998. *The lyrics are: Viva la virgen de aguas santas que en el nuestro pueblo tiene altar y que vive siempre infante cristo en este pueblo noble y leal siempre seremos su fieles hijos nuestra patrona siempre será y con tu ayuda madre querida derrotaremos a satana. Hoy que venimos con frescas flores para ponerlas sobre tu altar son tanto tanto nuestros dolores que no podemos flores cortar son tanto tanto nuestros dolores que no podemos flores cortar. Siempre seremos tu fieles hijos nuestra patrona siempre será y con tu ayuda nuestra señora derrotaremos a satana. Viva la virgen todos nos vamos madre querida y te dejamos en el corazón. Y recompensa solo esperamos que nos días tu madre tu bendición. Viva a la virgen de agua santa que en nuestro pueblo tiene altar. Son tanto y tanto nuestros dolores que no podemos flores cortar.*

228 Interview with Dorotea Mejía. The phrase *"se consumía entre el agua"* was translated as: submerge. The mine refers to a real old earth mine where other indigenous people (their spirits) have been seen.

were shorter, typically lasting for only four days. Until now, the life-size statue of San Isidro is found in the left corner of the Boyá church. His meaning for the community was further explained: "*San Isidro is a Saint of farmers, those who work on the land and you say 'San Isidro, the Farmer, remove the water, and bring the sun'. One day there were droughts and well we went to bring him to Arizao* (river), *(and we said) let's wash him and see if it is going to rain, and, Oh Lord, it started to get cloudy, and it was huge, it was a long time that we did not see such a strong rain. And this San Isidro had in one hand a coa and in another a hoe.*"[229] San Isidro as protector of the farmer is a popular saint in many other Dominican and Cuban locations as well. The Boyá image of San Isidro holding a *coa*, known in Boyá as an indigenous instrument for the cultivation of *conucos*. Similarly to the custom of Boyá, at other locations (provinces Puerto Plata, Monte Christi) patronal saints and virgins have been taken in procession to the river during droughts. Also in Cuba, Virgins and Saints have been taken out of the church and carried around in processions in order to ask for rain, and generally it is said that it started to rain before the procession was completed.[230] Besides being invoked in collective prayers, rains have been asked for or detained by individuals.[231]

During a year of drought, rain was prayed for at various locations; many people remembered its destructive power from the preceding years. There are different ways how to protect a harvest from the rain. Spiritual protection can be secured by the prayer of a specialist. Such a specialist, called Water Binder (*Amarrador del Agua*), has a gift or knows a special secret prayer to stop or remove the threat of rain.[232] Likewise, the fruits from trees can be protected from heavy rains by tying stones to their branches with white or red scarfs.[233] Houses may be protected from thunder by blessed *guano* leaves or other herbs, which are collected on Good Friday. Different herbs (*e.g.* leaves of mango, guanábana, piñón) would be collected early in the morning, without speaking

---

229 Interview no. 184.

230 See for details for example interview with Mrs Hernandez from Jiguaní or Mr. Mendoza from Guao next to Jiguaní. The latter narrates about the Spiritist called Buteca: *"Jiguaní was an indigenous settlement and some Bayamo peoples came here and said that here Jiguaní is the river of gold, and this river pass there, and it was gold river, and sometimes it gets angry (gets dangerous, se pone bravo) and it took many peoples away, this caused that in Jiguaní many things happened and among them was this gentleman. This gentleman lived there in (inteligble) I forgot his name, his nickname was Buteca, and it was a extraordinary person, he believed in spirits, and in Spiritism, his custom was to organize a reunion of adherents of Spiritism and give blessings (santiguaban) and everything. When it was not raining in the whole region he got this character to organize processions passing through the village and when the procession was done it started to rain. It is not known what it was that he had."*

231 Mrs. Candida Dominga Olivo, an agriculturalist from Jaiquí (prov. Monte Cristi) narrated how she prayed for rain: *"when I saw my harvest sad, I would enter in the middle of the harvest, open the arms and say: Gran Poder de Dios, don't let me lose the harvest, and I was believing a lot in this because, look, doing like this, opening my arms watching my harvest nearly lost, it was raining and my harvest did not vanish. I have had every time a good harvest."* Mrs. Olivo also warned that when praying, money should never be offered. She explained that: *"Once after coming from the field I was relaxing and told to Ana Luisa: don't hurry and it will rain soon. I bought water for 50 cent (*she laughs briefly*) and I was relaxed. Listen, that night felt a flood, and it destroyed the wells and everything, so she was angry with me and says: for what reason did you pay without a shame. I say: Ana Luisa, what do you think, if I bought water it was not even for a penny (chele), but there were many people who bought for fifty."* (Interview with Mrs. Olivo from Jaiquí).

232 Interview with Mr. Felipe Ortiz from Naranjo, Boyá.

233 The symbolism of the red and white scarf will be further discussed in relation to the protection of the crops against the evil eye. In general, red ribbons are used until now in Spain against evil eye. Red stands also often for Santa Barbara/Chango, who is the owner of the thunder.

to anyone. These herbs are successively kept in the house in order to protect it or they are dried and burned to drive the storm away with smoke.[234]

Offerings to the Earth

The wellbeing of the communities in rural areas is conditioned by a good harvest, which depends on nurturing the soil. Some contributors indicated that the care should be mutual. A conversation with Mr. Juan Pablo Rosario Araujó in Boca de Mana after the event of San Juan (see later) clarified with respect to food offerings to the earth that if a grain, yucca, batata or other crops accidentaly fell on the ground it is wise to leave it there because the earth asked for it. Familiar with the Dominican 21 Division, he did not believe that earth is or has a *lwa*, but was certain that the earth has to eat and that by nurturing her we induce her to nurture us. In another location, in Jaiquí, Dominga Olivo too remembered how people *"after the vela (*informal mass*) for a Saint obtained peanuts, and morro (*a dish made of rice and beans*). But people weren't eating it, it was without salt, they were taking it and giving it to the field. They were spraying it (throw the offering) in order it would give a good harvest."* To whom exactly the offerings were dedicated was not clear to this contributor because offerings were made individually without discussing it with others.

In other Dominican locations, Bánica and Pedro Santana, the earth was considered to be the domain of indigenous ancestors. Mr. Juan Abraham Rosario Jiménez explained that people of Bánica and Pedro Santana were offering the first fruits of the harvest. Corn, bread, peanuts, and beans were offered to fields, small streams, or other places. In more detail: *"Well, before, there were some people, not some, a large majority, all, who went to offer the harvest to an Indian, so when the harvest was before consuming, if it was a rice or whatever, the first meal was prepared for the neighbors, but before eating it, the first (portion) was thrown to the river in the ravine."* The first half of the offering was said to be given because of a previous commitment the person had made, while the second half was given in order to assure a positive relationship for the rest of the year. This can be done in every harvest. In Mr. Rosario's view, the earth has power and it has a (spiritual) ruler: the King of the Earth (*El Rey de la Tierra*). According to him, the status of this ruler is expressed in his name: the King of the Earth is more powerful than indigenous ancestors. He clarified that besides the King of the Earth, there is the King of the Wind, the King of the Water. He added that *"nearly everything has a king because it is as a bee that would disappear without a queen"*.[235] This is in accordance with the teaching of the 21 Division that every division has its own Master (*Jefe*).

In Cuba, Mrs. Celida Hernández Reyes, the oldest inhabitant of Jiguaní, also recalled the food offerings to the earth as an expression of gratitude for a successful harvest.[236] Mrs. Hernández recalled that after a harvest was collected and sold, people organized from the money a celebration that in itself was an offering. For this celebration, they would prepare specific meals and invite their friends and believers. To cite her own words:

---

234 The weather is to be prognosticated on the basis of general observations of the moon, wind, behavior of the animals or cabañuelas. The latter is a Spanish belief that the weather on the first twelve days of the year is indicative for the weather of the twelve months of the whole year.

235 Also others have mentioned the *Rey de la Tierra*. Altagracia Vargas says that Caonabo and Rey de la Tierra are brothers.

236 Interview no. 140726.

"*The aim of this was to show respect.*" In other locations, sharing the first crops from a harvest between neighbors by offering a small feast was also part of the collective work in a *junta*. For example, in Jiguaní the harvest was shared with the beings from the invisible world. Mrs. Hernández explained that some people from Jiguaní also brought food offerings to the field: *"A dish was prepared, which was later offered in the place where you cultivated your harvest, they have served it on plates, not old broken ones, but on plates, you put it in the corner of the place where you planted and there you left it and dedicate it to whom they were offering it…they did not say to whom, they were saying it for themselves and dedicate to whom it was."* Also, this contributor was not sure to whom the offerings were dedicated, but she suggested that *"they were not spirits but Saints"*.

One of the inhabitants from Chorro de Maíta in Cuba, Mr. Juan Gutiérrez recalled that in the past it was common to prepare offerings to the earth. Without much talking to anyone, the grandfathers and grandmothers put ñame, boniato, malanga in a basket (*jabita*), buried it in the ground while saying their prayers.[237] This contributor explained that it was a custom in the past when the harvest was still huge; now that the harvest is poor there is nothing to offer. Sometimes the appreciation for gifts received from the earth would not be communally driven but rather a matter of individuals expressing their personal gratitude. One Cuban contributor of Haitian origin said that one day she just went to do it because she felt it was a correct occasion: "*One day I gave the food to the earth, in a hole I put congrí and meat, and I dedicated some words. This is the reason I do not lack food, I gave it to the earth.*"[238]

The food offerings are one of the means to secure the balance between the invisible world and the visible world, which affects the wellbeing of rural communities. Other customs aim at protecting the fields and crops. One of these was restricting the entrance of women during their period to these fields.[239] Another widespread traditional practice is to protect one's crops against the evil eye, plant pests, for example: a specialist is called upon to combat these pests with secret prayers. In Jiguaní the remedies for plagues include tying up three points of a yucca plant.

Dominican fields are sometimes protected by beings called *bakás*. Bakás are mostly described as mostly taking the appearance of a domestic animal with supernatural powers. Their status varies from having intentions to protect one's property against evils, thieves, or other misfortunes to trespassing the accepted moral rules when doing so. Their agency is used to explain the quick enrichment of a person. Especially where there are animosity and resentment among neighbors some persons can be accused of having *baká*. Baká has been in views of a large part of contributors believed as rather harmful being that be obtained through a pact with evil or at least because of black magic. Multiple other rituals for protection of fields can be mentioned, but for now, it is clear that the harvest is the center of attention for wellbeing in rural communities.

237 Interview no. 144748.

238 Interview no. 140726.

239 In different Dominican locations it is believed that the characteristics of women would transfer to those crops. Mrs. Elia Torres from Villa Isabela explained that, although she does not personally believe it on the basis of her own experience, it has been said that: *"si uno se marchita las matas se marchitan, los plátanos no sé qué problema es el que tienen que los plátanos se dañan las cebollas, ajos, etc. se pudren."*

The indigenous heritage in the traditional ecological knowledge

This chapter was an introduction into ecological knowledge as displayed in foodways, crafts, house building, and agricultural activities. This ecological knowledge inherited from different generations and from diverse cultural backgrounds is being reactivated while dwelling in a particular environmental setting. The interpretation of traditional ecological knowledge in terms of indigenous cultural continuity remains a highly speculative and challenging endeavor in the Greater Antilles without definitive conclusions. The first step in the voyage of deciphering the history of traditional ecological knowledge within this domain is to review historical and ethnographic parallels.

The present-day foodways illustrate how the contemporary inhabitants connect to their ancestors. Paleo-/archeo-botanical research (Rodríguez Suárez & Pagán Jiménez 2006, 2008; Pagán Jiménez 2002, 2007; Pagán Jiménez & Oliver 2008; Newsom 2008) has confirmed the early colonial descriptions and suggests that some crops such as cotton, maize, beans (Fabaceae fam., *Phaseolus vulgaris*), higüera, guácima, jobo, ñame, maní/cacaguate, batatas/boniato, yautía/malanga, maví were already cultivated centuries and sometimes millennia prior to the European colonization.[240]

When compared to the Fernandéz de Oviedo´s description (2002 [1535]) the present-day use of native crops such as yucca displays certain continuities in ways of preparation, utensils included in its preparation and associated vocabulary (*burén, sibucán, jibe, naiboa*). The utensils for its preparation may have been slightly modified in the early stage of the colonial period, when Las Casas (2002[1527-1566]) mentions that "*prensillas de husillo*" were used. Similarly, a detailed comparison of contemporary consumption of guáyiga with archaeological evidence and historical sources (Rodríguez Suárez & Pagán Jiménez 2008; Pagán Jiménez 2016) offers a promising avenue for further research.

The distribution of crops like yucca and corn reflects the paths of the colonial voyages. Both crops were introduced in 16th century Africa. In the 1550s, cassava became a provision for the Portuguese ships bringing West African captives to the Americas. Corn cultivation was already well established in the Cape Verde islands by the 1540s (McCann 2001). At present, corn is used for dishes carrying New World indigenous names such as *guanimos, pinol,* or *tamales* but also *gofio* that have parallels in the Islas Canarias by the 1820s (Alonso de Herrera 1818, p. 210), and others like *chenchén, chaká* that are most likely related to the early incorporation of corn in the diet of enslaved people.

Other important crops like plantains in turn reveal the ancestral influences from Africa. Plantains (Musa paradiasaca, guineo Musa sapientum) were introduced to the Caribbean during the early colonial period and are components of various popular dishes: Dominican *mangú* (also *mofongo*), and Cuban *fufu* (mashed green plantains with yucca) seem to have a parallel in the West African dish called *fufu.* Similarly, yams, a

240 Among the plants that have been identified in the Caribbean archaeological records are: Spondias sp, Annona sp., Cresentia sp., Bixa Orellana, Hymenaea courbil, Inga sp., Piscida sp., Persea Americana, Malphigia sp., wild cherry, cotton, guayaba (Psidium guajava), Acrocomia media (corozo), Colubrina sp., Genipa Americana, Zanthoxylum sp. Chrysophyllum sp., Manilkara sp. Or Sieroxylon sp., Pouteria sp., Melicoccus bijugatus quenepa, Guazuma ulmifolia, Sterculia sp., Siphonoglossa (health care), Trianthema sp., Xanthosoma sp., Canna sp., Zamia sp., Arachas hypogaea, Phaseolus sp., Calanthea sp., Marantha sp., Oenothera sp., Setaria spp., Capsicum sp., Passieflora sp. (Newsom 2008).

common source of food on Portuguese ships, according to De Oviedo (Oviedo 2002 [1535]) were introduced with enslaved peoples from the African continent and formed an important part of their diet on the island since the early colonial period.

Like the inhabitants of the Old World, those of the New World integrated exotic crops into the local diet without anyone questioning their origin. The contemporary foodways display an integration of both native and exotic crops, combining those as dishes or products created or marked by a long process of transculturation.

A similar process of fusion of skills and ecological knowledge may be observed in crafts displayed in housing areas. Many aforementioned plants used in housing area have been described for their utility by different historical sources. Precious wood, like roble, *caoba*, mahogany, gained European attention from the beginning (Oviedo 2002 [1478-1557]).[241] Fruits of *higüeros* were used as vessels, plates and cups among indigenous peoples (Oviedo 2002 [1478-1557]). The know-how of preparing rope from the agave plant, for example, was documented by Oviedo (2002 [1478-1557]) and later among the Kalinago (Taylor 1948). Nowadays this technique is still known and used among the population of Cuba and the Dominican Republic (*e.g.* in Fray Benito and Boyá). Palm varieties were used for house construction (*cana, yarey* and *guano),* for furniture (*yagua)*, and basketry (Sánchez Valverde 1785 in Deive 2002). Other plants like sábila and peonía are of exotic origin (Acevedo-Rodríguez & Strong 2012) and possibly link present-day inhabitants with the African ancestry.

Basketry was in the past supposed to be an indigenous legacy. Several designs (*e.g.* Fig. 86) are similar to those found on the island of Dominica but others remind us of contemporary Spanish basketry. In Jiguaní, for example, the basketry has a long tradition and is a source of income of various Jiguaniceros until the present. Some of the employed vocabulary as *jaba* (a type of basket) seems to come from an indigenous language (*haba*). Magüey, bark of bixao (possibly bixa) were used as materials for indigenous basketry (Oviedo (2002 [1478-1557]). However, generalizations proceeding from the design or the type of material used may lead to hasty and unwarranted conclusions. In order to assess any continuities from pre-colonial times, more studies are needed to map the situation on both islands, taking into account as well the possible influences of ancestors of various backgrounds including those from Caribbean (Taylor & Moore 1948), Europe (cf. Moreno 1998 on Canarian basketry) and Africa (Rosengarten 2013).[242]

Another plant that connects the present-day Cuban and Dominican populations to their indigenous predecessors is the tobacco. Because of its importance in economic and religious life, there will be more comments on tobacco in the following chapters in order to analyse its multiple meanings from a historical perspective. Here I will just

241 Fernández de Oviedo wrote about roble and *caoba* used for furniture in the major church of Santo Domingo, which were so beautiful that they should be shipped to Spain. *Caoba* was also used in *trapiches* for the wheels and building material.

242 In Cuba the following plants were used as material for basketry making: *Trichostigma octandrum L. Arundo donax L., Paullinia fuscenscens, Clusia rosea, Saccarum officinarum L., Oryza sativa L., Zea mays, Stercuia apetal, Panicum maximum L., Acrocomia armentalis* (Moreno 1998). And in Dominica: *Gynerium saccharoides, Stigmatophyllum puberum, Merecuja sp., Thrinax sp., Bamboo, Heliconia bihai and H.*

make a short remark about some of the customs associated with its cultivation such as the work in *junta* and the use of the lunar calendar.

Similar patterns of labor exchange to *la junta* have been practiced among the peasants in other Caribbean islands as well as throughout Mesoamerica and the Andean region. In Haiti this custom is known as *combité* (personal communication Sony Jean 2016), in Dominica and St. Lucia as *koudeman*, from *coup de main* (Stancioff 2018). Barrow (1992) has argued that it has African antecedents.

The lunar calendar was used in European, West African and Caribbean agriculture. When cultivating (*e.g.* corn) indigenous peoples of Hispaniola took into account the moon. The sowing was done after the new moon until the full moon, but never when the moon is waning, because as the moon wanes also the crops (Oviedo 2002 [1478-1557]). When describing the caoba Oviedo indicates that this should be felled when the moon is waning. The same reasoning about that the fertility of the garden or field is influenced by the waxing moon is to be found among Dominican agriculturalist and was also registered among Kalinago (Layng 1983). There are numerous parallels for this in other parts of the Americas as well.

Pané´s and Breton's accounts demonstrate that the moon had a great symbolic importance in the indigenous worldviews. The cavern from which the sun and moon came forward was very much respected among indigenous ancestors in Hispaniola (Pané 2011 [1498]). Similarly, the Wayuú identify a cavern as the site of origin of the Sun, the Moon, and the first Wayuús. Among the Kalinago the Moon was the father of Hiali, the first forefather of the Kalinago nation. Again, the coincidence in the worldviews as to the importance of the moon for the agricultural cycle could create a point of encounter where indigenous thought merged with European and West African beliefs.

The same can be said about the concern to secure the source of the peasants' lives. Spaniards have been praying too to the Virgin of Holy Waters or San Isidro for centuries, asking them to regulate the weather conditions. Chapter 10 will analyze into more detail the connections and associations of the Virgin of the Holy Waters and her sanctuary with the indigenous ancestors.

The custom of sharing the fruits with the Earth and associated diving beings (King of the Earth) or spirits residing in the landscape expresses the common preoccupation of agriculturalists around the world with the outcome of their harvest. This study registered such customs in settlements or regions with long-term presence of indigenous descendants. Corn, yucca, batata, maní, beans, but also other meals (rice & beans) are offered to the earth in Boca de Mana, Jiguaní and Chorro de Maita or brought to the river or ravine in Bánica. Among the offerings there are native but also exotic crops. As this custom is common among indigenous peoples elsewhere in the Americas, one might consider it to have an immediate indigenous origin. In British Guyana, for example, before cassava-roots are going to be harvested, a drink is brewed out of the first batch and left on the field as an offering (De Goeje 1943). A libation is a common tradition in many West African religions.

In Boca de Mana these offerings are brought to the Earth, in Jaiquí to the field (after a *vela* to a Saint whose name is omitted), in Jiguaní to Saints, in Bánica to the Indigenous Ancestors and to the King of the Earth. In accordance with the teaching of the 21 Division every division has its own Master (*jefe*) and the Earth has its own King. These are literal translations of names of certain West Central African deities that are called Kings of specific domains (Macgaffey 2009; Herskovits & Herskovits 1933). Similarly, we find in Mesoamerican and South American contexts indigenous beliefs in divine beings called the Master, Owner, Lord or Lady, King or God identified with a specific domain. An example is the Mixtec *Iha Sau*, "Lord Rain", whose name is generally translated as the "God *of* Rain" (cf. Posselt Santoyo & Jiménez Osorio 2015). We should be aware that translations may have been influenced by Western epistemologies so that some details of the indigenous or West African worldviews are lost in the process.

The gratitude for a successful harvest would be expressed in offering a celebration on one's own costs to the neighbors, or those who have help carry out different tasks. This custom was found across different religions and seems to be related to the junta tradition, which was so widespread in the past. Cuban Regla de Ocha devotees present offerings to Ilé Ógéré, an *orisha* (spirit) representing the earth (Edmonds & Gonzalez 2010). The sacred biography of this *orisha* suggests that humans should give the earth an offering of fruits, just like the earth has given her fruits to them. Humans should show gratitude for the favor and affections that the earth gives them by producing materials that are used in daily life. Ilé nurtures people and after their death they nurture her with their bodies, which the earth has maintained for so many years.

Parallels to Dominican and Cuban earth offerings are found in Haitian customs. Before the rice was gathered from the fields in the Haitian part of the Aitibonito valley a small part was shared with the friends who helped during the cultivation family, with the unknown ancestors, with the Haitian and African dead, and furthermore the dead twins, albinos, and other deceased persons, for example those who drowned or were lost at sea (Herskovits 1937). Similarly, the corncobs of the first maize harvest would be offered to Jesus Christ, the Saints, the Twins, and the Dead by throwing them to the four cardinal directions (Herskovits 1937). Analogous harvest festivals for yams or rice have been celebrated throughout West Africa, *e.g.* by the Ashanti in Ghana (Herskovits 1937).

Epistemological and ontological overlaps may mask how divine and spiritual beings were originally honored or how their symbolism fused with belief systems introduced from elsewhere. Instead of devaluating these traditions as superstitions or foreign intromissions, we should take their long-term existence as an invitation to reflect upon the centrality of the ecological knowledge in the wellbeing of communities in rural areas around the world. This is also true for protective figures like Water Binder or for the religious specialists combating plants' pests, which have been documented in the Americas as well as in Spain (Christian 1989). *Bakás* (described as phantasms) are said to have correspondences with *bakru*, which might derive from the West African beliefs about little folk (Herskovits 1937). Courlander (1960) suggested that there is a possible link between them and the Congo-Guinée deity Bakulu Baka, or Bakaku Baka, who can devour persons, and who like the Haitian Baká sometimes live in the *mapou* tree. Customs aiming at protecting the fields and crops, for example by prescribing that women during their period should not enter the fields, have their parallels among the Kaliña (Artist 2016). The blessed *guano* leaves as protection of homes from thunder may equally be derived from the symbolism of the palm in Catholic beliefs, as from similar meanings in pre-colonial Caribbean religion (cf. the *mauriti* palm described by de Goeje 1943) or in Regla de Ocha and other Afro-Caribbean beliefs.[243]

These examples illustrate the complexity of the historical analysis of Dominican and Cuban traditional ecological knowledge. It cannot be overemphasized that indigenous heritage should not be seen as more traditional, rural or "primitive" than the European or African. Certain aspects of contemporary ecological knowledge clearly contain elements of ancient indigenous knowledge. On the other hand, it is clear that this traditional ecological knowledge is a composite of beliefs and observations that combine the pre-colonial legacy with elements introduced from Europe and Africa during the colonial period. It is telling that specific origins of contemporary ideas and practices often cannot be established. The syncretism has been intense: different ontologies have been merged to reinforce each other, forming a new unit, a true synergy of knowledge and symbolism from different cultural backgrounds.

Concluding remarks

This chapter revealed how ecological knowledge is central to the wellbeing of communities in rural areas. Furthermore, it illustrated how for the people the economic significance of flora, and in turn the communal wellbeing, cannot be separated from religious convictions. Regardless of the origin of these beliefs the present-day ecological knowledge is a testimony of how diverse Caribbean ancestors were able to adapt to the changing landscapes. The subsequent chapter will describe some facets of this ecological knowledge as employed in healing practices. Concretely, after presenting the general features of animated landscapes in the Dominican Republic and Cuba, it will introduce some etiologies and describe in general lines the roles of Dominican healers, and their interaction with medicinal plants before these are used as a remedy. All these daily activities take place in a landscape that is animated by forces that may influence the health and wellbeing of individuals and entire communities.

243 Another example is that of the protective power of thunderstones, which can be traced to West Africa but is equally present among the Kaliña of Suriname (Pernard 1907).

7

Healing in sacred and animated landscapes

The health of peoples living in agricultural settings depends on the ecological knowledge that they use in daily practices. For believers, health is influenced by divine agencies and spiritual entities, which can manifest their healing powers through different features of the surrounding natural environment including the embodiment of diverse spirits, *lwas*, *misterios*, spirits or *orishas* in the healers (be they mediums, *babalawo*, or *caballo del misterio*), through the illness but also healing virtues of plants, places and other landscape features. Different religious systems in Cuba and the Dominican Republic have their own theories about diseases, which are sometimes related to such divine manifestations in the surrounding landscape.

Adherents of 21 Division mentioned that everything that has existed is part of the creation of *Gran Dios*, The Supreme Creator, and therefore must be cherished. All living beings have a protective *misterio*. [240]As a result, *lwas*, are to be found in all of the four elements: water, air, earth and fire. The *lwas,* also frequently called *misterios,* are intermediaries of *Gran Dios*. There exist different divisions of *lwas*. Every division in 21 Division has its own element, which it dominates and works through. The most frequently mentioned groups/divisions of *lwas* are the following. The Legbá division with the main *lwa* Papa Legbá is the first to be asked for permission before any spiritual activity, and as such belongs to all elements. *Los Ogunes* (*e.g.* Ogún Balendjo), which are the warrior deities, and *Los Belies* (*e.g.* Belie Belcán), entities fighting against injustice, work through air. The fire element belongs to *Los Petroses* (Gran Buá), dreaded warrior deities, and *Los Candelos* (*e.g.* Papá Candelo), protective deities. *Los Candelos* with *Guedes* (*e.g. Barón del Cementerio*) are beneficial for business and belong to the earth. The Indian Division belongs to the water element. Other divisions, like Congo and Marassás, can work with all elements of nature.

In Cuban Regla de Ocha, the *ashé* is the vital energy of *Olodumare*, the God by whom the whole universe is created. *Orishas* and the dead also emerged from Olodumare, and are present in all four natural elements. The symbolism of specific landscape features is explained by their sacred biographies (*patakis*). These also clarify the relationships between the histories of *orishas*, and landscape symbolism, which often turns out to

---

240 For more on the 21 Division in the Dominican Republic see Tejeda Ortiz (2013).

play a role in the ceremonies. The symbolism expressed in the ceremonies often refers to links between *orishas.*

Together the orishas of the ritual specialists from *Regla de Ocha* specify the healing location and method of spiritual work during a consultation.[241] One of them, Ms. Eloisa Marina Peréz from Holguín explains: "*When I am going to do the spiritual work I ask where should I do it, whether at my home, at the four corners, at a plant, river, sea and so on. I ask and they give me signs and tell me where the work and cleansing should take place. This is also shown when doing the investigation with the shell (caracol): the shell gives you a song through Elegua. Every deity speaks to you through Elegua. And it tells you where it should be done, at the four corners, manigua (a uncultivated terrain of herbs, and shrubs), at the door entrance, to pass a dove around your body and throw it away on a hill and so on.*"[242] Guided by the consultation, ceremonies are then performed at different locations. Elegua, the principal messenger, the Bright Star, who has control over the roads and destiny, is sought at crossroads.[243] Prayers and spiritual works with the Obatalá can be performed at a mountain, with Ogún in hills and *manigua*, and Babalu-Ayé at hospitals or at El Rincón in Havana. Ritual baths invoking the power of Yemayá are carried out at the seashore, those of Oshún at river banks, and spiritual help of Oyá is sought at cemeteries. In addition, *orishas* can manifest themselves through different natural phenomena (see also James′ 1989 principle of multiple representation). For example, Oyá is the *orisha* of the four winds and lightning. Earth, parts of sacred trees, and plants from these places are brought to house-temple settings.

Famous Catholic pilgrimage shrines like the church of the Virgen of Charity, the church of the Virgen de Regla or El Rincón de San Lázaro are of great value for followers of Regla de Ocha because these three saints are seen as symbols of particular *orishas*, namely: Oshún, Yemayá, and Babalú-Ayé respectively. Devotees of Catholicism and Regla de Ocha visit in thousands the sanctuary of the Virgen of Charity and Oshún close to Santiago de Cuba. In Cuban East sacred places located in Havana such as El Rincón or Havana Bay are also well known. Thousands of pilgrims seek improvement of their health when praying to Babalú-Ayé and Saint Lazarus at El Rincón or when they come to fulfill their vows to the Virgen de Regla or Yemayá at Havana Bay.

Similarly, for Cuban *Espiritistas de Cordón* (Spiritists of the Cord) the visible world is parallel to the invisible plane from which the spirits of the deceased can intervene in the world through their medium, invoked individually or collectively through the *cordón* ceremony.[244] Dividing spirits into different groups (called *comisiones*) according to their nation, race, and profession, Cuban *Espiritistas* believe that in some places the

---

241 Ceremonies are initiated by paying homage to Oldumare, and his other manifestation, Olofi, the connection between the earth and sky). Then the sun is greeted, the owner of the heaven Olorun, and successively the great stars (Irabo) and moon (Shuwa). The rest of the ceremony is conducted as accustomed for the specific *orisha*.

242 Interview no. 49.

243 For more information on the symbolism within the Regla de Ocha see Cabrera (1954), James Figarola (1989), or Meighoo (2013).

244 For more on cordon ceremony see the work of Cordóva Martínez & Barzaga Sablón (2000).

contact with the spiritual world is more easily facilitated.[245] In the majority of cases, *Espiritistas* consult at centers/temples, but the connection can also be facilitated outside, at specific places where the spiritual presence is sensed. Special natural or historical places, like caves, mountains, and cemeteries are considered to be powerful spiritual places. Some places might be considered powerful because of a long tradition of the use. Inhabitants of Guao, a settlement close to Jiguaní, recalled a traditional healer and *espiritista*, Cecilia, who sent her patients to San Pedrucón, a Saint that represented himself as a rock, in order to make a vow and leave their offerings in the form of hair, nails, and money. The faith in the healing effect of San Pedrucón seemed to be lost, but when San Pedrucón was removed because of road construction, current inhabitants brought him back as a sign of respect to their parents and grandparents. Some places might also be represented through objects found there. For example, Jiguaniceros protect their houses with stones from the fortress that according to oral traditions was built by Spaniards and indigenous peoples. In the past, spiritual sessions were organized on the top of the hill close to the fortress.

Catholics and Protestants (Evangelistas) in both locations believe that, alongside traditional sacred places like churches, chapels or pilgrimage places, other elements of nature may also reveal divine signs; for example, a particular form of clouds may be related to the manifestation of a Saint in certain places, trees or plants. The dead too were sometimes seen as being able to influence wellbeing and health. Roman Catholics would search for spiritual help and cures in churches and chapels. Some of these might have been constructed at places of Marian manifestations in trees, like the Ceiba tree at the Templete in Havana or the Virgen de Higuey. Also other places where the miraclouse appearance of Virgen de Mercedes at Saint Hill near La Vega are until now the popular pilgrimage place. Many devotees ask the Saints and Virgins to cure illness and to help in different life struggles also at natural holy sites such as Cavern of Saint Francis in Bánica. Similarly, Evangelistas seek contact with God during the church services, but some of them such as Angel Montilla Guerrero from Boca de Yuma, following the example of Elijah, search for that contact in caves because of the privacy that such sites offer.

Cuban and Dominican religious traditions, in spite of the various differences between them, coincide in paying homage to ancestors and to the dead. Ancestors are considered to be those to whom one has a personal family linkage, but also those who are more remote. Ancestors and the dead in general have a central role in Cuban Spiritism.[246] At Dominican (popular) Catholic altars, photos of deceased loved ones

---

245 Josefina Pérez Yero from Cienfuegos described the cordón as follows: *"We make a circle, the outer part are the brothers, that ingrate the cord, the head man (leading figures) and the head women, the first finishes with a man and the second with a woman. They are four heads. Then there is the hammer that is the inner circle where the biggest potential resides, a place where they work the most. My grandmother left behind her songs calling for works (llamadas de trabajo) y to help those entities. There is only the tone, and the rest we add. It is how would l describe you this tone: "Lolelale, lolelaela", like this. Afterwards I have to add what I would like to ask for, how I will call the spirits. Like this we have these calling songs and we have the labor. When we speak about labor it means that the commission of spirits is already there. So you speak about llamada when you call the spirits and then commissions, you speak about labor when the commissions and calls are in the cord...."* A similar description was giving in Jiguaní; unfortunately, this was not recorded. The reader might find also different youtube videos made in Monte Oscuro in Cuba.

246 For more on the Spiritism of Cord see James Figarola (1993), Lago Vieito (1996), Córdova Martínez & Barzaga Sablón (2000).

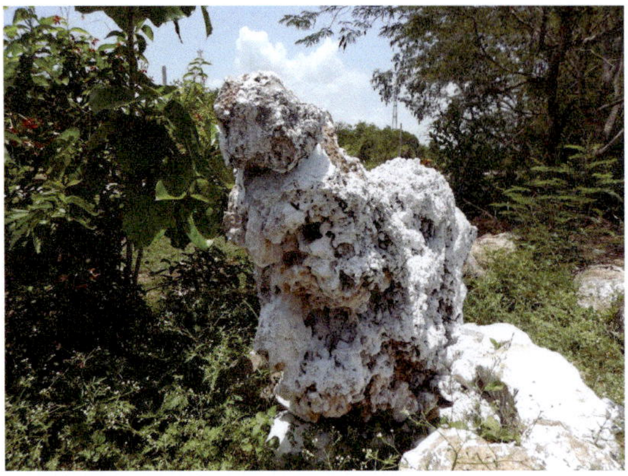

Figure 20 San Pedrucón in Guao near Jiguaní, Cuba.

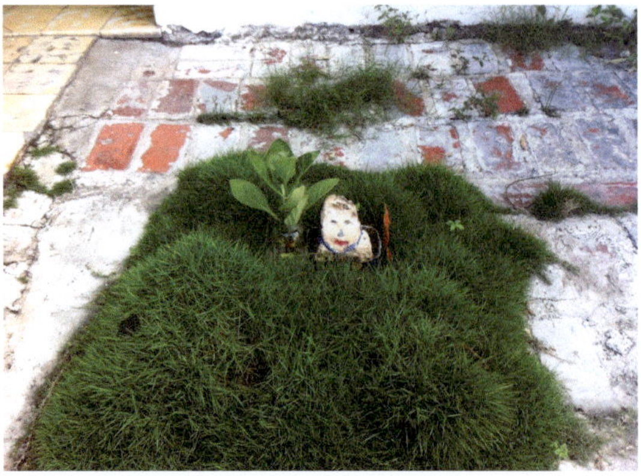

Figure 21 The protecting plant and stone at a house in Jiguaní, Cuba (right).

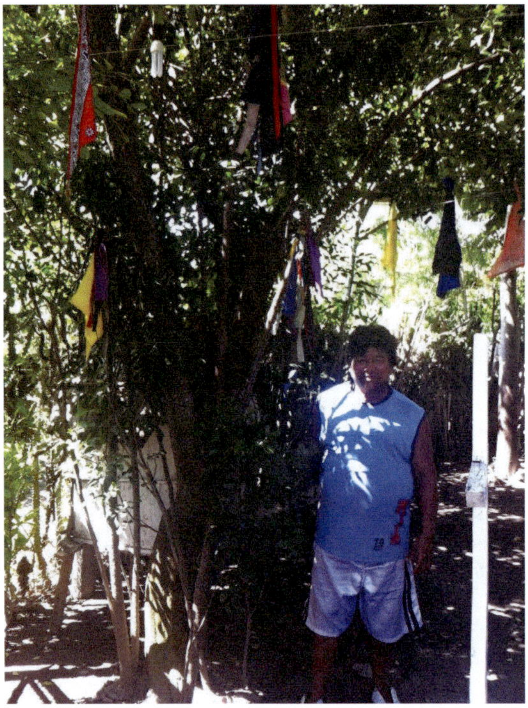

Figure 22 Siguaraya tree afront of a house-temple in Niquero, Cuba.

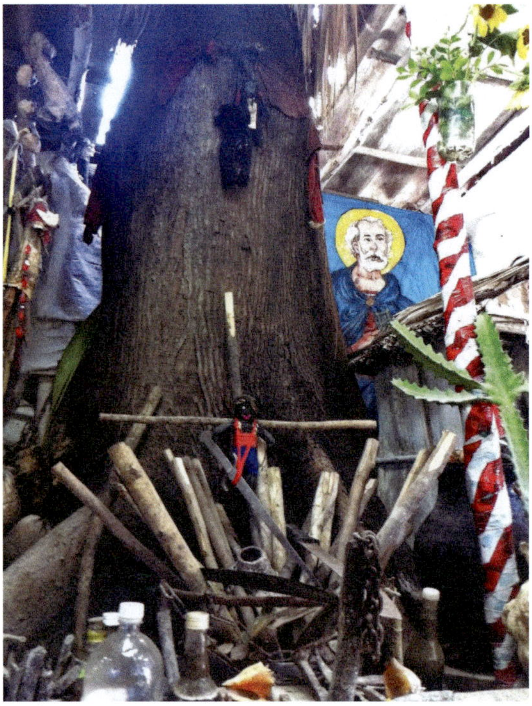

Figure 23 Ceiba and nganga in house-temple in Niquero, Cuba.

are often accompanied by a glass of water and a lit candle as an expression of devotees asking for guidance in times of personal need.[247] Ancestral agency is searched for in sites that are historically associated with their presence. The Egungun, remote ancestors in Regla de Ocha, reside at places of their heroic events, often palenques (fortified sett-

247 James Figarola has written more thoughts about the death in the Spiritism of Cord (1993a) and summarized some widespread Cuban beliefs (1993b).

lements) and other monuments commemorating their resistance to the colonial rule (*e.g.* the Maroon Monument in El Cobre).[248] Egungun reside also in manigua, on the hill, or at other places where their presence is perceived through material remains, even archeological sites, or where that presence is sensed by healers or devotees. Similarly, in the Dominican 21 Division, some historical places, such as La Negreta, the Cepi Cepi sugarmill, and some sites with visible material evidence of indigenous occupancy are locales where ancestral forces might be mobilized to enhance one's own or collective wellbeing. Lastly, particularly powerful healers from the Dominican past, like Liborio Mateo or Bibiana Rosa, are ritually commemorated and invoked in places associated with their life and work.

Other spiritual beings in Cuban and Dominican landscapes

Besides places that are recognized in different local religious traditions, there are other parts of the Cuban and Dominican landscapes that are animated by spiritual beings. These beings can frighten and incommode people, but in general are not thought to cause illnesses or severe harm. Among the beings that are said to appear sometimes in the Dominican countryside are the *galipotes*, described as men who transform themselves into an animal, plant, or object. Some have argued that they have, in general, malicious intentions, to steal, or to make trouble. The status of these beings differs, from beings seen as evil, or beings that just bother people.

These may be compared to the Cuban *cagüeyros* are described as men who can transform into animals, such as pigs, dogs and, birds, but also can mimic or transform into plants. *Cagüeyros* figures also in narratives about revolutions and during the war, wherein some men were able to transform themselves into a tree stump or a tree branch to escape dangerous situations in East Cuba.[249] Similarly, in Dominican Boca de Mana, Mr. Julian de la Rosa narrated about his uncle: "*I have heard stories about this, about the people who were able to receive spiritual entities (se montaban). I have heard a story about warriors who were here in this country, that when the guards were searching for them to imprison them, they transformed into a stump, a guineo plant with a one ripe fruit in the cluster of bananas. My grandfather was always telling this story. I also had an uncle that knew an eel's prayer, and who could transform into a fish to cross over the river. A person that transformed in a stone or an animal by means of spiritual invocation – these people were called brujos.*" Curiously, this uncle, who is said to be one of those "*brujos*", *i.e.* spiritual specialists practicing dark spells, was rescued at the end by his grandmother, the famous healer Bibiana de la Rosa. In few cases, such spiritual specialists were considered to have the ability to tie up or take away a soul.

---

248 See also Fernández Olmos & Paravisini-Gebert (1997).

249 One of the inhabitants of Barajagua, Rosalina Segura Hidalgo also described cagüyeros as causing troubles but also as offering help: *"It was said that an old man that worked at night building house on his own, that cagüeyros were helping him. These are being that throw stones and earth from trees. They climb and can make you troubles at nights. J: Do they live in trees? RS: They live in caves. J: So, were peoples afraid of caves? RS: Yes, people were afraid to go to these places, because they could tie you up, they throw earth at you, or to your meals when you were cooking. J: Into what cagüeyro can transform? RS: In dogs, or birds".*

Other frequently mentioned beings in Dominican rural areas are the *ciguapas*, described as naked indigenous women with their feet facing backwards. *Ciguapas* live in forests and on mountains; sometimes they come down to the village to steal salt (see below), and throw earth into the pot when people are cooking. Another kind of beings known from the Cuban countryside are the *jigües/güijes*, small human-like figures with dark skin who live in dark pools and parts of Cuban rivers. *Jigües* are said to frighten and trouble people, but in a playful way, rather than to cause real illnesses. On both islands, *cucuyos* (fireflies) are representations of the dead, and are therefore respected, and never killed.[250] Lastly, owls are respected for announcing the death of someone known to the observer in both regions of the study.

The visible and invisible worlds can interact in various ways through landscape symbolism, but within the scope of this study it is not possible to mention all the different examples collected during the fieldwork, especially as many of these do not have a direct link to healing practices in the present.[251] Now, before discussing the healers as one of the major components of the local healing landscapes, it is important to address the concept of illness itself.

Illness and cure

Beliefs concerning illness vary between and within cultural and religious systems. Many share the idea that illness is caused by a disturbance of the equilibrium between individual and external factors. In general, an illness may have material, human and/or divine causes. The material causes, like for example viruses, bad hygiene, and food poisoning, are considered to be the most common causes of an illness. Common illnesses such as flu, constipation, kidney infection, or stomach ache are often first treated at home. As these illnesses are common, medicinal herbs needed to cure them are well-known in the public sphere, and this knowledge is exchanged routinely between family members, neighbors and friends. For instance, the flu, is cured by a tea made of guanabana leaves; the fever by tea from ozua, quinoa, or mara; and for parasites, children are given guatapanal, guahabo, or apazote (for Latin names see the appendix).

Illnesses may be interpreted in line with culturally specific syndromes or religious explanations. As a result, new illnesses like *chikungunya*, an infectious disease that broke out in 2014, was interpreted by some as being caused by "bad air" (*mal aire*). Bad air can be a malicious spirit moving with the wind, which can penetrate the body of the patient. At the same time bad air can refer to air pollution, or diseases transmitted through the air. So it is both a culturally bounded syndrome, and also a culturally specific way to describe observable phenomena.

The equilibrium between the individual and external factors is also maintained through preserving an internal balance between conditions that are characterized as "hot"

250 Ms. Rosalina Segura Hidalgo told a narrative about the use of a cucuyo to light the journey at night: *"There was an old man who had caught a cucuyo to light his journey on the way home, but when he came and went to release him, el cucuyo said to him: and now you have to leave me where you took me from."*

251 One of the Cuban respondents suggested that to have bats at home was seen as a negative as they might take away the person. Others saw them as molesting people when cooking by throwing earth into the meal; they could even tie one up. This might be related to the pre-colonial worldview as bats are discussed by Pané and representations of bats appear as decorations of archaeological ceramics.

or "cold". These qualities are not necessarily related to actual temperatures, but stem from a cosmic categorization system that shows similarity to (and possibly a relationship with) the classical theory of humoral balance.[252] In order to keep the balance, people in Dominican border regions pay attention to which crops are cold or hot as imprudent consumption could be dangerous and might cause harm if the body is in the opposite state. Sometimes the hot and cold rule is applied for medicinal plants.[253] Accordingly, washing one's hair during a hot day with cold water is believed to cause illness.

Illness furthermore can be caused by social imbalance, *i.e.* by the disturbance of the good relationship of an individual with the community and humankind but also with the divine forces. Malfunctioning health could be an indication of a problem in the relationship with the divine beings, possibly caused by their whims, or their punishment for violating some social moral code. In 21 Division, the relationship with God was maintained through divine messengers, the *lwas*. Among Catholics, illness is often perceived as a divine punishment for not living up to the Holy Scriptures. Obviously, the explanation of illnesses as being caused by violating some social and moral behavior code is not applied indiscriminately to everyone.[254] In addition, divine messengers, and other invisible agents can cause an illness, like the dead, and the ancestors. Especially in Cuban Spiritism, the dead are important actors in wellbeing. Cures and ailments are all related to the agency of the dead. A case from Jiguaní may serve to illustrate this. Mr. de Los Santos narrated that one of his grandparents became sick and passed away because he chased away one of the dead from his place in a disrespectful way. The consequences of his threat were a high fever and later the grandfather's death.[255]

One of the cultural syndromes that will be discussed in a later paragraph is the concept of soul loss or capture. The experience was often described as the soul being

252 See on more this theory the work of Barbara Tedlock (1987) or Chevalier and Sánchez Bain (2003).

253 This custom was described earlier by Brendbekken (1998). In Mexico the idea is that the disturbance of equilibrium between the two (cf Yang / Yin), causes illness and that in order to restore the balance one needs to take cold herbs for hot diseases and vice versa (personal conversation with M. Jansen 2018). According to Prof. Jansen it is likely that the contemporary view is the consequence of synergy between an ancient dichotomy beween the influence of the Sun and that of the Rain and the hippocratic idea.

254 One of the examples to be mentioned is that a blindness of an individual from a Holguín province was interpreted as a punishment for the fact that he allegedly had violated an underage girl.

255 Mr. Los Santos (born 1929) Jiguaní told about what happened to his grandparents who were living in a small settlement called Caimanes: *"One day when the children were going to get water in the river, before they got there at a paddock they saw a man without a head. They were frightened and returned quickly home. Their father first did not believe them until he saw with his own eyes. His first reaction was to pray but when the dead did not want to leave he took a weapon, so the dead left, disappeared behind the cayo de guácimas. Soon after he went on pilgrimage to el Cobre. On their journey they had to overnight in a house where the day before someone passed away. That night the dead did not leave them a sleep. The day after, they again had to search for a water in house, where the lady when she saw the man asked him to come and to be seated. Under his chair a huge spider appeared and when it started to get to him, the woman told him: "Listen to what I am going to say, the threat you made you are going pay with your life, this is going to cost the life. When you arrive home, you will become sick and will not get better because the place where you have seen me, the place where you threatened me, this is mine, and I am there every time when I want, everything that you will take will turn into salt and tears, and you are going to die." Afterwards he was given also a protection (resguardo) for his son, that he would not pass away during the pilgrimage. And it seemed that the thing that he (the son) was carrying passed on the horse. Then they went to el Cobre to fulfill their vow, and when they returned, exactly as the one said the man arrived with 40 Celsius of fever and lay down into a bed from which he never woke up again. He passed away as the woman said because he has threatened the dead."*

tied up (*está amarrado*) or being taken away by a *misterio*, an *lwas*, or an ancestor (*el misterio se lo llevó*).[256] Soul loss is induced by divine beings like the *lwas*, or ancestors, but also by other dark spiritual specialists. The expression of being taken away refers to displacement of the soul, which can result in temporary or permanent illness, which may lead to death. Mental illnesses are often described in terms of the soul having been taken away. In a subsequent chapter, several cases will be discussed in which illness is related to the agency of the indigenous ancestors. The ailments induced by the indigenous ancestors are often described as a result of a misbalanced relationship, and the ancestors' whims.

In addition, illness can arise from a social imbalance caused by social conflicts.[257] The illnesses within this category are often described as induced by another man or ritual specialist through an evil eye, spell, or witchcraft. The evil eye refers to someone's gaze on another person with admiration or envy, which might lead to illness or even a death. For that reason, a compliment is often followed by the expression "May God bless you".

People are frequently frightened of becoming the object of different kinds of spells. For protection, they use different amulets (*resguardos*).[258] The objective of these amulets can be to harm the health or wellbeing of another person, to influence someone's behavior in terms of attracting the person, and influencing their decision processes. Spells harming others are referred to as witchcraft. Harmful spells can be induced by inserting some secret ingredients into the adversary's food or beverage. Mariano (from Guananico) gave a testimony about such an incident. About twenty years ago, Mariano brought his sister to a doctor because her belly was inflated. After visiting an official doctor who could not help, he brought her to a healer living near Santiago de Caballeros. The healer gave her a bath, and herbs which caused her to vomit the exogenous object that was in her body, which appeared to be a snake.[259] Mariano commented that his sister was carrying a snake because of something someone gave to her in a meal or beverage.

Healing specialists

Besides the official medical care, people in rural areas have remedied their health with traditional healing practices. In general, a patient combines and complements different treatments. Healing practices often draw on a wide cultural repertoire of possibilities

256 The Haitian Creole has a term for the soul loss: "*pran bonange*" (personal conversation with Sony Jean 2017). The technique of tying up someone to someone else is quite popular magic among Dominican and Cuban women who often practice tying up the name of their husband or lover to a small tree branch in order to keep him at home.

257 This model is to be compared with attributes ailments and illnesses to thoughts or emotions from oneself or from another person overlaps with the psychological explanations as being caused psychological stresses.

258 One of the more frequently mentioned *resguardos* was to take the water from seven different *tinajas* or to tie up a stone. Different seeds are used to make amulets. Especially popular are those of Dominican plants like azabache, framboyán, chakara, peonía, macramé, haba, or sambo. Popular in Cuba are: ojo buye, santa maría, jikí, jiba, cedro, moruro, úcaro, pionía, jala jala, guayacán, caguyrán and the before mentioned azabache (Sapindus saponaria L.).

259 The snake in this context could be interpreted as a symbol of the evil.

and creativity, assuring that if one remedy does not work out, new solutions are sought. When people in rural areas become sick, if the doctor is far away, unaffordable or not specialized in the illness, they often seek help of non-institutional care providers like religious specialists, healers, herbalists, *sobadores* (massagists), diviners, and other care givers providing home treatments. *Sobadores* are called upon especially for constipations (*empacho*), while *santiguadores* are approached for the evil eye, *culebrilla* (Herpes Zoster), or St. Anthony's fire. Traditional healers are consulted for a wide range of illnesses and issues concerning physical, mental and spiritual wellbeing.

People consult spiritual specialists when they want to improve their general wellbeing, like becoming luckier, getting a job, receiving more love, dominating a person, or attracting clients to a business. People seek the help of ritual specialists in other matters as well, before going to court or winning other types of personal disputes, or trying to ward off a negative spell from an adversary, or to return it to them. With the exception of one ritual specialist, none of the healers wanted be associated with malicious spells.

Dominican healers

Dominican healing experts are often referred to as *curanderos*, "healers". A few contributors have referred to them as *sabios,* "wise persons".[260] Those specialists who were formally initiated often referred to themselves as *caballos del misterio*, "horses of *lwas*". The latter name refers to the fact that the body of the healers, or more specifically the head, is the medium through which the *misterio* or *lwa* (terms used often interchangeably) descends. The *lwa* chooses his servant (*servidor*, a term used by the specialists themselves), not the other way around. If the healers are considered to practice spiritual works causing harm and illnesses, they would be called *brujos,* "witches". This pejorative denomination was used by people who, in general, despised the healers' belief system on the basis of prejudices and misunderstandings, rather than on the basis of knowledge of the kind of spiritual works that the healers perform.

Dominican healers work with one *misterio* who is their guarding *lwa*. The healers are said to be born with or receive the virtue to heal (*tiene don*). In the Dominican 21 Division, every person has a guardian angel / divine being that is his protector and guide during his entire life. Similarly, this is the case in Cuban Spiritism and *Regla de Ocha*. In all three systems there are specialists who have developed skills to communicate better with their guardian, and later developed further their ability to contact with the invisible world.

Before healers are initiated, they receive different signs, like revelations and dreams, which indicate the special virtue and calling of that person. Many of the healers are said to neglect, or to refuse to accept, the fact that they have been chosen by the *lwas* to serve. This denial can lead to incarnations of *lwas* at public places in unexpected moments. The virtue is often said to be more pronounced (through frequent revelations, and involuntarily incarnations of *lwas*) after a severe illness or loss of an important family member (often a mother or a grandmother). This period of their life would be a decisive moment for the prospective healers to further develop their gift to heal. The

260 Personally I would prefer this term instead of healer but only four contributors (out of hundreds) referred to them as *sabios*. None of them was a healer himself.

denial may also be related to the stigma of the 21 Division, as well as to the burden of the responsibility and the obligations that come with this task.[261] As a consequence, different Dominican healers mentioned that their initiation was preceded by their rejection of the gift of healing, but this rejection lead to an illness. The cure for the illness was only possible by accepting this virtue and dealing with the divine beings.

The narratives about events preceding the initiation have many overarching features in both regions. To mention just one example, Mr. Reyes from Jiguaní described the beginnings of his work as follows: *"I started as an Spiritist, developing myself in the spiritual realm. After, when I was about 18 years old, I started to travel to Havana because of my disease. I started to turn my back on my spiritual field, I did not want to work with this. I remember that I took my Saints and stored them, I think that I did it because of the fear of what other boys would say, I was in the process of adolescence. I began to reject that, and began to get sick. I had to go to Havana to treat my illness, I was hospitalized for two months at the Surgical Clinical Hospital of Rheumatology and then they sent me to the Oncology in El Almejeira. Then I began to visit spiritual people and santeras in Havana, and they told me that I have to develop the grace that I have, that I was afraid of, that afterwards I am going to be rid off all of this. So I went back to exercise the spiritual work and started to throw the cards. I began to improve and get out of the illness, and from there I succeeded in becoming a saint. Since then, the Yoruba rule, the rule of Osha entered into my life."* One of the shared themes in the narratives about becoming healers is that the denial led to an illness, which could be only cured by developing one's own gift in the spiritual domain.

On both islands people consider that neglecting the gift of healing can be dangerous for the individual. Mrs. Mayra Dominguez, a traditional healer from Villa Isabela, works with Belie Belcán lwa pertaining to the air domain, and Maria Lionza pertaining to the water domain. She works with Maria Lionza because through the family line she inherited "*el corriente del indio*"[262]: *"We Dominguez are under the protection of the Indian race, because the majority of the old people had el corriente indio."* The expression '*corriente del indio*' could be freely translated as a spiritual connection with the indigenous ancestors. This spiritual connection in some cases would be based on a presumed or real genealogical link, manifest in a few physical traits like color and type of hair, or other arbitrary aspects of racial categorization like skin color, but sometimes also on the person's interests in culture and the history of indigenous peoples. Mrs. Dominguez narrates further: *"When I was a young girl, I was afraid but then I spent three days in the river and my father and mother said that I was dead, but I was not, because I felt how they raised me up and I saw everything and everyone, all people and I spoke to them... This was in the river Yaque in Santiago, because, after I left school my mother sent me to bring food*

261 In one of the interviews with a ritual specialist from Monte Plata she described an involuntarily incarnation of Indigenous Misterio. The excerpt from this conversation is as follows. On my question where Indians live, the healer answered: *E: I have heard that they live below the water, but I think that it is not possible, because people are not fish, they have to live in caves. Actually, I have only seen one, in 2002, I was introduced, and I was about to die. JP: How did it go? E We were going to Bayaguna, it was around 1 am. I see a tall, strong man with long hair coming towards me. I lost consciousness and woke up after three days.*

262 For further information on *corriente del indio* see also the account of Mr Morillo from Caño Miguel, interview with healer Benito from Estero Hondo.

to my grandmother. She prepared me a bag with the meal and I went to the river and felt the river was pulling me inside... Yes, the river is dangerous but not for me anymore. I got lost and my parents were searching for me and my father angrily said: she will return, they will bring her back... ". In this excerpt, Mrs. Dominguez refers to the widespread belief that people who are guarded by the indigenous ancestors should avoid bodies of water because they run the risk of being *taken away* by the *misterios* that are living under water. Born with the gift of healing, for her this danger is even greater, and in order to be able to better direct this *corriente* Mrs. Dominguez had to be initiated.

Her case resembles others from other Dominican regions, where the initiation as a healer is linked with travelling into the invisible subaquatic world. In Bánica, a former healer called Cusha (since deceased) is said to have gone to a place of indigenous ancestors, and after her return became "another person", she could heal people.[263] In a similar vein, the grandfather of Mrs. Carmela Alcántara (78 years old) gained his healing grace by living under the water for seven years, after which he reemerged with a *misterio* and the power to cure. Not only healers but also Dominican midwifes were said to receive their skills after having been taken away by the indigenous spirits to their subaquatic kingdoms. In the past, midwives were said to have had such spiritual encounters with indigenous ancestors.[264]

In order to control these forces, which are like involuntarily possessions, healers have to be initiated or baptized by another, more experienced healer. An initiation is often referred to as a baptism, and normally takes place at the temple of more experienced healer, but it can also be performed outside of the healer's temple, like at a river, cave, sea, or one of the dwellings of the *lwas*. Thus, healers who are said to have indigenous *corriente* are first examined by a more experienced healer; their religious education culminates in a concrete ceremony during which they are prepared to receive

---

263 Interview with Hecfredes Gómez.

264 One narrative of midwives' spiritual encounters with indigenous ancestors was told by Santos Morillo Martinez from Caño Miguel (Puerto Plata province). Mr. Morillo narrated further about his great grandmother: *"I will tell you a very old story. This was told to me by my grandmother. Her name was Saturnia Fermin and they searched for her but I do not know at what place it was, maybe it was at Castillo. Her brother used to say that his mother was taken away (his brother Lindo inserts: The Indian lady) they took her to this cave and entered her into a deep water and took her on back. This was not a dream they took her to help with child labor. They took her to this cave and she stayed some time, I do not remember how long exactly, maybe it was a week or three days. They were counting it and she was there for some time. When she returned they gave her an object. I do not know if it was a lump of gold or some other golden thing... They brought her back because they were not allowed to keep her. It is possible that it was in a cave at Ranchette or in the sea. From there we have this Indian race or a branch of our family tree. From there we all have this corriente, that we are from this race we carry this. Now I am not doing it but when I pray to Indian forces I say it like this: I hope you will help me with these* people who are mistreating me and put them in front to stop seeing me." Sometimes the Morillo brothers gave the *indigenous misterios* a water offering on their small family altar in their bedroom like they use to do regularly for their deceased mother. The above family history fits within the widespread oral tradition about people from underwater who were searching help from midwives (e.g. in the location of Imbert). Also in the following version where the main characters have switched roles the river is a source of birth: *"Once upon a time there was a man who saw that his wife is in labor and searched for the midwife and found her in the river, come and I will go to deliver the baby and when she finished she told him to come bring me back and at the same place where he took her, she disappeared."* Here rivers are symbols of life, more specifically of birth. In this light, the previous narratives about being taken away by indigenous ancestors could be interpreted not as referring to a place of death in negative terms but as referring to a place where life continues for the dead who have "*corriente del indio*" in the subaquatic world.

the spiritual beings (*montarse*). For the indigenous *misterios*, this initiation takes place at altars, water pools or caves.

Consults at altars

The cause of illness is established during the consultation with the healer in his temple. A healer's altar is situated in a room in his/her house or in a small wooden house separated from the main house. Among initiated healers, it is custom to construct shrines following strict ceremonies in order to create good conditions for the *lwas* to operate. In every temple, there is a principal altar with images and other representations of the *lwas*. In the middle of the altar, patients find the main protector's image, a statue of the *lwa*, or objects representing them (*e.g.* a sea shell for Yemayá). The location of other *lwas* is often based on their family relations or hagiographies. The offerings are embodied in the lit candles, aromatic oils, flowers, perfumes, and ceremonial foods. Under the altar on the ground are *Guedes*, working with the earth element and a small human made water pool for indigenous *misterios*.

Healers can be consulted every day, but many healers prefer to work on Tuesdays and Fridays. During the consultation, the healer calls the *lwas* by smoking tobacco, blowing the smoke calmly up into the air, and consuming rum (depending on the *lwa*). Healers often light a candle or use a glass of water as a means of communication. When the *lwa* descends, and enters the body of the healer, he/she calls the patient by ringing on a small bell to enter the temple. The incarnation of the *lwa* leads to a transformation of the healer's identity. This identity shift is expressed materially through the clothing (*e.g.* the color of the scarf) and personality. The behavior of the *lwas* varies according to their personalities. Sometimes the *lwa* shows his power by extraordinary behavior like eating the glass, or drinking alcohol in a quantity that would be dangerous for a normal person. Based on the indications from the patient, the *lwa* establishes the cause of the illness and its remedy. The healer might receive the remedy from the *lwa* when dreaming. In Cuban Spiritism and *Regla de Ocha*, remedies are also obtained via divine beings and spiritual entities, when these incarnate in the bodies of intermediaries but also through their manifestation in the healer's dreams.

During the consultation, the patient might address different kinds of material, mental, spiritual, and physical health issues. Among the frequently suggested cures are baths, cleansing, and herbal mixtures. The herbal mixtures are frequently prepared as tea, or as a combination of different herbs preserved in bottles. Another common means of rehabilitation (physical and mental, balance between the patient and the divine world) is dedicating a prayer, making an offering, fulfilling a vow or participating in a celebration of *lwas*.

In Dominican 21 Division, the patients of the healers are expected to participate in the celebration of the patronal *lwa* of the healer. During these celebrations, the altar is cleaned and decorated with fresh flowers, and ceremonial meals, often including *moro* (rice and beans), peanuts, and corn, are served at the altar for the *lwas*. The *lwas* descend later, after having been called by a group of drummers using special *palo* drums and singing hymns. When the *lwas* descend, the devotees and the *lwas* dance, sing, drink, and eat together. In various celebrations that the author attended, after the principal *lwa* arrived at the celebration, other *lwas* of visiting *caballo del misterio* also arrived. Besides the *lwa* whose day was celebrated, other *lwas* would also be given offerings. By attending these collective celebrations of the *lwas*, patients publicly display their belief in these spirits, and their gratitude for being healed. Through their attendance and contribution – by helping with the organization of the ritual, by bringing alcohol, preferred meals and offerings, or by playing and singing for the *lwas* – the patients express their care for the *lwas* and their respect for the healer.

To a certain degree, the *lwas* may be considered to be specialized in certain problems. For example, Belié Belcán, (San Miguel), a popular protector, is consulted for all kinds of illnesses but especially to ward off malicious spells, while his wife Anaisa Pie (Santa Ana) is the queen of love, consulted in case of matrimonial problems. In a similar way, specialization can also be found in *Regla de Ocha*, where *orishas* like Yemayá are consulted for ritual cleansing, for travels, to open the ways, San Lázaro is consulted for curing sores, leprosy, and pain. The indigenous ancestors do not seem to have any specialization, rather in 21 Division they are in general associated with the power of the water element (both in its constructive and its destructive aspect), which is widely employed in different healing rituals in order to obtain positive wellbeing and for resolving health, relational (family, protection against enemies) and economic problems. Lwas together with healers are considerent important agents in healing practices passing on religious and often also of botanical knowledge. For more abou the botanical knowledge see the following section.

Healing Plants

Plants accompany people during their life from birth until the end. In fact, plants act upon people even before birth and continue to do so in the afterlife. Herbal mixtures are used to increase fertility, applied for cleansing the uterus after birth; they are used as amulets for the protection of children and given to babies as their first food. At the end of the corporal life, special meals and teas are prepared for the people assisting at the burial; other plants are used to help the spiritual essence to leave, and serve as offerings to the dead. Plants are particularly important in the countryside in times of illness when they are used for curing physical, mental and spiritual ailments.

Dominican healing plants

A wide range of diseases is treated with medicinal plants. Among the most frequently mentioned illnesses that are treated with herbal medicine are common illnesses like flu, gastrointestinal diseases (flatulence, indigestion, diarrhea, stomach ache, parasites), and urinary infections (*mal de orina*). Green medicine was also used for controlling blood pressure, cleaning kidney stones, or more broadly for inflammatory and infectious ailments.

Medicinal plants often have multiple uses, and are frequently used in combination with other plants in infusions such as teas, baths and *botellas*. *Botellas* (bottles) are popular Dominican herbal blends, named after the bottles in which they are kept. Different parts of the plants (mostly roots, barks, leaves, seeds) are cleaned, boiled (for a variable amount of time), flavored, and preserved with alcohol in a bottle. The exact composition of the recipe is kept as a secret within a family, or as a personal secret of the healer. Recipes for *botellas* vary according to whether the mixtures aim to cure a specific illness or whether they are prepared for a whole range of illnesses, for example when all the plants with an anti-inflammatory or laxative effect are combined.[265] Among the popular *botellas* are those for vaginal infections, cleaning blood, and for fertility for women and men. The number of the ingredients of *botellas* varies. On average, at least twenty different plants are used in one *botella*, but some contributors like Ms. Estela Sadí from Cruce de Guayacanes, mentioned more than sixty ingredients of her *botella*, which is used for a whole range of infectious diseases.

The usage of plants is based on long-term experimentation. In addition, the selection of plants seems to be guided by their perceived character. Plant qualities like flavor and scent, and their being categorized as warm or cold have implications for the choice of plants for a specific ailment, and the quantity in which they are used. The scent of the plants (bitter or sweet) seems to be decisive in their use in sweet and bitter baths, the former attracting positivity while the bitter smelling plants are used to drive off negativity. The cool and warm plants are characterized according to the environment in which they are grown, their properties, and their effect on the body (warming up or cooling down). These characteristics have consequences for their use: for example, the fresh cool plants found at the banks of rivers are used for inflammatory diseases. Likewise, the hot character of *anamú* or *sábila* affects the quantity of the plant that can be given as a remedy. The hot and warm distinction of plants is important in border regions for dietary restrictions. Some crops are considered hot (*e.g.* pineapple) and others cold, and they have to be eaten in balance to maintain good health. Sometimes the doctrine of signatures is followed, paying attention to the shape of different parts of plants in indications of their use. Lastly, when plants are dioecious, sometimes the gender is important.[266]

The existing rich knowledge of medicinal plants would fill several volumes. Many plants that were described by the first accounts for their economic use have in the present besides their economic also medicinal use. To mention one example, Oviedo (1535/2002) elaborates quite extensively on the importance of corn. However, he does not mention aspects that we find in the present-day uses: corn silk is a very popular ingredient in *botellas*, it is used as a remedy against stomach ache and fever, for cleansing the uterus after the childbirth, and for lowering cholesterol. The great variety in herbal uses across different regions, households and participants complicates historical reconstruction of the historical continuity of medicinal uses of specific plants. One of the first Caribbean plants that has fascinated Europe with its medicinal properties was guayacán, used then for curing syphilis. Nowadays, this plant is still used to treat rheumatism, skin infections (*rasquiña*) and to wash clothes. Furthermore, when comparing the first accounts of Caribbean flora with present-day accounts, the former often lack the information pertaining to what kind of illnesses these plants were used for. In spite of much incoherence in the data, the current use can at least partially help us to estimate past medicinal uses. This is also the case for plants that have been recorded among Afro-Caribbean healing specialists during the 17th century in the Cartagena trials, where their uses were not specified. To mention just three: *anamú* serves for catarrh, *botellas* for infections, warding off malicious spirits and the dead,

265 The herbal mixtures inducing purging (vomitive effect) were called *tomas*.

266 The gender might also indicate a different species as in the case of *broquelejo macho (Piper peltatum L.)* and *broquelejo hembra (Piper umbellatum L.),* both native to the Tropics.

and *tuatua*, known in the Dominican Republic as *tatúa*, is used for stomach ache.[267] Lastly, Pringamosa roots (*Urera baccifera*), in combination with other herbs, are used for bottles that combat infections.[268]

From historical sources, it is clear that the colonization of the Caribbean also implied the import of exotic flora to the region. Plants of exotic origin were used for both medicinal and ritual purposes. Following the study of Moret (2013), it has been hypothesized that the origin of the plants could provide insights into sociocultural histories. Following this study, it could be hypothesized further that also indigenous botanical knowledge was more likely to be preserved in the settlements in which the indigenous people and their descendants were present throughout the colonial history. In Boyá, it is clear that the majority of healing plants are from the New World (see attachment). Nearly eighteen percent of these plants were brought from the Old World, some of them, like cundeamor, *ajonjolí*, and *sábila*, from the African continent. Exotic plants were used in combination with native flora. For example, *ajonjolí, sábila, yerba de calentura* and a small bloom from *guano* were used for protection against malicious spells (witchcraft). *Guano*, native to the West Indies (Coccothrinax spp.), still popular for construction and weaving, was already used by ritual specialists in the Caribbean in the 17th century (Gómez 2017). *Guano* replaced palms known from Europe and Africa. Following Catholic teachings, in Boyá now *guano* is also called Saint Guano; it is blessed on Palm Sunday and later used to ward off the storms, which would harm homes and harvests. Another popular category of plants in Boyá includes those mentioned earlier by Oviedo (1535/2002) as plants that were similar to Spanish plants, but existing in Hispaniola before their arrival. In Boyá, *albahaca morada* was added to baths for protection against malicious spells, and *verdolaga* was used in teas against stomach ache and flatulence. *Vervena*, the sacred plant from Calvario, was used for indigestion. All three plants were recognized on the genus level (Ocimum spp.), and are believed to be of pantropical origin (*Trianthema portulacastrum* L.): the Spaniards considered them the same as those known at home. Another exotic plant, cundeamor (*Momordica charantia* L.), also used as an abortive in other locations, is used for treating diseases like smallpox, introduced during early colonial period. Smallpox was also treated in this location with *bruca hembra* (*Senna obtusifolia),* and *piñón* (*Erythrina berteroana* Urb. or *Jatropha curcas* L.), all native to the New World. A similar tendency to treat new exotic diseases with local plants was clear during the *chiqunguya* epidemic, which was treated in this location with *Juan Prieto* (*Varronia curassavica*). This supports the argument that remedies for introduced diseases might be also found in local flora during the early colonial period.

As in Boyá, in many other Dominican locations we find plants of exotic origins being used in ritual contexts. This is especially the case for plants used for protection in early modern Europe, like *albehaca, artemisa, mejorana, mostaza, pachulí, romero, ruda,* and *sangre cristo,* which are also very popular plants in the present-day, for protection, cleaning from spells, malignant spirits, and bad luck, or bringing good luck, success,

267 Cuban Catholics explain that as this plant has its own *misterio*, the remedy from tuatua is related to the collection process: when the leaves are gathered in the upward direction they are used against vomit, and when gathered in the downward direction against diarrhea.

268 Although Gómez identified this plant as Urtica dioica the author is convinced that in the Dominican Republic pringamosa is Urera baccifera (L.), which unlike the first is also native to the West Indies.

and love in the Dominican Republic (see Table 6). The widespread use of plants like rue, basil and the orange tree is related to the fact that all three plants are still used during baptism. The orange tree (exotic) is a prominent sacred tree, related to the manifestation of the Virgen de las Aguas Santas and also regionally thought to be related to the manifestation of the Virgin of Higüey. Again, exotic plants are used in combination with others – for example in order to drive away the malicious spirits azahar, lemon flowers and orange tree leaves are used. This combination would be used in baths with ingredients like water, holy water, floral waters and perfumes bought at *botánicas*.[269]

Regardless of religious affiliation, many contributors agreed that plants of use, and especially medicinal plants, were to be respected and protected. Mr. Benjamin Alcántara, a converted *evangelista* from Bánica, told about an accident that occurred many years ago to a former inhabitant of Bánica. According to his words, every large-size, beautiful tree has a *misterio*. A narrative about one of these, a *jobo* tree, illustrates how the agency of the *misterio* residing in this tree can be also detrimental to the human health. Instead of following the warning to leave this tree in its place, this Baniquero went to cut the *jobo* tree and consequently was fatally injured. *Jobo*, *ceiba* and *higo* are associated with a *misterio*, and as such cutting them down is prohibited among Baniqueros.[270] The *jobo* tree (Spondias spp.) was used to treat smallpox in this particular location. This is just one example among many trees that are inhabited by divine beings or spiritual entities. Across different locations, trees like almácigo, mango, *naranja*, *guano santo*, *piñón*, palm, ceiba, *caña brava*/bamboo, *jabílla*, and *higo* were regarded as having *misterio*.

Dominican landscapes are empowered by different miraculous plants. The power of plants is explained by sacred scriptures and teachings based on the underpinning beliefs of Catholicism, and 21 Division. One of the frequently mentioned trees was *Guano*, which is blessed on Palm Sunday. Orange tree and *pino* are also said to have miraculous properties on Holy Friday. Others like *cedro*, together with plants like *verbena* and *Rosa de Jericho,* are described in the Bible and were used for protection. Other trees were known in local religious histories as places of Marian manifestations. As the Virgin of Higuey appeared in the orange tree, the people in the surrounding area also used the leaves of orange trees for protection, bringing good luck and for curing cold, flu, anemia, and hepatitis. The hierophanies of Virgins in flora also occurred more recently. In Mamey, the Virgen de Altagracia appeared in a plant and so an altar was built on the property of the owner of the plant. In Loma Cabrera, the Virgin Mary appeared in

269 Azahar is popular in Spanish cleansing rituals until present. Certain species, registered as having ritual purposes among the Kalinago in Dominica (Hodge 1957) have also been used in Boyá and Jiguaní.

270 Benjamin Alcántara, who has been working in agriculture his whole life, narrated about the prohibition to cut the *jobo* tree: *"Look this tree is prohibited to be felled, it is tamarindo, it produces things, and the other you can cut because it does not. J: Was there a tree that had a mystery (misterio)? A: Yes, there are trees with misterio. Every huge tree full of leaves and branches (frondoso) every trees that is beautiful. There was a tree called and a man that went to cut it during the clearing of the forest in a ravine. This man already cut down the forest, the field (conuco) is already enclosed, only the huge jobo tree is left. He got a boy, because listen to me that the misterio really exist, and when he says tomorrow we are going to fell this jobo tree. When he wakes up in the morning, a guy arrives. The man arrives and greets him and they start to have a conversation and there is this old man until the sun is high in the sky and this man still there. He gets the boy and says come here, get the ax and go cut the tree because the man is still here. The boy went and goes to cut the tree with the ax, prú prú prú. And the man goes out and the other follows him, and the ...*

a mango tree. The media news items confirm that these manifestations were reported in different locations prior to the fieldwork. As such, the Marian revelation in a palm in Hoya Grande de Licey, the Virgen de Mercedes in a palm sector in La Gina in San Francisco de Macoris (2011), and the Virgen de Guadalupe in a Jabilla tree in San Juan (2014), entered into the memory of the wider public.

Some trees like ceiba, *jabílla*, bamboo, and palm were also agreed to have a *misterio* associated with them in 21 Division. However, there was often disagreement about the character of the *misterio*. As some of the *lwas* can be both detrimental and beneficial, followers of other Dominican religions emphasized the negative character of the *lwas*. For some Catholics and Evangelists Ceiba and Jabílla would be trees of the devil. The same trees are ultimately powerful and also miraculous for adherents of 21 Division. From their testimonies, it is clear that the ritual in which the agency of the *lwas* residing in these trees is invoked can be applied with different aims. These rituals are often directed at the removal of negative spells and at recovering one's wellbeing and health in general.

Activating the Healing Virtue of Dominican Plants

The healing virtue of plants is conditioned by following certain rules that apply to their collection. The collection of plants typically is done in accordance with the lunar cycle. Plants collected during the new moon are considered to be useless. Tree bark is preferably collected from the east side of the tree, the side on which the sun shines in the morning.[271] During the collection of medicinal plants with Luperona at Villa Isabella Mr. Lucillo Torres explained to me that medicinal plants can heal only if permission is asked. In his case, he asked permission silently before gathering each plant for his *botella*. This custom was widespread in the Dominican Republic and was practiced by both adherents of 21 Division and Catholics. The permission had to be asked not only for the plants used in ritual baths like *salvia*, *albahaca*, and *vencedor*, but also in the case of plants that were to be collected for *botellas*, in order to cure physical ailments.

In the Dominican Republic, unlike in Cuba, the person collecting the plant addressed the plant by the plants name, followed by a short explanation of the objective of the gathering, for example: "marjoram (mejorana), marjoram, marjoram, give me the permission to take you with me and use you for a bath". Mr. Hecfredes Gómez from Bánica also suggested that if leaves are collected before daybreak, it is necessary to shake the plant a bit, talk to it in order to wake the plant up: "*Wake up if you are*

...other tries to distract him, says this and that, but the first man says this is not possible already, go away, ay ay. When the boy cuts it, the man leaves, and the old man goes to where the boy is, and when he arrives he says him give me the axe, and when he goes to give a tree a blow like this pá´ and there at the same spot he starts to scream ah ah ah and the boy he brake his spine. R: did the tree felt? E: the boy already cut it, but the old man went to cut it in pieces... and they bring him home and there he stayed crippled until he passed away with the broken spine. So it was he who tried that did not go the one who hit him. R: he was avoiding him to go, and he kept avoiding to go. J: Let´s say that it was punishment? A: Yes, it was a punishment. There he stayed until he passed away. J: do you remember it or have you heard this? A: I knew this man he was the husband of Mamita who already passed away. J: Look, do people say about the ceiba that it is prohibited to cut? A: Yes, it is said you cannot fell it. J: Why? A: Because it is a tree that they say that has a un misterio hecho, this was a tree how the story says holy. J: Do you know what kind of misterio was living there? A: Yes, this misterio of a saint. I have not believed in this. J: But it is not important if you really believed it, I am interested in what is said. A: And it was really existing and it still exists really in higo it exists."

271 The contributors from Bánica and Sabana Larga suggested both West and East.

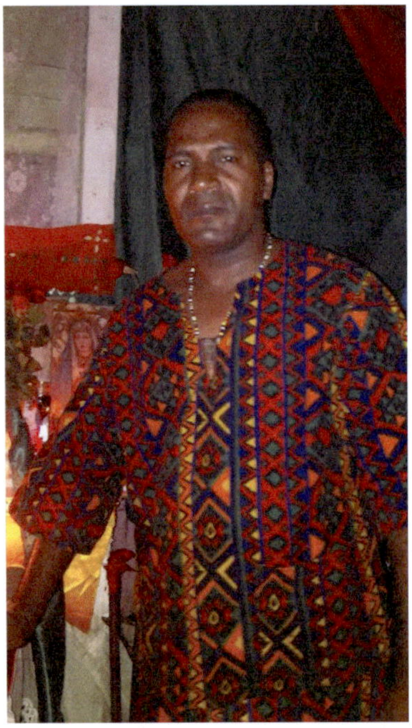

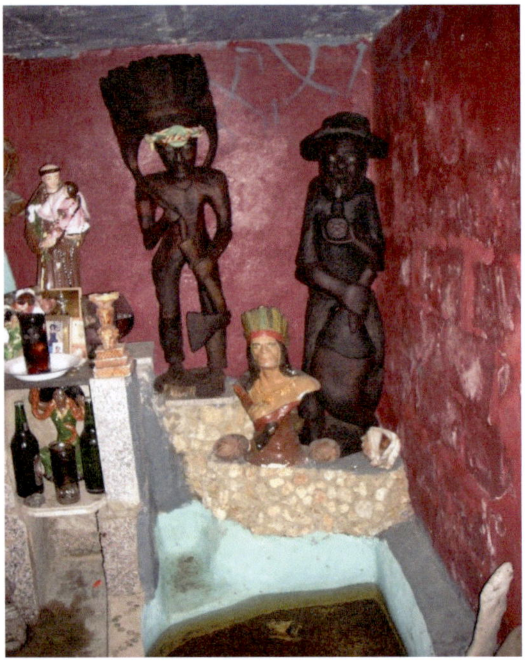

Figure 24 Giovani Guzman from Bajo de Haina, Dominican Republic.

Figure 25 A part of Giovani's altar dedicated to the indigenous lwa, in Bajo de Haina, Dominican Republic.

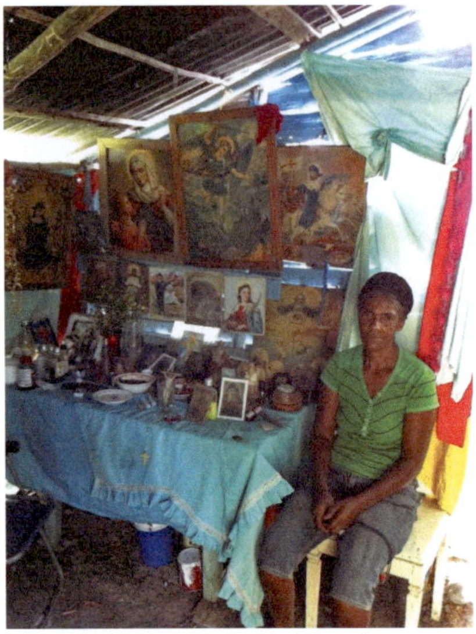

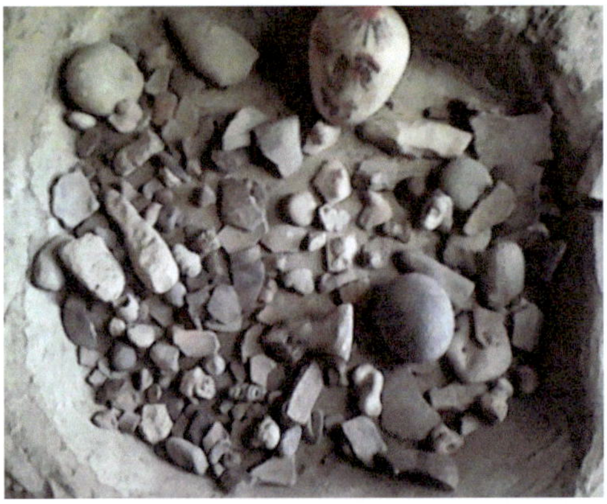

Figure 27 Ancestral indigenous objects at the altar of Estela Pérez from Arroyo de Agua. This is normally covered by water.

Figure 26 Estela Peréz, healer with her house-altar, Loma de Guayacánes, closeby to Mamey, Dominican Republic.

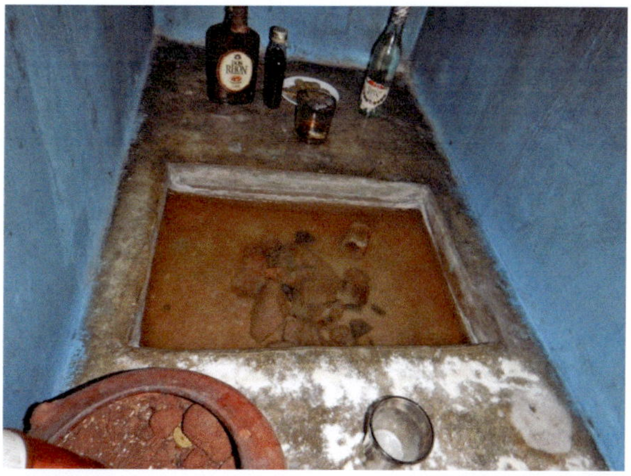

Figure 28 A part of an altar dedicated to indigenous misterios, region Boyá, Monte Plata.

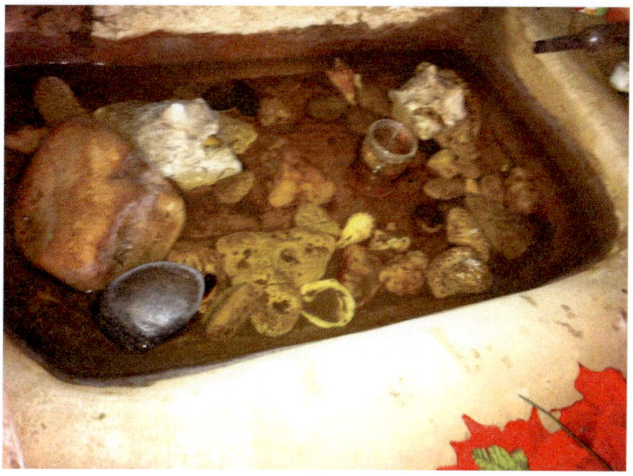

Figure 29 A part of an altar dedicated to indigenous misterios, in the left corner alive turtle, Monte Christi, Dominican Republic.

sleeping, I need you for this thing, and then she wakes up."[272] The prayers are often said quietly or just internally without uttering them.

Some contributors were convinced that every plant has a virtue and a *misterio*. One of the contributors, Mrs. Dorotea Mejía, a former traditional healer from Boyá explained further: "*Every plant has a misterio, every plant like we who are born in this world, because for sure you think that you do not have a misterio, but you do have because this misterio have chosen you to have this work that you are doing, so you have this misterio because everyone who is born on this world is born with a misterio. There are people who say that it is not the case but, if they had not their misterio they would not come to this world, isn't it true? They would stay in the space, lost there."*[273]

By asking the plant for its consent to be collected the healing virtue is activated. Mrs. Dorotea Mejía asked for permission in the following way: "*Maria de los Remedios I need this plant for… (makes a pause), in my hand I receive this in the name of the Father, the Son, and Holy Spirit."* And she added: "*If you take such a thing without praying to the God and the Virgen to whom do you think this can be beneficial? To nobody. Everything*

272 Interview with Hecfredez Bánica. He suggests that this has a scientific explanation because when touching it the process of the acquisition of the oxygen changes.

273 Interview with Mrs. Dorotea Mejía from Boyá.

comes because the Lords permits it." She also remembered that people have been asking for permission directly to the plants and clarified that this was done because: *"I had the faith in the plant, that the plant could help me and do what I wanted her to do, so I was asking her to provide me the permission... And this is done with every plant. If this one I am going to take for the bath, I will take it for bath, If am going to take it for the bottle, I take it for the bottle, I take it with the misterio she has, because she has a misterio, maybe I do not know what misterio it is, but if you think of her when wanting to prepare the bottle she herself gives me the strength and power. This is because of the misterio that she has."*

Cuban Medicinal Plants

The medicinal use of plants in Cuba is as rich as in the Dominican Republic. In general, herbal mixtures for oral use are prepared in the form of teas and contain fewer ingredients than the Dominican *botellas*. To illustrate some of the medicinal uses, the data from Jiguaní are summarized in the appendix. As previously indicated (chapter 5), Jiguaní is a location with a long presence of indigenous people. Like in the Boyá case, it is clear that the majority of plants used in this location were native to the New World while others were of Old World origins (25%, including 8% which were of both origins, or could be recognized on the level of taxa). Many plants mentioned in Boyá are also used in Jiguaní, and sometimes they are used in a similar way (see *e.g. apasote, albahaca, anamú, guanábana, guyaba, higüero, bejuco indio, piñón, ruda*, and tobacco). Roman Catholicism and *Espiritismo del Cordón* are the two major religious affiliations in Jiguaní. In local *Espiritismo* every commission has its own plant. These vary according to the teachings of different centers and associations. Several plants that are exotic to the regions were used in the ritual realm too. For purifying baths, we also find plants native to the New World like *amansaguapo, quebracho, espante muerto, hierba de aura*, and *caimito de cimarrón*, but also exotic plants like *vencedor*. For clearing the mind, one combines three *albahacas, mentas*, and *vervenas*, and drinks these together with clear water from different sources. Some contributors (*e.g.* Mr. Orestes Iganacio Zalazar Gonzáles) use aromatic herbs like *vencedor, salvia, quebracho, caimito*, and *yagruma* in ritual baths because of their aromatic character. Again, similar to what is the case in Boyá, the scent of certain plants is considered to attract positivity or ward off negativity, so for example baths of *anamú* (which has a strong, rather unpleasant smell) were used to remove dark spirits of the dead, which were sent to harm their victims. In the case of a whole household being persecuted by malicious spirits, seven branches of *anamú* are tied up with a red ribbon and placed behind the door.

The religious diversity in Cuban society implies that certain features of the Cuban landscape have multiple meanings. The ceiba tree is one example. As in the Dominican Republic, in Jiguaní and also other locations the ceiba was said to have a dark and a clear side, where rituals for the improvement of general wellbeing take place. The ceiba is said to fulfill all kinds of wishes, good and bad. The latter concern also are said to be asked for by ritual means after midnight. This fits within a broad national belief that the ceiba is a sacred tree: in Cuba it is widely acknowledged that the ceiba tree should be treated with respect and should not be cut. As the lifespan of the ceiba spans several generations, it is also widely believed that it is the place where the dead go. For some, the ceiba is a place where all *orishas* go, or at least some like Changó and Yemayá.

Among Catholics in rural areas of the East, the ceiba is believed to have offered refuge to the Virgin Mary. When the Virgin was a fugitive, the ceiba opened to shelter her, and covered her with spines to protect her and Jesus in Cuba. Both Catholics and Espiritistas have respect for the ceiba. As Mrs. Rosalina Segura Hidalgo from Barajagua puts it: *"The ceiba everyone respects, because she has saved the Virgin. People were putting candles there and were leaving yellow flowers."* At the foot of the ceibas we may indeed find candle holders, images of San Lázaro, bundles of plants, fruits, coins, corn, peanuts, the rest of the cocoa, and calabashes, all product of continuing ritual practices. A combination of different plants in a bundle is usually deposited at this sacred tree in Barajagua. The example of the ceiba shows that symbols from local flora sometimes synthesize different meanings from diverse religions. The status of local ceibas is reinforced by the fame of one ceiba at a *templete* in Havana where, on the night of 15th December, just before the day when Diego Velazquez established the city of Havana at this place reportedly celebrated the first mass on the island, pilgrims circle the trunk of a ceiba three times while praying with love and faith and offering coins. For followers of *Regla de Ocha*, the ceiba is the most sacred, it is the mayor tree of *monte*, the main force, a place where different *orishas* can gather. Firstly, the ceiba represents *Iroko*, the female materialization of Obatalá: *"Obatalá has various paths, there is female and male, ceiba represent Iroko, the female denomination of Obatalá. There is Obatalá Ayaguna, who is a warrior. Obatalá Osaliñan, Ochalá (female), Obamoró (male)."* For some, the ceiba is a place where all *orishas* go, or at least some like Changó and Yemayá. [274] The example of the ceiba shows that symbols from local flora sometimes synthesize different meanings from diverse religions.

The diversity of the interpretations of landscapes further increases when we consider Palo de Monte, Catholicism, and in some zones, Haitian Vudu.[275] In short, trees such as *guano santo, palmera, cedro, anacagüita*, and *piñón* were perceived to be the domain of divine beings and spiritual entities across Cuban religions. In addition, herbs of exotic origin such as *albahaca, artemisa, anamú, sábila, vencedor, vervena, mejorana*, and *ruda* are used across different religious affiliations for ritual purposes.[276]

In religious contexts, the selection and the application of plants are related to the narratives of their origin and hagiographies. Some of these are described according to principles of *Regla de Ocha*. During consultations, plants are advised as remedies that can be ingested, or be used in baths, served as offerings, and be used for the preparation of amulets and sacred objects. The selection of plants is based on the (spiritual) "owners" of the plant, the *orishas*. These *orishas* have different specializations for curing illness, and different preferences regarding offerings. The intrinsic characteristics of the plant, its medicinal properties, its growth form, color, scent, the hardness of the wood, the life cycle, including the durability, are often associated with the character and specializations of their *orishas*. The color of the flowers, for example, can be linked symbolically to attributes such as dress. Ochún, associated with the Virgen of Charity and like her dressed in gold, is offered yellow flowers like *marilope* or *botón de oro*. Similarly, red and white flowers are offered to Changó (palm), associated with

274 Interview no. 190331.

275 Cuban Haitians consider also mapú, higuero, ceiba, higo, bambú, jabía to be sacred trees.

276 There are more cases, for example: the sunflower in Espiritismo del Cordon in Jiguaní represents the Indigenous commission, but it represents Shango (Santa Bárbara) in Regla de Ocha in the same location.

Santa Bárbara. The hardness of wood is seen as crucial and is associated with personal characteristics of *orishas*, symbolizing the resistance of Ogún the Warrior. The name of the plant may also indicate its use as well as its patron *orisha*: *abre camino* is of Elegua, *vencedor* of Changó. As for the form of growth: a plant whose parts get entangled with others could be used for a spell on another person in order to entangle his or her endeavors. It is possible that the association of the plants and deities in this way functions as a mnemonic tool, to remember what plant serves for what ailment, as the deities are often specialized in specific illnesses. As San Lázaro helps to cure sores and leprosy, his plants are those that serve this purpose.

The knowledge of what each plant is and of the *orisha* to which it belongs is transmitted during initiation. This knowledge is important for healing ailments, but also for distinct ceremonies in which herbs play a role. According to Mr. Harvin Ramírez Reyes from Jiguaní, *bayoneta* and *pionia* (pueriyeye) have to be present during all ceremonies. Each *orisha* has its own group of plants. Ogún's plants are *yerbafina*, *rompesaraguey*, *atipola*, *peregún*, *aguacate*, *caña santa*, and *cortacalentura*. Ogún's vessel is a bath with *verdolaga*, *hierba fina*, *mastuerzo*, *peregún*, *buereyeye*, and *bleo blanco*. *Marpacífico*, *embeleso* (a blue colour), *orosún*, and *cucaracha morada*, all belong to Yemayá, an *orisha* who protects travellers and opens the roads. In the case of *marpacífico*, it is the name that indicates its use instead of its color (red flowers). Lastly, among the plants that belong to Obatalá, the owner of all ideas who lives on the top of the mountain, are *guanábana*, *almendro*, *seso vegetal*, *algodón*, and the ceiba. Offerings to Obatalá can be made at a mountain but also at the foot of the ceiba tree.

Knowledge of the religious underpinnings for the selection of the plants is of importance when preparing offerings that are to be served to *orishas* during celebrations. For Santa Bárbara: *harina de maíz* with meat, Yemayá: *natílla*, and again tobacco are popular offerings.

Bambú is used for a ceremony to Anatu, for whom a knife is used later for an animal sacrifice. These are just a few examples of the multiple meanings of Cuban flora for adherents of *Regla de Ocha*.

Collecting Healing Plants in Cuba

Among adherents of the Roman Catholic church and the Cuban *Espiritismo*, some of the plants like *romero* and *mejorana*, are offered a coin (or are rewarded by coin) if later used in baths. Many of the prayers and requests for permission are specific to the particular moment, when the plants are collected with a particular objective (mentioned in the prayer). In *Espiritismo Cruzado*, the healing virtue of the ceiba, being a sacred tree, was addressed in the following chant, accompanied by ringing a small iron bell: "*They baptized me in La Cañambo, in La Cañambo they baptized me, all Saints you have to come to this ceiba tree, Mother Ceiba is my godmother and my godfather is the caguayran tree. They baptized me in La Cañambo, in La Cañambo they baptized me. All saints must come to this ceiba. Glory to God, glory to the Orishas!*"[277] In general, trees that are famous

277 Interview with the healer from the temple of Charity and Peace in Niquero.

for being used for rituals in other religious traditions (*e.g.* the use of the palm oil tree in *Regla de Ocha*) are also respected or avoided in those religious traditions.[278]

In the realm of *Regla de Ocha*, it is believed that not everyone can collect the plants used for healing. In order to be able to collect plants, one has to undergo liturgical and philosophical training. One of these specialists is the *osainista*, a specialist who has profound knowledge of the medicinal and other sacred properties of the plants. Before the collection he performs a ceremony that prepares the plant for the specific problem that it is going to be used for. This ceremony begins with a ritual dedicated to Osain, the *orisha* of all herbs, and nature itself, considered by some to be the Lord of the Mountain, *Dueño del Monte* (*manigua*), who is asked to give his consent to enter. The reason for the visit is explained to him and offerings (tobacco) are given. Afterwards, a specific *orisha* to whom the plant belongs is asked for permission. These plants are used as offerings to these divine powers or as a cure in which the corresponding *orisha* is invoked. Orishas have their own histories, characters, and preferences regarding the plant offerings. Some plants are manifestations/representations of the *orishas* themselves. Every herb has its own song, which empowers the plant and helps with the specific problem that the patient has.[279] The objective of the collection of the plants is crucial. Thus, for example, when gathering a plant that will later be used for the protection of one's home, after praying to Osain, one would ask permission also from Ogún del Monte, San Silvestre del Monte, and Santa Inés del Monte. As plants like *yaya*, and *yagruma* belong to Changó, a prayer would also be dedicated to this *orisha*.[280]

Poetic remembering of flora

The transfer of knowledge about the medicinal and ritual use of plants does not seem to be restricted to specialists. Healers, however, have an important role in their communities, as they are the ones who usually have a more profound and detailed knowledge about the variety of medicinal uses and rich symbolism that the flora can have. As well as healers, herbalists, therapists, and midwives, also agriculturalists, caretakers, patients, participants of collective celebrations, and other members of the broader community can acquire (snippets of) knowledge about the ritual and medicinal value of plants. As for the means of transmitting botanical knowledge, in addition to traditional means like oral tradition or participation in healing consultations, one should consider collective ceremonies (*cordón*, celebrations dedicated to *lwas*, *orishas*, and Saints) as well as the role of institutions and available literature. Especially in Cuba, Radio Rebelde's programs explaining the specific characteristics of medicinal plants contribute to the valorization and preservation of the medicinal flora. Also, research into the medicinal properties of plants together with the affordability of books and the distribution of herbal remedies through official institutions, like green pharmacies, all seem to contribute to the preservation of botanical knowledge in Cuba.

278 Close to Niquero there is a popular ritual place where a huge ceiba tree is surrounded by palm trees. Before we entered this place together, one of the local devotees of Spiritism said: "Give me the license to be able to reach you and to be able to see and recognize the capacity, and the things that you have there in your depository, we are going to visit you, a group of people who are here for research purposes, nothing religious, please give us the license to enter."

279 Interview with initiated person of Regla de Ocha in Holguín.

280 Interview with initiated person of Regla de Ocha in Holguín.

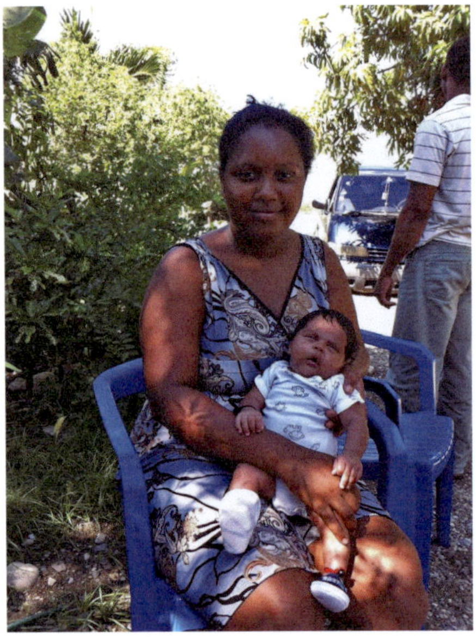

Figure 30 Mrs. Torres with her daughter who is protected with a bracelet against the evil eye, Proyecto, Mamey, Dominican Republic.

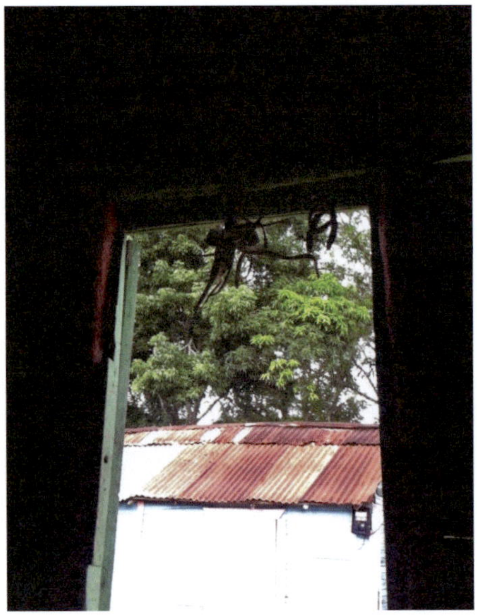

Figure 31 Aloe Vera and horseshoe protecting an entrance of a house in Cacique, closeby Boyá, Dominican Republic.

The centrality of the flora in the daily life of humans also offers itself as a theme for oral poetry. In this way, oral poetry is a means of remembering and transmitting knowledge. This can take the form of sacred speech, invoking the powers of the *orishas*, but can also be designed with the aim of teaching the broader public. The latter possibility seems to explain the popularity of the *siguaraya* tree. The *siguaraya* was recognized as sacred, and was respected across different religious affiliations. Some of the contributors immediately recalled this tree as the first or as the only one that needs to be paid before taking its leaves and even referred to a song from Oscar de Leon which talks about its power. This tree cannot be cut down without asking permission beforehand, because it is an *orisha*.[281] In *Regla de Ocha*, the *siguaraya*, as well as other trees like palm, belongs to Chango, but also to Ellegua, important *orishas*. It is considered to be a tree for the *fundamento*, and for *nganga*.[282] *Nganga* is an animated subject represented in an iron vessel with a combination of secret ingredients, *i.e.* human remains, and parts of specific kinds of trees.[283] Details such as which specific *orisha* is associated with this tree were not known among the contributors, who were not familiar with the teachings of this specific religion.

281 Similarly, also Puerto Rican singer Héctor Lavoe has written a song "Rompezaraüey", with similar lyrics indicating that one should be cautious of the Saints and do the ritual bathing.

282 Interview no. 19033.

283 Secret ingredients including human remains are brought together to create a new sacred and powerfull object, *nganga*. Among the powerful trees used for *nganga* are: la ciguaraya, el jibá, la yaya, la cuaba, el jiquí, el caguairán, la guácima, el carbonero, la algarroba, la guajaca. Interview no. 190331. For more information see Dodson et al. (2008).

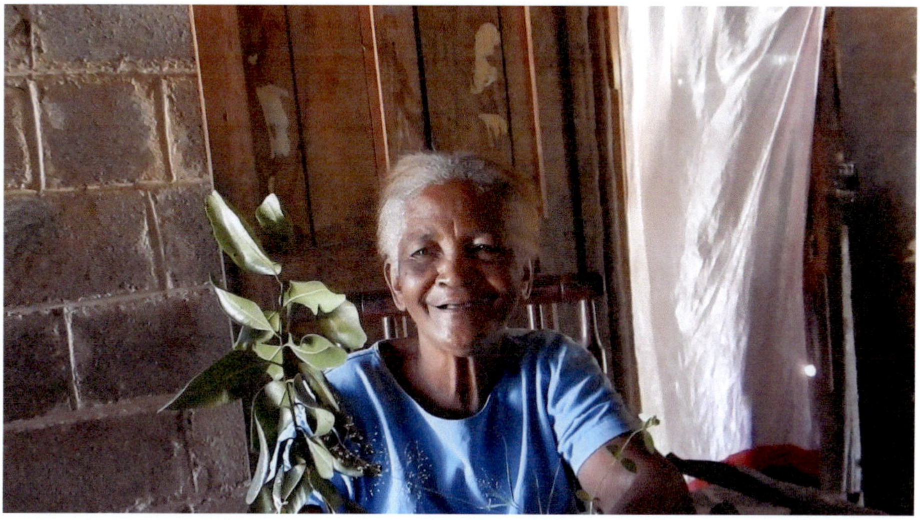

Figure 32 Mrs. Dorotea Mejía, former traditional healer from Boyá, Dominican Republic.

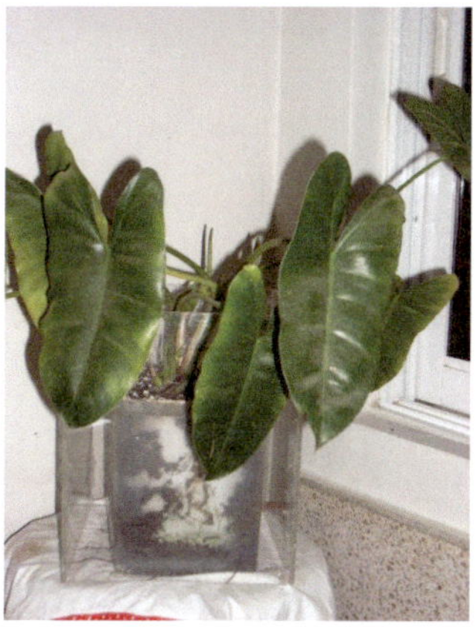

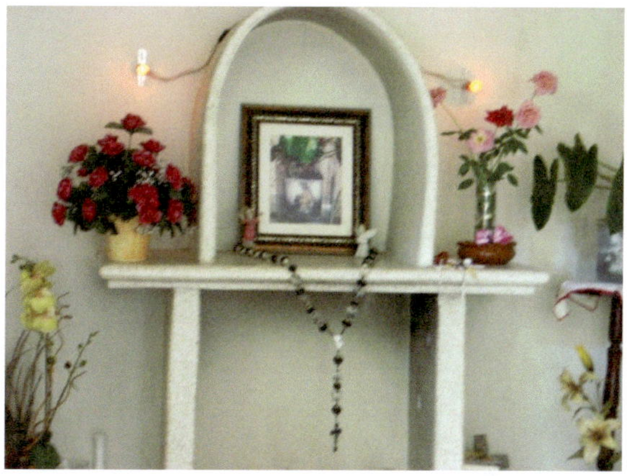

Figure 33 Left: The Virgen manifested in this plant in Mamey, Dominican Republic. Right: a small altar built to remember this manifestation the photograph of which is in the middle.

From Jiguaní there is clear evidence that the knowledge of the spiritual importance of plants is transferred through religious music at healing ceremonies in Cuban *Espiritismo del Cordón* and *Espiritismo Cruzado*, but also through songs that are sung in a secular context. The latter songs may transmit certain information about the spiritual importance of specific landscape features. Mr. Anaya, a renowned *decimero* in Jiguaní, who grow up in spiritualist tradition, sang us this song[284]:

284 *Decimero* is a type of singer or poet who is reciting or singing *décimas*, which are ten-line stanzas. Some of these are sung for amusement. The topics of these *décimas* can vary from love to politics. They are often improvised and include ambiguous cues, critique or jokes.

Voy a contarle una cosa que muy admirable es,
Voy a contarle una cosa que muy admirable es,
De una calabaza que he cosechado en mi choza.
Una ceiba portentosa la guía,
Podré igualar para empezarle a contar de la calabaza mía.
Partí y adentro tenía diez máquinas y un central,
La calabaza tenía una mina de oro y plata,
Y muchísima fruta y mata que ni yo la conocía,
Una arboleda tenia de marañones y zapote
Una iglesia y su sacerdote y un pastor y muchas ovejas
Y en cada esquina una vieja empinando papalote.
La calabaza tenía algunos misterios más,
De diez cordeles y un majá y más de cien mil jutias,
Cerca de mampostería, un cuartel y su escuadrón,
Y allá por mediación, ramal de una carretera,
Y si no me equivoco era la catedral de Japón.
En una semilla había más de mil habitaciones,
Quinientos puercos cebones y mil objetos de cría,
Una luz también había cambiante como la luna,
Y el que quiera tener una Santo que se la mande, (Santo soy yo)
Que calabaza grande como esa no hay ninguna.

This song contains playful references not only to a powerful ceiba tree but also to an admirable *calabaza* full of miraculous symbols of richness and fertility. In *Regla de Ocha*, the *calabaza* (*Curcubita maxima* or *Curcubita pepo*) is also used in rituals for attracting good fortune and positive developments when praying to God and Ochún, who is said to be the (spiritual) owner (*Dueña*) of the pumpkin.[285] Cubans also use pumpkin seeds against parasites and for the prostate. Similarly, Dominican *Auyama* (*Curcubita pepo*) is believed to be a symbol of fertility. Mrs. Elia Torres from Villa Isabela recalls: "*It is said that when a pregnant woman moves with the plant leaves there are going to be more auyamas. Other people say that when the auyama has many flowers these are collected, and spread over the street where people step on them like this there will be more auyamas, but I am not sure if it is the truth.*" Auyama is also medicinal, for cleaning the uterus after childbirth; the seeds are used for eyesight, and are also said to be good for constipation, against parasites, and for the heart.[286]

Oral poetry, as an important means of transfer of information, can be vital for the preservation of knowledge, not only concerning medicinal uses but also concerning other uses. Mr. Santos Anaya knew another song about a *maraca* made from *güira*:

En el mundo se desata, oye el canto que me inspira
Ahora te voy a explicar como se hace la maraca
Se coge la güira, se le abre un hoyito, se le sacan las tripas y se pone a secar
Y ahora por buenas razones se le echan las municiones

---

285 Interview no. 152257.

286 Farmers in Jiguaní use to tie the tip of yucca in three parts so that the plague does not affect them (María Palmares from Jiguaní).

Se coge un palito, se le abre un hoyito y ya está, óyela como resuena ya
Pobre mi maraquita, óyela como re resuena ya.

Maracas are still one of the major traditional instruments used in Cuban and Dominican music. During fieldwork I could observe their use only twice, in both cases in Cuban centers of *Espiritismo* (one in Barajagua and the other in Niquero) and I saw them on altars in Pedro Santana and Bánica. As Mr. Anaya suggests, *maracas* are made of *güira* (*Crescentia cujete)*, which has also been used for the preparation of another traditional musical instrument of a similar name: *Güiro* and in the Dominican Republic *Güira.* While Dominican *Güiras* are now placed by *Guayo* (metallic graters), they are also an important component in sacred chants for making the *lwas* descend. In both islands, *Crescentia cujete* (C: *Güiro, Higüero,* D: *Jigüero, Higüero, Jícara*) has been an important material for domestic utensils like plates, spoons, and water receptacles (of a different type, but still called *higüero* (*Lagenaria siceraria* or *Agenaria vulgaris*). Like *Curcubita maxima, Crescentia cujete* has also medicinal uses. The inner part is used in *botellas* for cleansing vaginal infections, and cleansing after giving birth. Leaves are also used for bruises, and blood circulation.

Ancestral roots and rhizomes

Having presented the general features of animated landscapes in the Dominican Republic and Cuba, some etiologies, the roles of healers, and their interaction with medicinal plants, we may observe several similarities when reading these in relation to historical descriptions or more recent ethnographic accounts.

The above-mentioned healers fulfilled a whole series of ritual services to their communities like spiritual protection, life advice, guarding the life and wellbeing of the community at large. Their multifunctional role could be compared to that of other religious specialists, *e.g.* shamans in Siberia, the *pyjai* of the Kaliña people, different ritual specialists among the Wolof, or Spanish healers. The first more detailed written reference to Caribbean indigenous persons who cured other people (Pané 1498) calls them *behiques* (or *bohuti*, in Las Casas: *bohique*). According to that source, *behiques* are intermediaries between the living and the dead, and between the living and divine beings. A healing session was initiated by an action in which the *behique* and the patient purged themselves (with a plant called gueio, gioia, gueio, or zacón), chanted (ritual prayers) and inhaled cohoba (snuff).[287] Similarly, Kalinago ritual specialists, called *boyé* (*boyáicou, niboyeiri*), contacted the invisible world through tobacco smoke and chanting (Breton 1665). More specifically, *boyé's* made "*the god descend, after which the deity is to be seated and to have a meal and drink*" in times of illness and at other occasions (Breton 1665). The contemporary use of tobacco by Dominican and Cuban healing practitioners as a means of communication with the invisible world resembles the one described by Breton. One of the documents dated to the end of the 16th century when discussing the habits of indigenous peoples of Hispaniola explicitly says that this plant was considered to be sacred (AGI, Patronato 18, N.1, R. 13). The ritual

287 In this identification, Arrom (the editor/commentator of Pané's text) followed Ortiz who suggested that this plant could be a plant used in the Guyanas called *weya*.

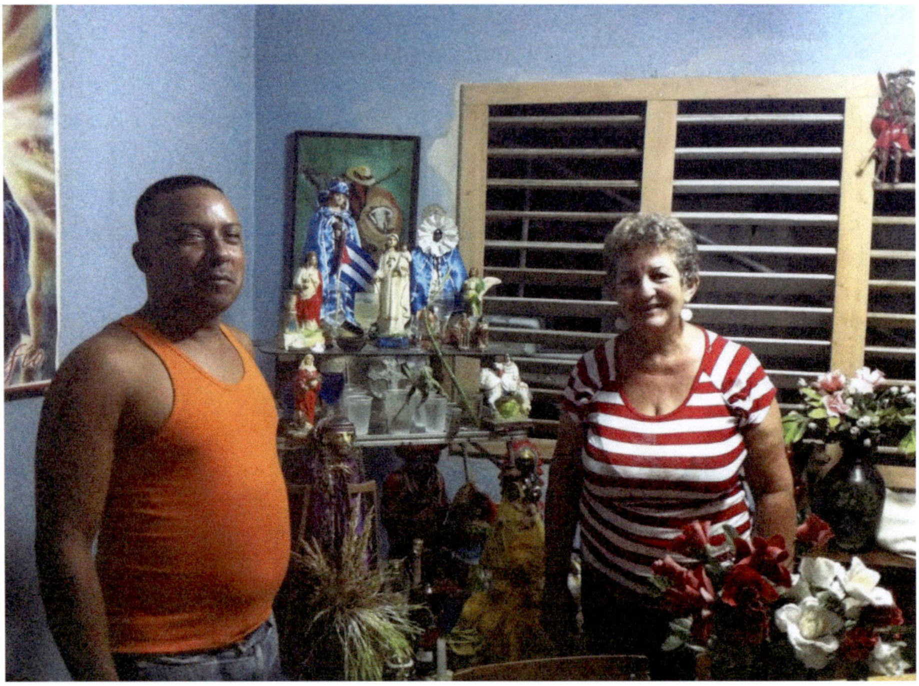

Figure 34 Mr. Harvin Ramírez Reyes, initiated in Regla de Ocha and Mrs. María Palomares, my guide from Jiguaní, Cuba.

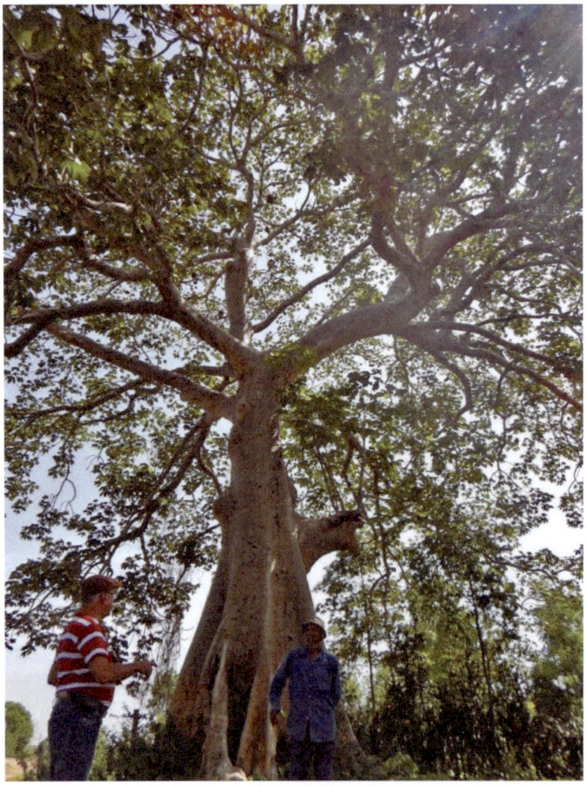

Figure 35 Mr. Armas and Mendoza under the mysterious anacaüita in Guao, Jiguaní, Cuba.

importance returns in the origin narrative about Maruka and Siniimari who received arrowroot from the Master Boa to make their charms. The exhalation of air or tobacco smoke in the process of saying a prayer or chant intended to facilitate the arrival of positive spiritual entities was also registered among indigenous peoples of Suriname (De Goeje 1943; Henfrey 2002).

The communication with the invisible world that takes form through dreams, visions, and an embodiment of divine entities and spirits in 21 Division, Regla de Ocha and in Cord Spiritism have their parallels in other parts of the world.[288] There isn´t consensus about whether the soul (or one of the different souls a person may have) leaves the body during a dream but the general idea is that when asleep the devotees – also those who have not been initiated – might sometimes communicate with the spirits of the deceased or with divine entities. Again, this type of experience can be found across different worldviews including those of the Wayuú (Perrin 1987).

The interaction with the divine being may also occur through its incarnation or embodiment in the medium, *caballo del misterio* or *babalawo*. Århem (2016) compared this with the ideas of Amazon perspectivism and South-East Asian animism, where it is characterized by the occurrence of a particular set of cultural expressions. In animism the spirit possession, ancestor worship, animal sacrifice and attention to a panoply of nature spirits were seen as normally accompanying each other. In perspectivism the magical flight and metamorphosis were argued to be the predominant elements of the altered state of consciousness. Within perspectivism, shapeshifting is seen as necessary for adopting the other point of view that is important in order to harness the wellbeing of the community. According to Århem's model the present-day Caribbean expressions of this relation fit more into the South East Asian model of animism while the shapeshifting resembles transformations in the origin narratives described by Pané or those from the mainland by de Goeje (1943).

Following strictly Århem´s model it would be unlikely to find Cuban and Dominican shapeshifters such as *galipotes*, *cagüeyros* or *bakás* whose major characteristics was their ability to transform from a person into an animal or object in a system where also ritual specialists may incarnate or embody a spiritual entity. Yet, both are common in the Cuban and Dominican context.

Based on the fragmentary sources it is difficult to reconstruct how the communication with the invisible world was experienced and articulated by the indigenous *behiques*. Both Pané and Breton suggest that this specialist approached the invisible world in an altered state of consciousness, and that the divine entities were believed to be present at the location. Among the Kalinago these divine beings were believed to be seated – and in one occasion also to enter – in the body of the men and to speak through them (Breton 1665, p. 6).[289] Breton´s interpretation might have been influenced by Catholic beliefs about demons, which could possess human bodies but which also could be exorcised.

---

288 While in 21 Division and Regla de Ocha the ritual specialist is the person that voice and incarnate, in the Cord Spiritism the medium that falls into trance passes the spiritual entity to a medium that can voice it.

289 See also Du Tetre 1650.

Many West African deities and semi-divine beings have multiple representations/ manifestations and may transform their appearances, and so may the religious specialists, which in the colonial idiom are typically referred to as "witches", *i.e.* persons considered to exercise "black magic" (Herskovits 1938). The present-day dominant incarnations of *lwas*, spirits and orishas (*e.g.* the focus on the head) display West African influences. Among the Yoruba (Bascom 1969) or Fon (Herkovists 1933) the body can be a vessel or medium for the spiritual beings.[290] Among the Garifuna (Bianchi 1989), who are seen as carriers of both African and indigenous heritage, this relation is described as "possession".

In spite of the constant demonization of the agents of such transformations in Europe and the Caribbean, the idea of shapeshifting was not completely alien to non-Christian European worldviews (*e.g.* the Norse Loki, the Greek Proteus and the *Metamorphoses* of Ovidius), and it has persisted through the centuries. Future investigations that would collect more information on the ritual specialists that articulate these relations as physical transformations and incarnations of the divine and spiritual entities have great potential to contribute to the studies of these religious expressions worldwide.

Parallels with the aforementioned concepts of illness may be also observed in other cultures. Some of these concepts such as the evil eye or soul loss are ways how the experience of the illness is described across different cultures, including Fon, Spanish, or Garifuna (Herskovits 1933, Christian 1989, Bianchi 1989).[291] The coral beads along with a jet bead commonly used in 16th Spain for protection against evil eye was found in a indigenous child's burial in Chorro de Maíta (Valcárcel Rojas 2013). The presence of these objects might also be explained as an integration of popular Catholic beliefs (with North African influences prior to 1492) among the indigenous ancestors. Such integration might be even more likely as it fitted easily within the indigenous or African worldviews, which held similar ideas. The fact that multiple plants and amulets, like the Sapondus saponaria (jaboncillo, mate negro) is also called called jet, are used for spiritual protection until today, suggests that this concern about one´s protection is an intrinsic part of the Cuban and Dominican religious traditions.

Soul loss as a possible explanation of illness is also found in West Africa and in Spain, where sorcerers were said to be responsible for soul capture (Hoyos Sainz 1947). In Spain the soul of a deceased person may roam around, return to the place the person once lived, and in this condition it may be harmful; as a remedy sometimes food is placed in the grave-yard (Machado 1886). The capture of one of the souls has also been described in the Dahomean context, the idea of a double-soul being widespread in West Africa. Also in the Americas the notion of soul loss, fright (susto) or of the soul being taken by a spirit of the earth is a common part of the theory of illness.

Locally, the analysis of details about soul loss may follow various lines of interpretation. One of the Baniqueros explained that the incarnation of 'Carib spirits' is an experience that feels like being devoured from inside. This description might be

---

290 Among Fon and Yoruba the deity enters into the head. This resembles the present-day ritual incarnation of *lwas* and *orishas* explained to me during fieldwork.

291 In the light of research that correlates the emotion of envy with the psychological and physical well-being of the envying person (Smith et al. 2010), the evil eye concept may summarize the ancestral insights about how such feelings can disturb social relations and one's own mental health.

derived from the stereotypical image of Caribs as cannibals that are believed to have violently attacked the peaceful Arawaks. The phrasing of this explanation may have been influenced by the Haitian Creole concept of *lwakapmanje.* My colleague Sony Jean commented on this (in 2018)*:"Lwa kap manje, literally translates as: the lwa is eating him/her. In Haiti this expression is used to refer to sick people who are troubled by lwas. It could be a person who has an arrangement with the lwa to protect the family, to improve economic problems, or something else. When the person doesn't fulfill the promise, if he/her doesn't make ceremonies for the lwa, or doesn't offer the lwa food, the lwa as a revenge can attack this person or a member of his family. There is another meaning of this expression. A person can force a lwa to eat another, because of the dispute between these persons. The hater can force a lwa to make the other sick until this person passes away. This is considered an act of sorcery.*" In this context the cannibalism refers to the soul, or part of the soul, which is consumed, and thus does not encompass physical cannibalism, as suggested by Chanca and as illustrated by Bry´s infamous images of persons eating a fellow human.[292] Descola has confirmed that the cannibalistic ingestion is executed by Masters of Animals who punish Jívaro for their excessive hunting (1996). Similarly, the Araweté believe that components of the soul are eaten and immortalized by the gods (Viveiros de Castro 1992; see also Århem 2016).

Among various peoples that speak an Arawakan language as well as among other indigenous peoples of the Americas illness and death were commonly seen as a result of neglecting certain prohibitions, disrespecting certain places, or of an imbalance between the natural environment and people.

The prohibitions of felling certain sacred trees have in the past often been interpreted as guarding and enhancing the ecological diversity. In the context of healing practices it is clear that the violation of these prohibitions can have negative consequences for health. The powers residing in the flora are both potentially detrimental and beneficial to humans. The customs to ask the tree, plant, or their keepers or spiritual beings that are residing inside for allowance to cut them down or collect them is one of the cultural referents to the importance of a respectful relation between man and natural forces. Similar practices may also be found in both the Americas and Africa. When a tree has a spiritual power this has to be placated before cutting it (for example when clearing the fields, cf. De Goeje 1943). In Regla de Ocha there are similar views, which are likely to have originated in West Africa and which may have fused later with ideas already existing in the Caribbean.

Injuries, illness or bad luck can also result of violating the prohibition to fell ceiba trees in the Cuban context. In Cuba and the Dominican Republic the *ceiba pentandra* or 'silk cotton tree' is protected in this manner. Also among Caribs speaking groups in Suriname it is forbidden to cut the silk cotton tree because it harbors different spiritual beings including the Amarari serpent, snake grandfather, who is a powerful helper of

---

292 A Dominican contributor referred to the devouring being as a person, in this case just "Caribs". This could provoke misunderstandings, as to whether the statement refers to a person or to spirits. Like in other interviews, this contributor confirmed that he is referring to spirits. Without convincing archaeological evidence to support European reports about cannibalism in the Lesser Antilles, one of the possible avenues to understanding past descriptions of such acts is to consider the flaws of intercultural communication. Arens (1979) and Sued Badillo (1978) has previously deconstructed the historical portrayals of cannibalism among the Kalinago of Lesser Antilles.

the healers (Van Andel & Ruysschaert 2011). Many Cubans consider the ceiba a sacred tree, one that protects the Virgin and is the marker of the place where all deceased depart. As in Cuba, the ceiba is a sacred tree for many indigenous peoples in Middle and South America. For Patamuna (Guyanas) and Mayas this silk cotton tree is a connection between sky and earth, between divinities and humans. For Patamunas it is the First Tree. It was also the beginning of the creation of the first animals by the first ancestors. At the same time, it is also the place where bush spirits and dark shamans can conceal themselves (Whitehead 2003).

The ceiba is widespread throughout the tropics so that the enslaved people coming to the Caribbean likely recognized the tree (Voeks & Rashford 2013; Stedman 2013).[293] In Ghana there is also a prohibition to fell this tree and it is thought to be inhabited by various spiritual beings, while in Benin and Gabon the ceiba is a sacred tree too (Quiroz 2015). For followers of *Regla de Ocha*, the ceiba is the most sacred, it is the mayor tree of *monte*, the main force, a place where all *orishas* can gather including *Irokó,* Changó, and Yemayá.[294] In Benin and Gabon another sacred tree is known: *iroko* (milicia excelsa), which like the ceiba is a very large tree (Quiroz 2015).

Another example of an injury that was a consequence of a violation of the prohibition to cut the *jobo* tree (the hog plum) was in Bánica. The parallels in the symbolism of the plum-tree among the indigenous peoples of the Caribbean and those of Guyanas offer us also new light on the sacred narratives as analyzed by Pané. The first women of the Arawaks, Makushi and Warao were fashioned from a hog-plum tree, a tree that has an extreme vegetative power (De Goeje 1943). In one of the Arawakan narratives, Nahakoboni, an ancestor healer, carved his daughter out of a plum-tree. The healer cut and carved the timber so skillfully that his daughter became a woman lovely to gaze upon.[295] Even Yar, the sun himself, wanted that daughter as his wife (De Goeje 1943). In Suriname, this tree is the dwelling of the Serpent Spirit (probably Amarari, like in the case of the ceiba tree), which is the reason to not cut this tree (Van Andel & Ruysschaert 2011). In Pané´s narrative about the origin of the women who descended from trees, the quadruplets with their coarse hands caught them and tied an *inriri*, a woodpecker, to them, which thought they were wooden beams and subsequently carved out their sex. Although Pané did not specify what type of tree these were, they may well have been *jobo* trees as these were most likely considered powerful or sacred: later they figure in his text as the trees wherein primordial man was transformed into by the Sun.

The sacred value of the hog plum tree can also be seen in its medicinal and ritual use. The *jobo* tree (Spondias spp.) was used to treat smallpox in this particular location and in Jiguaní the same tree was used for baths and cleansing. In North-West Guyana its leaves are used as an abortifacient and to cure sores. The Kalinago from Dominica

---

293 Different lines of evidence like morphological divergence within African Ceiba, fossil pollen of Ceiba 13 000 old in Ghana, trade of a cultivated form of C. pentandra from West Africa dating to the 10th century indicate that Ceiba was not introduced into Africa by European traders (Dick et al. 2007).

294 Interview no. 190331.

295 Across the two islands a poem about a woodpecker or carpenter which made his woman of wood is retold for amusement of the public. This poem later tells about the infidelity of the woman and the naiveté of the man, and may also mock the hagiography of the biblical carpenter Saint Joseph. While the trope of woodpecker/carpenter also returns here it will remain an enigma as to whether this poem can be considered the remains of a desacralized origin narrative or if it is just a result of a local poetic creation.

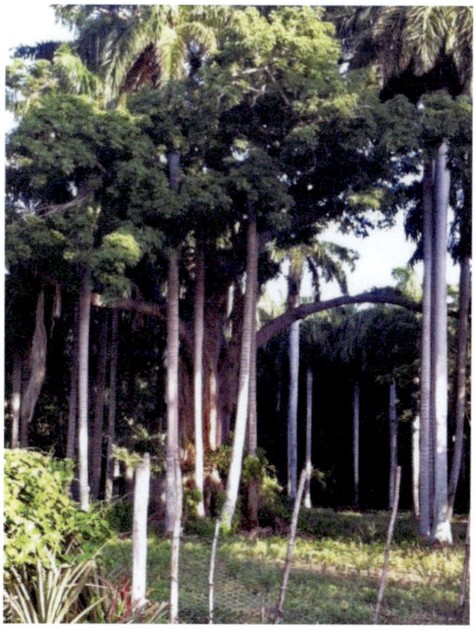

Figure 36 A sacred ceiba surrounded by palms in Niquero, Cuba.

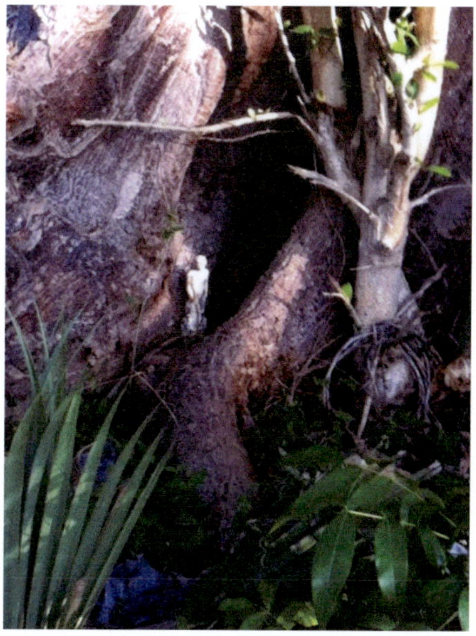

Figure 37 The statue of San Lázaro/Babalú Ayé at the foot of the ceiba in Niquero, Cuba.

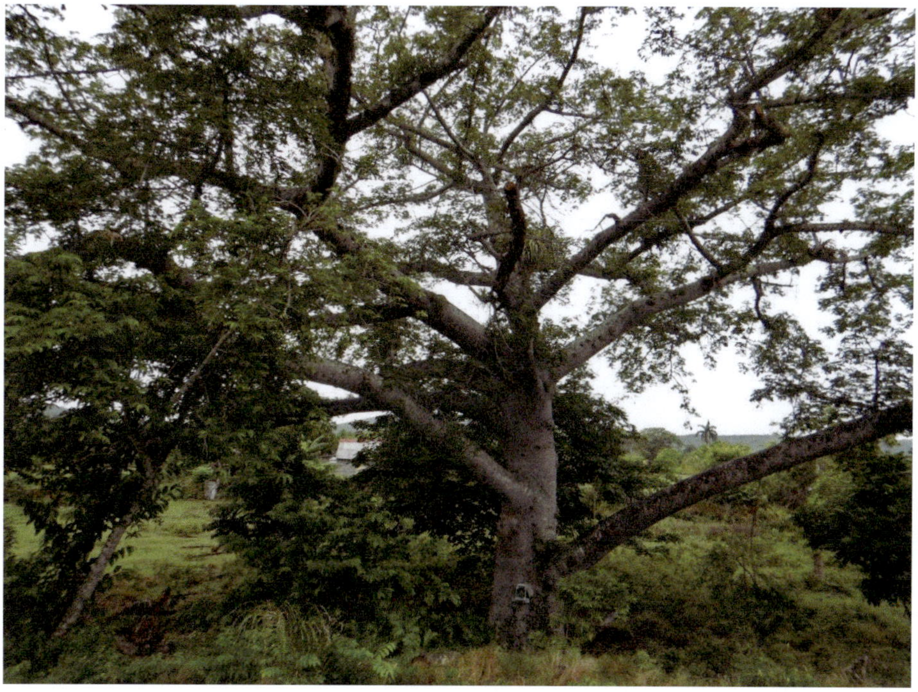

Figure 38 Ceiba with the image of Virgin of Charity hung on its trunk close to Managuaco, Cuba.

used Spondias mombin for a fermented drink, a tea to treat a sore throat, to purge after parturition, and induce lactation (Hodge & Taylor 1957). Like the ceiba also *Spondias mombin* has a pantropical distribution. At present, in Benin it is used for spiritual protection against weapons.

If we consider that the indigenous and African meaning of trees like jobo or ceiba played a role in their integration into the Caribbean religions including Catholicism, the selection of the ceiba tree as the first place of Catholic mass in Cuba seems not to be accidental but rather a skillful manipulation of power on the part of the colonizer. From this perspective, ceibas with images of the Virgin as encountered in rural areas of Eastern Cuba are unique testimonies of the synergy of Catholic, indigenous and African beliefs.

Archaeological evidence suggests that the *guayacán* is yet another tree that may have had special religious significance in indigenous worldview. The majority of wooden objects found in the Greater Antilles were carved from the *Guaiacum sp.* and some found in Hispaniola also from *Carapa sp.* (Ostapkowicz et al. 2012). Together with the *palo sancto*, the *guayacán* was used *in early colonial times* as a remedy for syphilis (mal de buás, mal francés); furthermore it figures as one of the trees used by AfroCaribbean ritual specialists in the 17th century (Gómez 2017). Nowadays it is used as a remedy for rheumatism, syphilis, and blood toxins while it is also for spiritual protection and for packing the amulets of Eshu/Elegba in Regla de Ocha (Quiros-Moran 2009).

The expressions of gratitude, devotion, vows, and care for a balanced relationship between the visible and invisible world through (votive) offerings occur in many different worldviews including those unrelated to the Caribbean region. While the details about the aim of these offerings are left undescribed in Caribbean historical records, Pané and Breton mention that offerings were brought to divine beings to the house of *cimiche* or a cavern, on ceremonial days. The Catalonian friar mentioned that those ritual offerings were dedicated to the *zemí*, with which people engaged after the healing rituals while Breton explains that before the start of the ritual the divine beings that had arrived were to be seated and received with a meal and drinks. Among the indigenous peoples of Guadalupe and Dominica *"at the beginning of every revel or feast, they offer him the first morsels of the banquet. In a corner they put amatoutou (which is a sort of low stool made of rushes like their baskets) for him and place the best cassava they have upon it, along with gourds full of ouicou /a kind of beer/, which is their usual drink. They do the same when they clear a wood to make a garden. They believe that this god eats what they offer him*" (Breton 1929, p. 5 [information from Dominica and Guadalupe 1635-1647]).

Concluding remarks

The final part of Chapter 6 indicated that tracing the roots of present-day beliefs and customs is a highly challenging task, especially in the Cuban and Dominican context. According to Ortiz, the main output of a completed transculturation is characterized by a change of character. Can we however chart the lines of these developments as chronological relations of cause and effect within such a complex reality characterized by a ceaseless synergy of connections and mutual influences? Do we find below the surface roots or rhizomes that are typified by nomadic growth, heterogeneity and semiotic chains, the origins of which are not traceable?

Human insights into the flora, the environment and the miraculous working of nature have led the different peoples worldwide to speculate about the source of life and have become a point of departure for human spirituality across different cultures. Consequently, sacred landscapes, soul loss, spiritual incarnation and metamorphosis could be recognized and "translated" between different symbolic universes in their historical exchange, but at the same time this interaction gave rise to changes of meanings and destruction of cultural memory, so that new elements may seem to have no relationship with the indigenous worldview.

Likely the reference to the soul(s) as part of indigenous medicine and local symbol systems should be understood as a parallel to the role of psychology in therapy in modern western culture. Soul loss then may be compared to trauma, for example, and the role of spirits to that of memories, values, symbols, archetypes and emotional connections. In the indigenous healing traditions of the Americas and Africa these spiritual or psychological aspects were completely integrated with herbal medicine and other physical treatments.

This Chapter introduced some forces of the universe that manifest themselves in healers, plants and other natural elements, which together form the Dominican and Cuban healing landscapes. The following Chapter 8 will highlight the role of the indigenous ancestors in the healing practices at Dominican water pools. Cuban examples (in *Regla de Ocha* and *Espiritismo*) will be investigated in order to advance our understanding of the importance of the indigenous ancestors in the broader regional context.

8

The subaquatic realm of ancestors and other beings

In many rural areas, surface water sources have been the only source of drinking and utility water until relatively recently (the 1960s in Cuba; 1990s in the Dominican Republic[300]). These water sources have also been a center of subsistence-related and cultural activities. According to international reports, in spite of many improvements the access to water supply remains insufficient in Dominican rural areas (JMP 2017). Simultaneously, droughts during 2014- 2016 and the following severe floods have made the potable water scarce. In some locations, the long-lasting droughts have caused food shortages and were a motivation for people to move to urban areas (*e.g.* Loma Atravesada, province of Monte Cristi).

In regions historically related to the Cuban and Dominican landscape biography, sweet water sources symbolize *i.e.* fertility, life progression, and cleansing from sin; they are seen as a house of birth and death (see chapter 3). The universal value of water raises questions about how its symbolism has been constructed in contexts with a multicultural background. The subsequent section has a threefold objective. Firstly, it explores the explicit association of sweet water sources with indigenous ancestors in the context of the multiple meanings of places.[301] This enables us to observe how the concept of health is often related to ancestral subaquatic dwellings and later to analyze how the diverse cultural historical backgrounds have been woven into the cultural memory. This chapter elaborates on the nexus between oral tradition and ritual engagement with water sources. Even though some narratives, tales, and testimonies might seem to have no clear or direct relationship with healing practices, they may be informative about how and why specific bodies of water were selected in the past for healing practices and were given specific (though fluid) meanings. Narratives are an important part of the broader knowledge of epistemic communities about the indigenous past and as such show about how the past is currently interpreted. These results will be assessed later in

300 Again also this information is based on the interviews and conversation in the region. For the current status of the access of the drinking water in the region of the study see https://washdata.org/data.

301 The term Indigenous Ancestors was used as translation to the term "indio". The term "Indian" was avoided as it carries for many of Indigenous Peoples of Americas negative connotations. Future studies could verify whether the same negative connotations are perceived by indigenous descedants in Cuba (e.g. in La Rancheria, in Manuel Tames Municipality, Guantanamo Province or Fray Benito, Holguín Province. If the contributor used the term misterio this was also left as such.

the light of the local history and educational discursive practices (discussed in previous chapters), which are replicated in practices such as healing rituals.

Dominican Ancestral Subaquatic Dwellings

The rich Dominican history is reflected in the diversity of divine beings that are represented by or associated with water sources. Among these divine beings are: *Rey del Agua* ("King of the Water"), the Divine Twins, Simbi (D'lo from de l'eau). In two interviews *lwas* such as Ogún and Santa Marta or Catholic Saints such as Saint John or the Virgin Mary were associated with rivers and waterpools.[302]

Most frequently, rivers and parts of rivers are seen as domains of Indigenous *Misterios*. Ancestral and divine forces residing in rivers, waterfalls, and pools are potentially beneficial or detrimental to human health. As dwellings of indigenous antecedents living in subaquatic houses or kingdoms they are potentially risky places for children and people with *corriente del indio*: these might experience soul loss, which could ultimately lead to their death. These water areas are also sites where the gift to heal can be developed.

Dominican devotees express their devotion to *indigenous misterios* at different water sources. *indigenous misterios* are approached as a part of annual celebrations of *lwas*. This was the case of the feast of Belie Belcán/San Miguel in La Jaiba, during celebrations of Saint John in El Hombre Parado closeby to Mana or the feast of the Virgen de las Mercedes, or Christmas or after the harvest in the Bánica region. In addition, waterfalls and pools Hombre Parado in Mana, Enchanted Well at El Burén (Estero Hondo), as well as springs La Descubiera, pool La Zurza (closeby to Bánica), Charco de los Mellizos and Charco de los Indios (Chacuey), or Waterfall Socoa (close to Boyá) are loci of ritual baths and healing rituals wherein ancestral powers are invoked. *Indigenous misterios* are sought at some of these sweet water sources for the initiation of healers working with their powers. At some like places in Charco del Indio in Marmolejos, people dedicated offerings to Indigenous *misterios*, but these traditions have discontinued. Even more frequently, water sources are a setting for oral traditions about indigenous people living in these places. A few examples of such accounts are described below.

Recovering through remembering at La Descubierta

The recovery of Mr. Javier De Los Santos at La Descubierta spring will serve as an example of how the relationship between humans, health, and landscape is experienced

302 One of the wells in the quarter el Pozito in Guayubín was the site of an appearance of the Catholic Virgen. She is said to have performed different miracles and also to have cured diseases of those who have visited her well. Dominican rivers were considered to be empowered on the day of Saint John through the whole island. Many people woke up early in the morning and without speaking to anyone bathed in the river, which was considered by many to bring wellbeing. The bodies of water are places of manifestations of *lwas* and Saints. For the traditional healer Mrs. Esperanza from Guananico the rivers are places where both Santa Marta and Anacaona can incarnate: "*When Anacaona arrived to me it was through the river…and my children were afraid that I would drown…and when Santa Marta arrived this was shameful I was crying when I saw this girl (*referring to herself when looking on a video later*), she was rolling down in the river.*" Her former patient adds: "like a snake crawling." The *lwas* impersonated in the healer gave consult to people seeking their help.

and articulated. Also it will introduce the complexity of place meanings and illustrate how healing practices are informed by oral traditions.

When discussing the composition (*botella*) of herbal mixtures for curing at his house yard in Pedro Santana, Mr. De Los Santos (born and raised in Bánica) stated that approximately one week earlier he had fallen from his donkey and suffered bruises. In addition to the herbal treatment, another remedy was suggested. Returning to the origin of the injury, Mr. De Los Santos described himself as *"being fastened by them"*.[303] This adverse situation could be improved by reestablishing positive relations with divinities living in a spring near his former house in La Descubierta.

This spring is a sweet water spring located at the abandoned rural settlement called La Descubierta, which is approximately nine kilometers from Bánica. This settlement, composed of few houses of *teja de maní,* had been abandoned by the couple of Los Santos approximately three years ago when moving to into a walled house with running water and electricity in Pedro Santana (2,5 km from neighboring to Bánica). The spring is located at the foot of the hill of their former house. The spring flows as a stream through a ravine and further into the fields. It has been used as a source for drinking water and baths. In spite of the long-term droughts that have affected the region the spring preserved water.

The journey for the recovery was started with the preparation of offerings, which consist of coffee, peanuts, bread, corn, and bonbons. After a one and a half hour walk the married couple De Los Santos, me and my personal guard Richard Peña together we arrived at the foot of the hill of the abandoned settlement La Descubierta. Upon our arrival, Mr. De Los Santos went directly to the spring where the couple purified themselves with the water they had brought. Mr. De Los Santos took off the cap, kneeled in front of the offerings that were deposited in a container of calabash. While he lit the candles, his spouse poured the water in a circle around the spring in a counterclockwise fashion. Mr. De Los Santos offered coffee while saying: *"Dorsú, Twins, and* (his wife added: *the King of the Water) and the King of the Water, come and receive this offering. To Dorsú, Twins and to the King of the Water."* Afterwards, I myself and Richard were also invited to offer the corn and *maní*. On our journey back, when asked whether he felt alleviated and if he sensed the presence of indigenous *misterios*, Mr. De los Santos confirmed that he got a chill and goose skin and therefore was convinced that he would quickly recover.

The question regarding the *indigenous misterios* was derived from our conversation that preceded the healing encounter: in that conversation Mr. De Los Santos associated different divine beings including *indigenous misterios* with water sources. His answer as to what the people in the past used to say about Indians or *Ciguapas* was: *"I have heard about Indians, but I have never seen them. It was said that they were walking in water; they were walking under the water. They belong there … People were preparing them food, because they were teasing them, so they were giving them corn to avoid that they would bother. In those times, some people knew them but not anymore. They were calling them with their names and then they came out. If you do not call their name, they will not come… I do not know where they were living… I can only tell you that they were taking away twins, because twins are from the water. I am dorsú, born after twins, so I am from*

303 Being fastened is used as translation for expressions like *"me tienen amarrado"*.

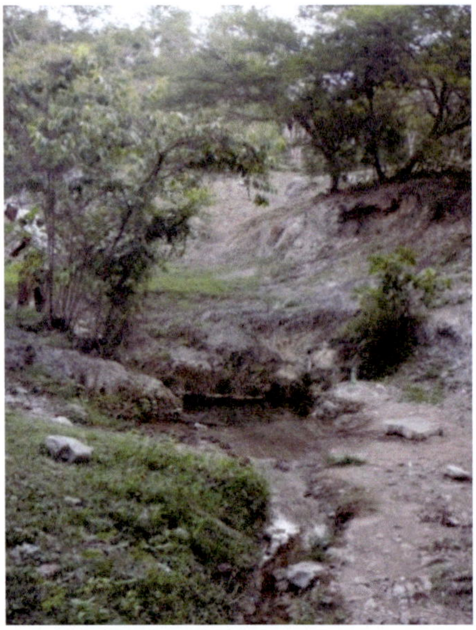

Figure 39 (left) Front view of the pool at La Descubierta, taken during the drought.

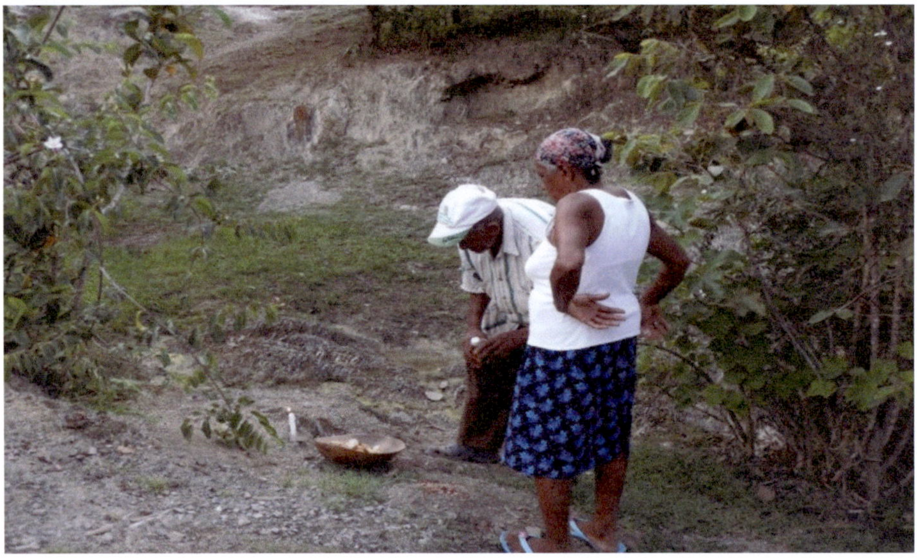

Figure 40 (above) Married couple De Los Santos making an offering at La Descubierta.

water… To Dorsú, you have to also give food. They tease a person who then feels sick and so you have to give them food. You roast corn and peanuts. I will do it soon. You go to the river and call him…" From the further conversation it became clear that he was born after twin siblings who passed away at birth. Mr. De Los Santos is therefore forever related to them, and to the water domains to which they belong.

Mr. De Los Santos' account indicates that the establishment of a balance between humans and beings living in the water pool is a central concept of health recovery and health maintenance. The affected health can be recuperated by taking care of the relations with ancestral and spiritual forces at places where one can easily communicate with them. This is clearly not only his personal view, but part of traditions inherited from previous generations, which consider that *lwas*, including indigenous ancestors, can be a "nuisance" if not dealt with properly.

The King of Water, Twins, Dorsú and indigenous ancestors are all associated with the water domain. In our conversation Mr. De los Santos associated these beings with each other. Although he did not provide us with more details on these spiritual entities, his relation to the deceased Twin siblings should be understood within the widespread Dominican belief that twins are born with the gift to heal, which if properly developed (by following some dietary restrictions, excluding vegetable and salt and maintaining their relations through the protecting Divine Twins) these persons can cure others. The figure of Dosú is integral to the twin cult in Haitian Voodoo, where Dorsú is a child born after the *Marasá*, the twins (Pressly-Sanon 2013).

The water symbolism in Bánica landscape

The Divine Twins are called *Marasá* in Bánica (approximately 4,5km from Pedro Santana). Also Mr. León Alcántara associated Marasás with indigenous ancestors when describing how these are paid tribute to during the celebration of the Virgen del Carmen after which offerings are brought to the river: "*This is done for marasás, marasás, it is called Indian from below the earth, from below the water. This you receive from up, you feel it up but it is not you, it is when you have it in your mind, in your head, you received it and you are turning. All this maní, maíz, ajonjolí, bolón, mint, egg, and they make this mixture. You have it there, and you throw it and give it to people, and then you take the rest that is remaining and you take it and go to the river to throw the remaining into the river. And who was the Marasá? This was invented by the God... They throw it there, in the yard, in the bohío.*"[304] From this account, it is also clear that not only the water domain but also the earth domain is shared by Marasá and indigenous ancestors. Also Hecfredes Gómez, spiritual leader and the organizer of the feast of the Virgen del Carmen, when asked whether ritual offerings are brought to Indigenous Ancestors, confirmed that these are occasionally made during the celebrations of Carmen, Saint Francis, and Christmas in an effort to enhance the communal wellbeing. During the feasts of Christmas and Carmen: "*the food is brought to the river. I also go and bring food offerings there, and more people bring food, almost all people who are doing here a feast the next day bring a dish to the river.*"[305] Other Baniqueros confirmed this custom and suggested that the offerings were brought also to the twins at a specific part of the river where there are watermills. For Mr. Gómez, who was also officially initiated in 21 Division, rivers are the domain also of Simbi an dlo, who belongs to the fresh water, in contrast to Simbi Macaya who is from the salt water.

The river of Artibonito or other specific places in the river like Las Tres Piedras or La Chorrera are areas where inhabitants of Bánica seek improvement of their individual or communal wellbeing. Testimonies about the agency of deities at these places

304 In this conversation, Mr. Alcántara seemed to mispronounce *marasás* as *majasás*. Given the fact that the *majá* (boa cubana) was found only in Cuba and not in the Dominican Republic I have considered that he meant *marasás* because he spoke at different occasions also about twins. Future interviews should verify whether he did not really mean *majasás*, the serpents that might be linked to the narrative about the Great Serpent – see later (Interview with Mr. Alcántara, no. 170).

305 Interview no. 171314.

are related to healing rituals. One of them is told by Mr. Benjamin Alcántara, who attended one of the healing rituals before he converted to Protestantism:[306] "*There was a lady, Ana María, who became sick and said: let's go make a petition to the river and throw food to the saints. The people arrived at a great pool with a waterfall, she placed a stone, the people started to make petitions asking to forgive this woman and they offered a lot of food, sweets. The lady suddenly drowned in the water and she was lost and nobody could see her. All of the people thought she drowned, they searched for her and in half an hour she appeared there (at the river) playing with the water, healthy.*"

Another cleansing ritual is described by Mr. Filomeno Mateo Alcántara who was raised and educated by his grandmother. When discussing the baths in the rivers, he commented on how there is a vow that you make with your twin: "*For the bath, you take three bonbons, and bring them to the river, three bonbons, you eat and you wash with soap, when assessing your problem. You eat and call the King of the Water and go in the middle of the river and throw it down and up, every time when you take a brush you throw it upstream and downstream...and you take it and when you finished you take the soap and wash with it... You throw it saying what you would like to say for this disease or this problem and when you have finished the bath the last piece of the soap which is left you do not take it back home, no, you throw it with the flow of the river and like this also your problems will flow away.*"[307]

The meanings attributed to the spring at La Descubierta or the Artibonito river suggest that ancestral forces manifest in distinct water sources in the surroundings of Bánica. Besides the spring at La Descubierta, there is another renowned spring called La Zurza, which is situated under a small cavern at the north side of the Saint Francis hill in Bánica. Sulphur springs in Bánica have been well known and used for cures in this community since the end of 18th century (Moreau de Saint-Méry 1796). La Zurza is a sulfur spring that is appreciated for the cure of skin diseases but also for obtaining or maintaining spiritual health.[308] The healing water of the spring and its location next to the cave was seen as evidence of the powers of indigenous ancestors. While the material remains (candles, coins), encountered at the spring, indicate that ritual bathing is still being performed, residents of Bánica and Pedro Santana observed that La Zurza has lost its importance compared to one or two generations ago.[309]

Also another spring close to Bánica was included among the places where one may mobilize the ancestral forces. For Mr. Arturo Valenzuela, grandson of a former healer in Pedro Santana, these traditions are only part of his memory: "*The grandfathers had a belief about this water source. They used to say that it was here where the Indians lived. This was their belief, their culture, it was here where they were making their penance and it was fulfilling. They watered a lot of animals and designated a part of them to comply with the vow in order that the animals will not get sick and will multiply. They were making a feast on 21st January at the day of the Virgen de Altagracia and came and toss meals. I was already lurking from behind the bushes and when they threw the plate I came and to ate it. They tossed roasted maní, corn, bonbons, mint, killed black*

306 Interview with Benjamin Alcántara (no. 162).
307 Filomeno Mateo Alcántara (no. 171314).
308 Interview with Hecfredes Gómes, Bánica.
309 Interview with Hermania Alcántara.

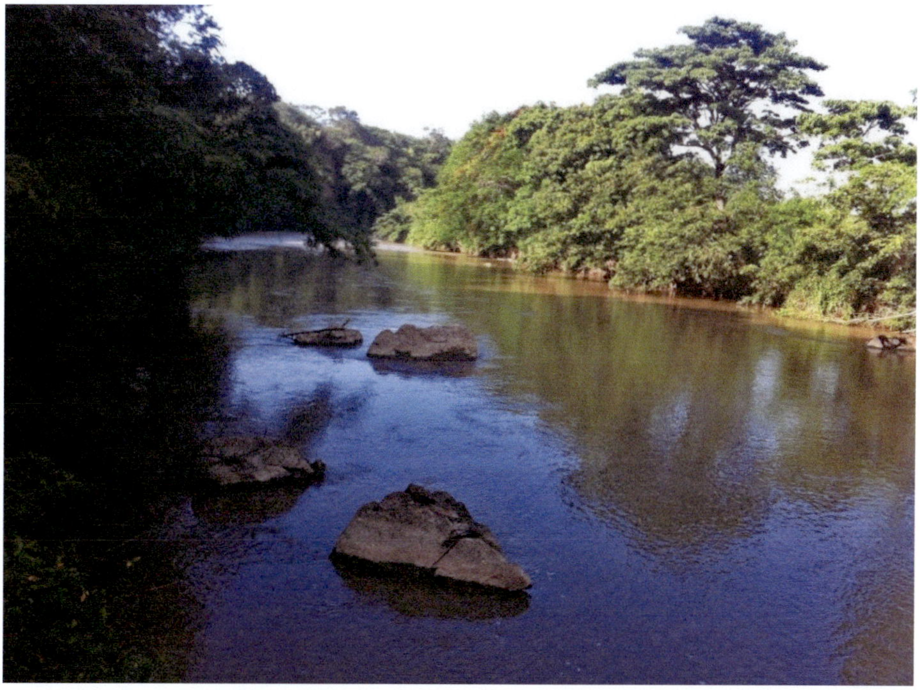

Figure 41 Aitibonito Tres Piedras.

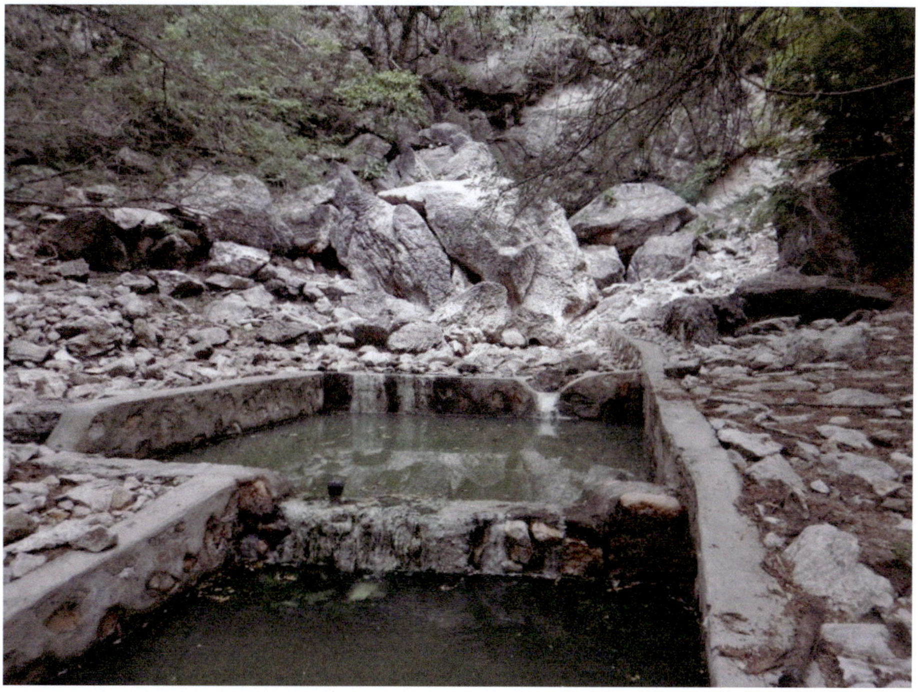

Figure 42 La Zurza closeby to Bánica.

*goats, hen, and made a great banquet. I was doing this (*pointing with his hand to a direction) *and hiding. In two or three hours I ate the food. For me, that was a religion that they had and their wishes fulfilled."*

The Valenzuela family comes from one of the founding families of Pedro Santana but he is uncertain whether this traditional activity was carried out before his grandmother. Mr. Valenzuela is sure that this tradition ceased when his grandmother passed away. The spring is no longer visited and cannot be visited anymore by outsiders because it is located within the area of the Valenzuela's property.

Different water sources were said to be the domain of indigenous ancestors but also of divine beings. As Mr. De La Rosa de Oro suggested, Indigenous *Lwas* are some of the "Saints" living in the subaquatic world, which were created during God's creation of land and waters. *"God poured a lot of water into pools and rivers so every pool and river has a lot of saints who live underneath."* In Mr. De La Rosa's account, the subaquatic world of rivers is not only a place of the Saints but also a place where the dead continue to live.[310] The selection of the place is often motivated by healer's revelations, the character of the place, the privacy to conduct the ritual or the patient's faith in the presence of water deities.

The interrelation between different divine beings living in sweet water sources is sometimes ambiguous and needs more description. Symbolically, water is clearly a powerful vital source for renewal of health and wellbeing; it is an integral part of ceremonial places where vows are made or cleansing ceremonies are performed. Some of the springs, like La Zurza, seem to have been used in curing for more than 200 years. In general, the rich amount of examples from Bánica seems to be related to the fact that here this topic was a taboo but of a lesser degree than in the following case of La Jaiba. The ritual engagement with ancestral forces at some of the water bodies in La Jaiba will help us to understand how meaning and knowledge are transmitted in a context where the value of these practices is strongly contested.

Contested landscape of La Jaiba

La Jaiba is a municipality of Villa Isabela, situated in the Puerto Plata province. The inhabitant of La Jaiba sought to improve their health and wellbeing not only in the shrines of the healers but also at Charco Tamare, La Poza Encantada and Cueva Iglesia at El Burén, all in the surroundings of La Jaiba.

Charco Tamare

The pool of Tamare is a highly contested place.[311] The followers of traditional healers, influenced by 21 Division, perceive the pool as a dwelling of indigenous ancestors. They believe that the ancestors, if they are taken properly care of, will be beneficial to individual and communal wellbeing. Representatives of a local evangelist church have condemned the offerings to the ancestors as acts of witchcraft. The residents of La

310 Interview with Carmelita de La Rosa Oro (her native language is Haitian Creole). *CR: "Indigenous is a saint, when the Lord made the earth, after making the earth he poured water in pools (noria) and rivers, but from that when he made it, he made a lot in noria, so every pool, every river has a Saint who lives underneath and that is why rivers and pools have a lot of Saints."*

311 The information about the possibly religious importance of Charco Tamare was kindly facilitated by Dr. Ulloa Hung.

Jaiba were hesitant to speak openly about the pool's current spiritual significance. This hesitance could be explained by the fact that I failed to establish a trustful relationship with the healer who was the main cultural carrier of traditions at this pool. Yet, from different conversations it became clear that there are many religious conflicts in the community. This situation leads me to reflect upon the pool's significance in the past, as remembered by the current population, and upon the importance of hearsay as a mode of cultural memory in the context of contested heritage.

Hearsay and other accounts facilitate useful information about the perception of outsiders and their role in the transfer of knowledge in the context of ongoing demonization of popular religion. The water pool Tamare is situated within a ten minutes' walk from the village La Jaiba. This water pool is named after an abandoned sector of La Jaiba called Tamare at the bank of one of the creeks that flows into the Rio Encantado ("Enchanted River"). The former inhabitants of Tamare have moved to La Jaiba because when the stream rose they were cut off from the main road. Even though residents did not provide more details on the name of Tamare they suggested that it is an indigenous name.

Since it opened approximately four years ago, the evangelical church has been gaining in popularity amongst the villagers, and with that the Charco Tamare has become a point of conflict. In fact, the ongoing religious disputes in the village have been literally inscribed onto the place as the evangelist father painted on rock walls around the pool the following text: "*The Blood of Jesus breaks all satanic pacts. The devil came to kill and to destroy but Jesus came to undo all the devil's work. Jesus is coming. Rescue me Jesus.*" During an informal conversation a representative of the evangelist church explained that the place itself and the river have been used for the baptism of newborn children because of the analogy with the river Jordan. Similarly, one of evangelist fathers saw a connection to God the Father also in natural places like one of the caves in the neighborhood. However, in his opinion the custom of bringing ritual offerings at Charco de Tamare should be abandoned because these are acts of heresy. It is clear that people who have previously attended the ceremonies at the pool have withdrawn from the participation in these rituals after their conversion.

In general, for many residents of La Jaiba the spiritual importance of the pool at Tamare has diminished, but there are some individuals who currently bring offerings at this pool to the indigenous ancestors as part of the celebration of the feast of Belie Belcán /San Miguel (28th of October), who is the patron of many Dominican healers. At one such occasion it was possible to observe generational differences in the perception of the value of this place. During the San Miguel celebration the healer sent twin brothers to take part in the ceremonial meal as an offering to the Indigenous spirits living in the pool at Tamare. This confirms the belief in ancestral agency. But the ceremonial meal sometimes did not reach the pool because these brothers thought it a waste to leave it there and instead they ate it. The twin brothers were aware of their potential to heal, but never developed this gift. They themselves never made an explicit link between themselves and the water domain, but the healer's selection of them as those that had to bring the offering to the pool does not seem accidental.

The present-day offerings are seen as continuation of a long tradition, which goes back to the time of Julio Tejada, the mayor of La Jaiba and himself a healer, who lived around 1900.[312] People recall that this healer used to perform healing rituals and religious celebrations. The accounts of past celebrations at Tamare resemble the descriptions of rituals for the *lwas* in Dominican rural areas. Also, Rafael, an agriculturalist from La Jaiba recalled past celebrations. Living close by the pool he and his family prepared a ceremonial meal (including rice, goat, chicken, potatoes, coffee, and sweets). He described these beings as *"Saints from the water spring, from the Indians".* After Rafael converted to evangelism he stopped bringing offerings to the pool, but confirms that: "*there are people that bring them still, people that believe a lot in the Saints, these are Saints they believe in, they prepare them dishes, bring them rum and candles.*" This particular person gave his consent to discuss this topic after encouragement by his friends, who assured him that the author was already familiar with the custom.

Regarding the celebrations at the pool, other residents only had reminiscences from their childhood. It is clear that those who were excluded from the celebration also had some knowledge of these happenings. One of the contributors living in the settlement of Tamare never personally attended the celebrations, because, according to her, her parents were too strict and did not let her attend; but she knew that one of the key elements of the celebration was that dishes were offered to Indians living below the surface of the pool. In addition, she commented: *"I knew that this place was something sacred for the people because there was a pool that belongs to the Indians, you understand, their houses because you could see a lot of their things, a lot of their dolls... Because they continued in La Tina my father told me."* This contributor drew a relation between the remains of indigenous ancestors and their agency: "*They saw the Indians as well, they were not doing this without the faith because sometimes people do something because they believe that it exists but this was not the case, they were presenting themselves. Where I lived there, there were a lot of things left by them as they were before in this world... so you could see a lot of things, cups, and it was the Indians who made the items... We girls took these plates in order to play with them (the ceramics).*" Until recently, the previously mentioned objects could be found at different locations in the villages and in their surroundings (see for the exact location Ulloa Hung 2014).

For some residents, the indigenous artefacts found around La Jaiba had a spiritual significance. Some inhabitants cherished and kept these objects at altars with other icons of the Saints. One person highlighted their healing power. During my first visit to the pool of Tamare the following account was told to me: *"This was the place where they were baptizing (initiation of new healers)...this was the place where they were curing... it is just a special group of people who come here... lwas incarnated in people (gente montada) still come here, because here they have seen Indians seated in the stone, they have seen people with long hair sitting here and still sometimes you can see a woman seated with braids in her hair. So if they emerge there they toss their hair here and there and every time the hair becomes braided"* And he continues: *"Up there was a house where a boy who was fourteen years old and never could walk and in the small field (conuco) he found a Virgin of the Indians. Hear this, the boy stands up and starts walking, and says: mom look, mom look. So his mother moved from there and in the time of San Miguel she was organizing vela*

312 In the village one of Tejada's descendants is believed to have inherited his gift to heal.

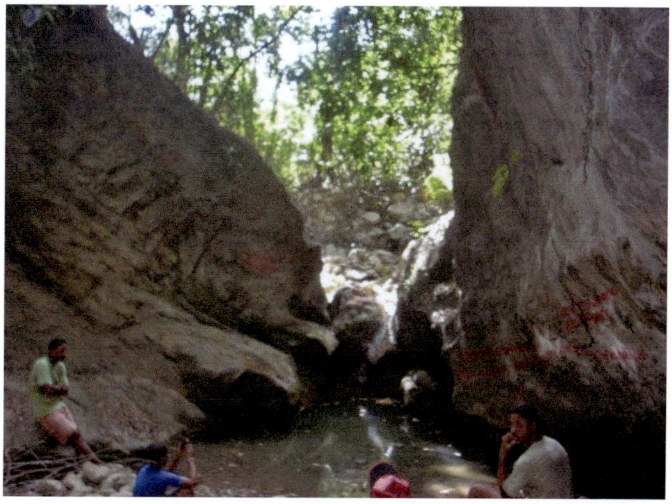

Figure 43 Charco Tamare in La Jaiba.

for nine days and this Virgin was sweating there (on an altar). But, they stole her, someone came, and stole her."[313]

The healing power of this particular statue has remained in wider public consciousness in the village. Mr. Eloi Cruz, an agriculturalist from La Jaiba, confirmed that this image was highly esteemed years after its rediscovery. The statue was venerated during *velaciones* (velations, vigils) organized around an altar at the family house. The figure was valued *"for prayers because it was from the Indians."* One of the inhabitants described this statue as *"a doll made from a dark stone. This statue was later stolen and sold to the national brewery for 500 pesos".*[314] He compared its meaning with another case he knew about: *"In Arroyo Caña there is a man that has two dolls and will not sell them… I do not know if he has them on an altar but he does not sell them because these dolls protect him."* Following up on my comment about pottery sherds gaining spiritual meaning, Mr. Eloi Cruz said: *"It reminds us of the Indians, we did not know them but this brings us together. As we did not know them and it was ours, you know, and one could not know it, so you keep it there. I remember I found a very beautiful one* (decorated ceramic) *and I brought it to my mother in law."*

One member of the community took special interest in ancestral objects. He explained that his past search for ancestral objects and enchanted treasures was motivated not just economically but also spiritually, because he has *corriente del indio*. This meant he was advised and protected by indigenous ancestors. They indicated archaeological sites to him in a dream and guided him to avoid danger: *"some nights I was lying down and they took me to many places and they warn you, this is good. The only good thing about this is that it you can see a problem that is going to happen. You see it first, for example when someone wants to hurt you, one night before you dream about it and see that there are people who want to hurt you and the next day you will not go out or want to walk there."*

313 Interview no. 20140101.

314 I have decided to not reveal the name of this contributor as he might not be fully aware of the negative consequences that his testimony might have for him. From an informal conversation with one of the private collectors from Santiago (May 2019) it became clear that «The Virgen» or for the collector: «the piece or artefact» is still part of his collection.

He experienced not only the protective role of the indigenous ancestors but also their healing agency through a dream: *"I have been in their (of indigenous misterios) church... In a dream they took me, and I stayed frightened where there was a priest, I did not dare to go because I got goose skin. There were more than one thousand candles and it was twice as big as the church but under the ground... When my mother was going to die I woke up because I also smoke and I got a strong stomach ache. I had like fifteen or twenty days, without eating, and one night my stomach was tied up. One night there came like five girls and women who already passed away and they went one by one and the last one untied the thing... and now I do not have anything (any sickness), thanks God..."* The formulation of the experience of disease as being tied up and the health recovery as being untied, released, is also common in other regions.

In contrast to the idea of a spiritual relationship, which is materialized in rituals or dreaming of ancestors and places associated with them, some evangelists see Charco Tamare as a place of invocation of the Devil. The contested nature of such traditions does not necessarily lead to their total discontinuity but seems to influence the process of transmitting and interpreting them. In fact, the secrecy surrounding the traditions and the conflictive opinions about them may be one of the reasons to conceal them from public eyes but to keep them in memory. In this manner they might even reach more people in the form of hearsay. Furthermore, the contestation may lead to discontinuity of practice but that does not mean direct oblivion. On the contrary, some of the converted contributors still believe that the agency of indigenous ancestors may be experienced in some places. However, after their conversion they considered it incorrect to continue the ancestral worship. The cultural memory about the indigenous past in this particular location seems to be supported by the materiality of the place, with archaeological remains functioning as mnemonic tools.

Enchanted Well and The Church Cave in Burén

Charco Tamare is not the only place associated with indigenous ancestors and sought for the reestablishment of wellbeing. Some inhabitants of La Jaiba, especially women, were told to do ritual bathing for good luck at Poza Encantada on the north side of the hill called Burén, approximately 6 km from La Jaiba.[315] Poza Encantada ("Enchanted Well") is a pool at the foot of a rock shelter. The pool is located close to another ritual place, a cavern called La Iglesia (also called Holy Cave or Indian Cave) situated on the same hill. Both places were associated with indigenous ancestors by the specialists and the public at large.[316]

---

315 Some elderly residents of Estero Hondo confirmed they were coming to the cave La Iglesia "to pray and bring meals to Indians".

316 Juan Cruz, a former teacher from La Jaiba, reacted in the following manner to my statement about a lot of people thinking that there are spirits living in the caverns: *"This was teaching of the past, this was one of the things that was taught by the Spanish, that people think that in the darkness are hidden the spirits, for this reason the cavern has this value, people still think this, including they were thinking that they were living in the water pool, so you were explaining and people were telling you: you are crazy to think this and my answer is no. Everyone who enters into the pool drowns, this was said. Everyone who says Cave of Indian should say Cave of Dominican..."* And he continues: *"But this was everything that they taught us. From the beginning because the history is written every time in the name of those who pay for it, that's why the history is almost never real. There is a relation between the history and reality but the history is as they pay for it."*

As one of the contributors commented on the hesitance of La Jaiba's residents to be formally interviewed on the topic: "*There are many people who practice this but never say so... But sometimes they are seen at the cave.*" Also here the offerings are brought to *"God and spirits of Indigenous Peoples."* Mr. Cundo added: *"There are women and men who go to this pool, bring meals, and bath but they do not like that it is said. Also when you go to the healer you cannot tell that you are going there... but now people almost never go, they do not believe in this."* In both places the presence of remains of offerings indicates that ritual activities took place recently.[317] A traditional healer from Estero Hondo confirmed that these rituals have a certain level of secrecy. This secrecy seems to be related to the social stigma surrounding these practices rather than to a prohibition to transmit the meaning of this place to outsiders.

During our visit to the place, the traditional healer Mr. Benito described its meaning. Before going to conduct ritual baths with his patients at La Poza Encantada, he eventually went to the cavern *La Iglesia del Indio* ("the church of the Indian"), to direct prayers there to the indigenous ancestors. He described it in the following manner: *"for them this was like a church, there was a Virgin of Altagracia which was painted on the ceiling of the church. There is an altar where there are many Saints, Saint Lazarus which is also portrayed there. There is also a Saint called Capú who has been husband of Anacaona, afterwards there is a Caonao... Capú was known for making miracles and spiritual works. Another Saint that we have used and that has done invisible operations was Saint Gregory/Saint Doctor. There is also Saint Roch/Saint pilgrim. They all are in the Church but it is characterized mainly by the old things that are indigenous (spirits/peoples), and you know that before they were walking around here. Including they* (some people from Santo Domingo maybe archaeologists) *have found here their little stick (tarito) and they took it to the museum that buys these things for a lot of money, and also a golden medal was found.*" Mr. Benito explained further the historical connection of this cavern with indigenous ancestors, which is said also to be the reason why prayers are directed to them here. This ancestral link might also be derived from the water symbolism as the bottom of the Church is covered by approx. 50 cm of water.

Poza Encantada is a pool partially covered by a rock shelter that is situated at the south site of hill from the cavern La Iglesia. Like La Iglesia, the Poza Encantada is not exclusively an ancestral place but belongs to "many Saints". Mr. Benito invokes here personally with divine help his patron Ogún.[318] In his view, *lwas* like Ogún, Anaisa Pie, Metreselí, and the *indigenous misterios* (Anacaona, Capú, Caonao) relate to the Division of water. For Mr. Benito, the presence of Ogún is perceived the most and there are clear signs of Ogún in the form of colored marks on the rock walls above the pool and reflections in the water. In a special song dedicated to Ogún, he asks him to come to help him in his work, *"and after all others enter, if you want talk to them you can do so in the language they spoke in before."*

According to Mr. Benito, many people still visit La Poza, including his patients, having different occupations and social statuses (he was proud to say he was here with

317 At La Poza rests of candles and tobacco were found, whereas in La Iglesia the offerings included bottles of flowers, tobacco and decomposed dishes, including bread, maní and sweets.

318 As Tejeda Ortiz (2013) suggested, the *lwas* may have Catholic patron Saints. Some devotees would consider them the same while many initiated healers would not.

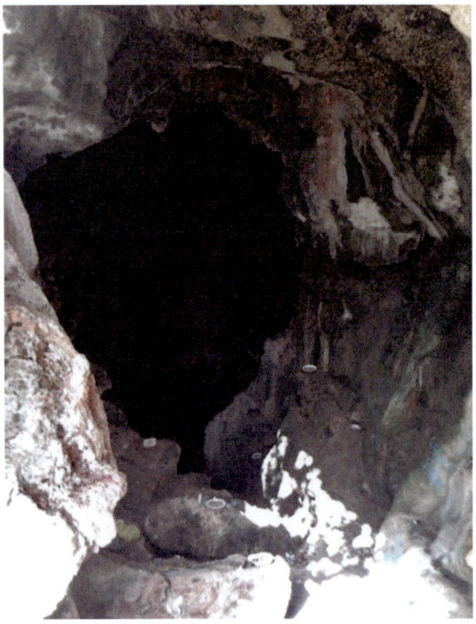

Figure 44 Cavern called La Iglesia close to Estero Hondo.

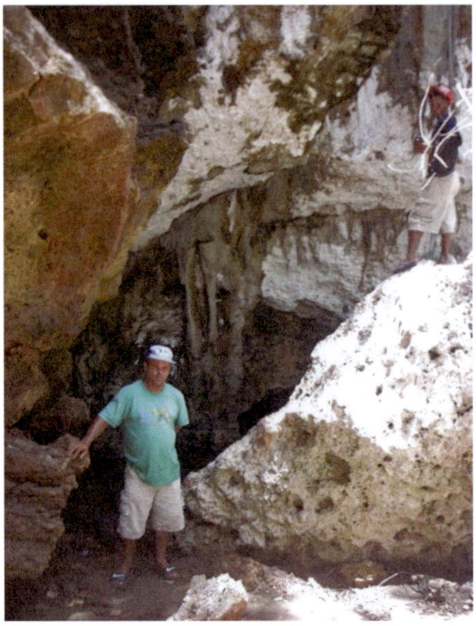

Figure 45 Mr. Benito in front of La Poza Encantada.

a civil judge), even people coming from distant locations such as San Juan. The ritual baths at La Poza are motivated by a variety of therapeutic purposes, such as warding off the negative spirits or resolving matrimonial problems. The function of bathing is to activate the good luck that is given by the gods. As he explains: *"It also depends on the god, because if you have good luck because a god gives it to you... the god also says, help yourself first then I will help."* It is through the knowledge that the Divine Father has given him and through botanical knowledge that he can treat different corporal diseases, like infections, kidney stones, asthma, and anemia, using a mixture (*botella*) of different herbs. For the cleansing rituals, Mr. Benito indicated that one should light *"candles of seven powers"*, while chanting to "Small Saint Virgin", asking her to *"take away all the bad, take away all the bad and take it to the sea and throw it into the sea."* The components of the ritual bath are frequently: "*sunflower to guide your good luck through the solar passage, pachulí, flores libertad, albahaca, rosa de piru, hierba luisa, hierba buena, mix from honey, coco de indio, perfume from the oriental wood, one perfume for home"*.

Both Ogún and the Virgin are invoked during the rituals; the well is associated with indigenous ancestors. Regarding my question about how God made the "Indians" live under the water, Mr. Benito answered: *"because they were old people, they were people like us...they decided to get into the water, you understand, because the Indians were living here before, ... because they were from the water..."* The last reference to the indigenous peoples as emerging from the water could be easily linked to origin narratives from the South-American mainland of various linguistically related groups (see chapter ten). At a different occasion he answered the same question with the following clarification: *"they owned this territory and were walking here on earth but also in the water and when Colón continued to attack them they went into the water"* The water here turns into a dwelling place of the dead.

Mr. Benito elaborated further on the spiritual relation with indigenous peoples: "*We are children of Indians and Spaniards. The Spaniards called this island Santo Domingo and the Indians called it Kiskeya. So they married and therefore we have race of Spaniards and Indian. There are people who do not feel this relation with the past. There are some people who are descendants but do not feel this relation, my wife has corriente del indio, la morena (dark hair, light skin) you have seen her. She receives Indian women if you want she will talk to you but she does not speak well, it is like in Latin... She has something from Indian because Indians had brown skin with good long hair and Spanish people were of your color but there is a lot of secrets, you know.*" In his view then, the *corriente* is a spiritual connection, which is also linked to one's physical appearance and ancestry. This interpretation is clearly embedded in his historical knowledge, which repeats concepts from the official historical discourse, *e.g.* the name for the island or the reference to Caonao, one of the glorified heroes of national history and the category of the Indian race based on skin complexion and type of hair.[319] In short, the spiritual experience of the contributor is strongly informed by the official discourse about the past as well as by broader oral traditions wherein *lwas* and ancestral powers can be invoked at certain places and mobilized for own benefits. The fact that multiple saints, *misterios* and *lwas* are sought and used in cleansing ceremonies shows the fluid meanings of some of these sanctuaries. Again, the material remains and broader oral traditions about these places seem to contribute to the continuous association of water pools, and in this case also caverns, with indigenous ancestors.

Indigenous ancestors at Dominican Altars

The association of indigenous forefathers with water is clearly displayed in Dominican altars, where they are represented in various forms, including icons bought at local botanical shops, objects like decorated artifacts, fossils, and stones of different shapes and colors that are placed in man-made wells. These items represent *indigenous misterios* and facilitate contact with them, other objects gain on special importance and uses because they proceed from ancestral sites.[320] Some of these objects, like a stone in the shape of a dove, encountered at Poza Encantada, is used for Mr. Benito's personal protection. Powder from the Charco Tamare is used as one of the ingredients of a *botella* in La Jaiba. The stones and calcic powders from caverns in Bánica and Boca de Mana are also considered to have protective properties and their water has healing powers. Popular artefacts founds at altars and households are also: thunder axes (petaloid axes), which are kept for their power to protect the household against thunder or for keeping water fresh. This is part of a broader worldview in which people can transform into intangible objects as well as into flora and fauna.

Corrientes and ciguapas: counterpoint of the self and the collective

The relation between the agency of ancestors and health should be seen within the horizon of knowledge that epistemological communities have gained through informal

319 Note that the "Indian race" is also one of the categories implying skin color on Dominican id-cards (see Moya Pons 2009).

320 Interview no. 30. The contributor answered my question "why do people put the ceramics in the water?" in the following way: *"Ah God, to give them drink, to keep them in fresh cold environment."*

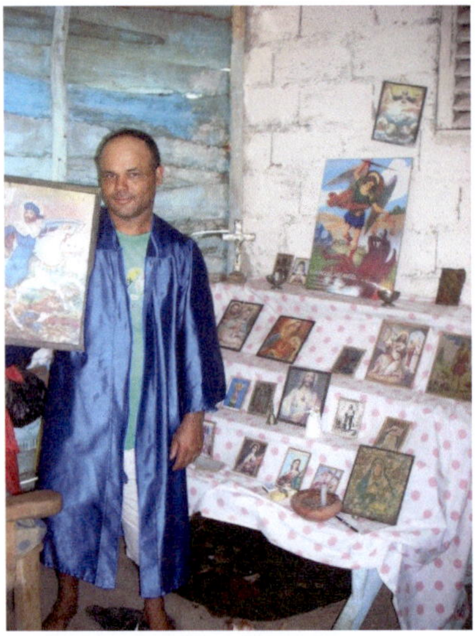

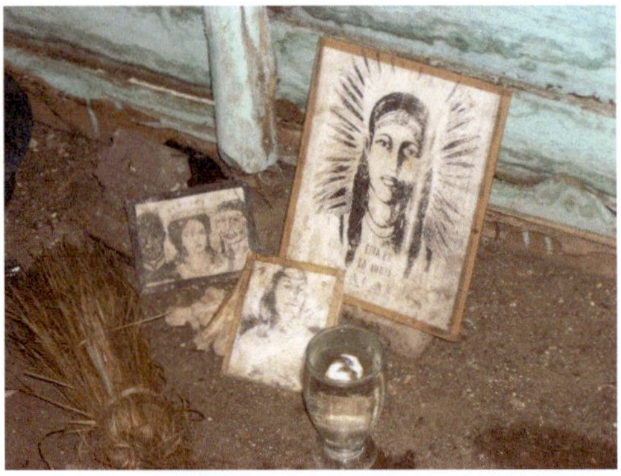

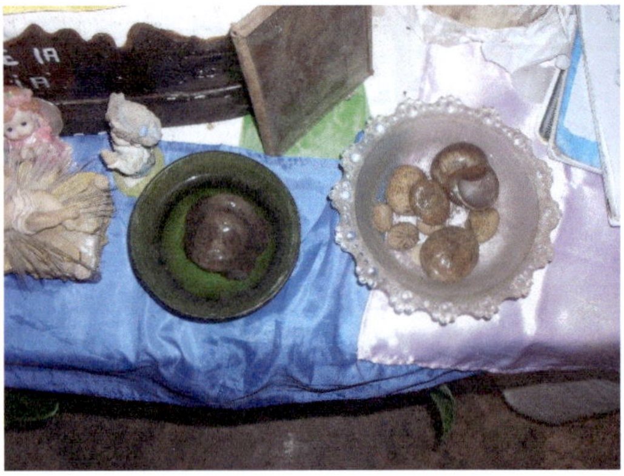

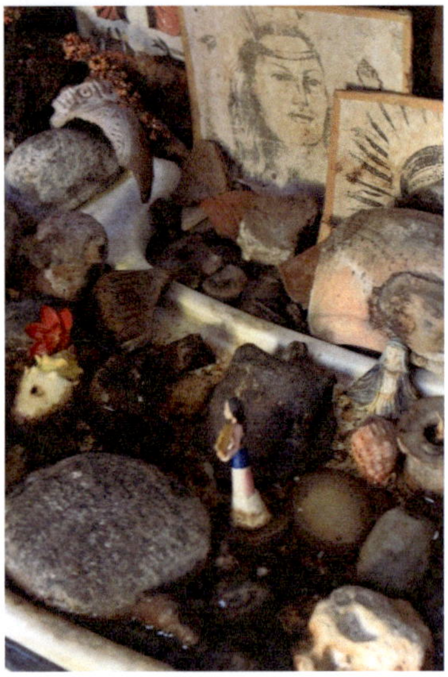

Figure 46 (upper row, left) Mr. Benito in front of his altar, holding the image of Ogún in his hand. Below the altar lies a man-made pool for Indigenous ancestors.

Figure 47 (upper row, right) The Image of Anacaona and Venezuelan Trinity at Mr. Benito's altar.

Figure 48 (lower row, left) Ancestral indigenous objects on an altar in Marmolejos, Puerto Plata.

Figure 49 (lower row, right) One of altars in Guananico, Puerto Plata.

education. Personal identification with indigenous ancestors is not just characteristic of traditional healers but also of individuals who might not develop this *corriente* further but are very aware of protection and different restrictions that this *corriente* implies.[321]

321 As earlier mentioned healer Benito´s suggested that to have "*corriente del Indio*" implies to have a spiritual connection of indigenous ancestors which is also linked to one's physical appearance and ancestry. This interpretation of corriente as a grace which is accompanied with different restrictions was also formulated by one of the contributors from La Jaiba. This contributor suggested that people with this *corriente* have to maintain well hygiene, regularly bath in perfumed waters and avoid some places in river because they are more likely to be taken away: *"at night they take you to the river, they fall in love with you, throw you into the water, and you will not get wet, to be taken away to the pool is to die from being frightened."*

The head of one of my hosting families also had this awareness of having a *corriente*. The person visited the Catholic church almost on a daily basis, but on one occasion confessed not to be able to enter the river alone because of getting a feeling of dizziness and of being pulled by the river. Similarly, my guide Abel Gonzáles (from Monte Cristi) would not believe in 21 Division, but to a certain degree admitted the possibility of having the *corriente*. This was diagnosed when he suffered as a child from respirational problems described as an experience of drowning (*ahogado*). Since Abel's childhood, his parents have been converted to Protestantism but they still were very concerned when he went diving because they believed this to be a particularly dangerous activity for him because of this *corriente*.

One recurring theme in Dominican oral tradition is water as a source of life and death, having both vital and dangerous potentials. The paragraphs above emphasized its vital force, but this is not to be disconnected from its dangerous aspect. There are several testimonies and narratives that might be interpreted as warnings to be cautious and act with respect towards bodies of water. This applies especially to children and people with *corriente* would run a greater risk of being "kidnapped" or "taken away" at the springs or when swimming in deep pools. Some people who are abducted learn from the ancestral lesson, develop their gift to heal, or are rewarded in material ways. Others stay forever in the realm of the dead in their subaquatic world. This is also the case of the subsequent testimony about the violent death of a grandson of Mrs. Felicia Ulloa.

During my visit to the Ulloa family from La Trinchera (close to Villa Vasquez, province of Monte Cristi), Mrs. Ulloa shared her pain caused by the loss of her beloved grandson. His violent murder several months ago was described in terms of him having been taken away because of having the *corriente del indio*. While showing me the picture of her grandson, Elia, she described this tragedy with a shaking voice: "*He knew he should not go to the river and that's why he never did. So, when his friends invited him to the river, he did not know how to swim. He had the corriente, poor boy, his name was Elia, and I just got goose skin, he had the corriente... They (the indigenous misterios) keep these people. So it could be that they took him away. They are secluded in the river Yaque.*"[322] This account was not unique, neither in referring to a murderer who had not been punished because of the corruption or failures in implementing the justice system, nor in referring to the realm of indigenous ancestors being a resting place for people with *corriente*.[323] Similarly, different members of the Torres and Rojas families interpreted the death of drowned children in a small stream at La Peña, a zone of Marmolejos near Mamey, as the result of ancestral agency.

At another occasion, the *indigenous misterios* appear as givers of healing power to members of the Ulloa family. Like in the case of Elia, Mrs. Felicia's sister Lola and her nephew (who passed away at young age) also had this *corriente*. In the description of Lola's initiation we find elements that are common in oral traditions about the indigenous peoples. Mrs. Ulloa recalls (but not as a direct testimony) that her sister was taken away by Indians to a cave where there was a green pool. They combed her hair with a golden comb and immersed her into the water to recognize her *corriente*. Afterwards

322 Interview with Mrs. Ulloa.
323 A similar case was recorded in Boyá.

she was able to work with fifty-seven indigenous ancestors, who were invoked to heal, to assist with childbirth, and to act as a seer.

Many quotidian activities of the past such as washing clothes, bathing, or just swimming were done at rivers. Their daily importance is also reflected in oral traditions. In this light, narratives about the indigenous ancestors, which is spread throughout the entire island, call for being cautious at water sources. In Boca de Yuma, a former resident of La Gran Chorra (the settlement near the archaeological site La Aleta) described how in the past the people were going to wash clothes in a spring called Escalera: *"In this spring you could hear water sounds/rings and when you came down you could feel that something sprung into the water because it splashed but we do not know what it was... Well the old people said that it was Indians of the Water but we have never seen them. People were frightened by this... You know the people, you know the old people talk like this."* This contributor remarks bear witness to the mixed feeling that some of the contributors had about these narratives. Many of them regarded the narratives about indigenous peoples as tales or stories (*cuentos*). Many of these narratives included also stereotypical representations, indicating dissociation on the part of the narrators. The status of tales and the corresponding stereotypical representations is informative. In a certain sense "tales about Indians" might seem to be positioned on the opposite end of the continuum of the identification with the indigenous ancestors. This could to a certain degree be considered as forming a contrast with the above mentioned spiritual or a genealogical link formulated in the concept of *corriente del indio*. As much as these attitudes might seem divergent, they still constitute the cultural memory of the indigenous past in the broader societal context.

In some locations, instead of the character of *indigenous misterios* we encounter *stories* about beautiful Indian women similar to Sirens/Mermaids. The setting or the manner in which such a narrative is told, indicate that these are stories for amusement of the audience. Referring to the place Charco de India near to Imbert, Mr. Bonilla, told us: *"This legend says that since 1800 people were living here and the legend says that an Indian woman was sitting on a stone combing her hair with a golden comb* (Mr. Rivera filled in: seated on the rock), *yes on the rock, when she heard people she went into hiding but some people were able to see her but they were scared because there were not many inhabitants here and this was before the railway..."* Mr. Rivera added that this particular indigenous woman was seducing one of the male passersby who fell in love with her. The danger here is impersonated as the deceiving beauty of this woman, who is described as well formed, long haired, and naked. This often, slightly erotic account of a beautiful lady seducing a passerby is comparable to stories about sirens, other mermaid-like creatures and *ciguapas*. The latter are naked creatures, depicted as half indigenous women but with the distinguishing inhuman feature of feet turned backwards. The *ciguapas* have been incorporated into folk culture throughout the island as eroticized, dangerous, and deceitful creatures. In Marmolejos, the story of a *ciguapa* has been encoded into a popular song; Martin Nuesis recited its contents as follows: "*In Nava, Samberes' land they made a song about her. On the way from Marmolejos in the land of Samberes they captured a ciguapa, they captured one because she stopped, when a man captures/takes ciguapa and she gave a birth in the cave, the man went there and there were like one hundred ciguapas and all of them jump on him and tear him into pieces and there they found him dead."*[324] Ciguapas are "the Others", for which the folk tales warn us. During my fieldwork, I did not meet anyone who would identify with *ciguapas* or would bring them offerings.

Dominican water sources are domains of a variety of ancestral and divine beings that can be salutary or detrimental to human health. Simultaneously, they also figure as settings for rich oral traditions. Similarly, in Cuba the cultural and religious diversity has been translated into a gamma of meanings attributed to the sweet water sources. Specific landmarks, like the subsequent example, function as places of memory that integrate this multifaceted symbolism.

Beyond the written history: multiple meaning of Waterfall in Barajagua

Saltadero is a small waterfall in the river Barajagua, which passes through the village that carries its name. Its multiple meanings speak about dynamics of the religious diversity, which is characteristic for this region. Both the waterfall and the village are intimately related to the history of the Virgen of Charity from Cobre, the patron Saint of Cuba. The importance of the waterfall as a sanctuary of this Virgin is evident when we listen to the testimonies of the contemporary inhabitants, which provide us with details that complement and expand upon the official historical version.

According to local history, the Virgen of Charity was brought from Bahía de Nipe to Barajagua before being relocated to her current location in El Cobre at the end of 16th century. In accordance with data collected by Peña et al. (2014), oral history about the Virgin at this location is often more detailed and situated within the local landscape, in which Saltadero is an important landmark. Mrs. Caridad Portelles from Barajagua explained the importance of this small waterfall: *"When they brought the Virgin here to Barajagua, they came navigating over the river from the beach Mabiseña of Nipe. So it was there where the waterfall is that they brought her, and it was here where she passed by. There at the waterfall they made her a small house. Since then barges sailed here because this river was traversable.... Three Juans brought her,... well they look like they are depicted on the picture."*[325] The waterfall is currently a place for spiritual reflection and pilgrimage, where people may direct prayers and offerings to the Virgin, seeking her help, protection and spiritual support.[326] At the waterfall there are no material remains of the above-mentioned shrine. Its current occasional use seems to rely on the oral history and continuous performances of acts of devotion.

The Virgen of Charity is kept in high esteem, especially among the older generation that still recalls her miracles and patronal celebrations. During droughts or other crises in the community the Virgin was taken out in a ceremonial procession and carried by community members to the church of Cueto, while people were praying, singing and publicly performing penance, showing their commitment to the Virgin. Besides being

---

324 Interview with Martin Nuesis.

325 Her testimony includes some details (such as that the waterfall was the place of the first shrine and river was passable by boat) that are not included in the historical sources. In contrast, his reference to the ethnic origin of the founders is likely to derive from the images of the Virgen depicted together with three Juans.

326 Interview with Caridad Portelles (no. 112355).

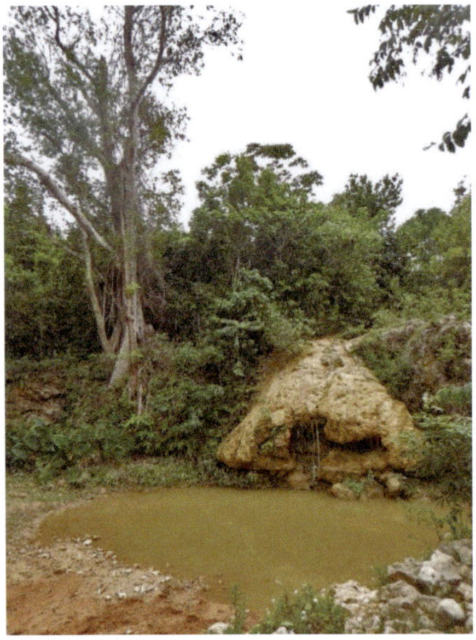

Figure 50 El Saltadero where the Virgin was located soon after her discovery.

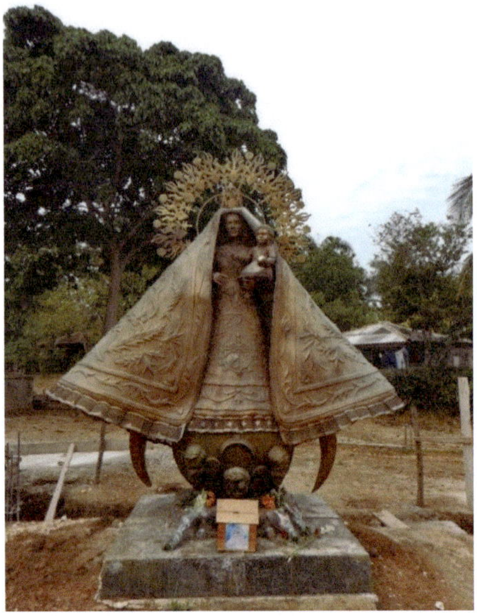

Figure 51 Virgen of Charity afront of the church (during its reconstruction) in Barajagua.

invoked at her natural shrine, the Virgin was worshipped in the church (which has been inaccessible for a long period) and in family homes, where masses were celebrated.

The Virgin is accepted as a patron both by descendants of funding families and by people of migrant background until now. [327] The testimony of Mr. Escalona Galán, however, provides us with an exceptional information about how certain landscape features may be perceived and reinterpreted by new migrants and fused with pre-existing symbolism. This young healer of mixed Cuban-Haitian origins described the various meanings of Saltadero.[328] As he has grown up with the knowledge of *Regla de Ocha*, Haitian 21 Division, *Espiritismo Cruzado* and Catholicism, this waterfall has for him multiple significances, a place where candles are lit to the Virgen de Caridad: *"Every time the Virgen de Caridad is the Saint of water, for Catholics it is the Virgen from Cobre, for Africans, Santería, it is Ochún and for Haitians it is Simbi, the queen of water. There it exists in (form of) a majá (Boa Cubana). El majá is mentioned as Majá of Saint Mary."*

While the whole river is representing Oshún, in the past people came also to Saltadero specifically to bring offerings to her. According to this healing specialist,

327 The narrative and the devotion to the Virgen are also well known among members of migrant families. Rosalina Segura Hidalgo, born and raised in Barajagua (origin: Spanish mother and Jamaican father; history related to the Cueto) adds: *"My father was telling us a lot of stories. It was said that the Virgin was brought from Bánica, they took her in Saltadero, it is a camp and soon they hid it in Loma Saíto. Some black gentlemen hid her, one of them was called Juan....."* This again embeds the official narrative in the local landscape and adds background information about her appearance. I could not find a Cuban location for Bánica; it is possible that the Dominican town Bánica is referred to, where the knowledge about the serpent narrative is still alive.

328 Interview no. 122930.

Oshún is *"a goddess of love, richness, gold, of virtue of health, of women, and of twins. It represents women, the mother, that has her son, a lot of women pray for their children and mankind... many come to ask for cleansing, to pray, as part of complying with a vow and when they go to a foreign country, others who are getting married."*[329] The sacred narrative connects the waterfall and the river with other domains of deities like the sea, because *"Virgen de Caridad and Virgen de Regla, which is Yemayá, are sisters. That's why it is said that the river flows into the sea, therefore when everyone who is going to travel and is going to cross the sea, we invoke both Virgen de Caridad and Virgen de Regla as a protection."*[330]

The Twins, called *Jimaguas* or *Ibeyes*, are messengers of the Virgin, doctors curing with herbs and protectors of children.[331] As they are children of Changó one may direct oneself to them through the álamo tree, and their place is the Palma Real. In addition, they are accompanying the river, which is the domain of their mother, Oshun.

Another divine being associated with the Saltadero is Simbi, the queen of the water, the guardian of sweet water sources, said to manifest herself as a *majá* (boa cubana).[332] Mr. Escalona continued about the figure of the *majá*: *"It is said that when a majá turns old, it sings as a rooster and goes to the sea... This is because it is a pact between the sky and earth. It is an animal that was walking but made a lot of incest which should not happen so God condemned it and said that so long as it will live on earth it will live dragging and when it turns into a adult age it will sing as a rooster and go to the water."*

The meaning of Saltadero within the broader Cuban and Dominican landscapes

This narrative about the *majá* is not particular to the Haitian 21 Division. Other contributors from Barajagua narrated about a mysterious giant serpent living in Saltadero. Ms. Segura Hidalgo suggested that some people were coming to see the *majá* in Saltadero, about which *"it was said that he was singing like a rooster...and after singing he would disappear."* The *majá* living in the pool was related to the level of the water: when the *majá* left the water level would decrease. Another resident, Mrs. Caridad Portelle, called this majá the Mother of the Water and said that she saw it when people were drawing the water from the last pool, the river where it was hidden.[333]

The personage of the serpent that sings as a rooster before leaving to the sea, was registered also at other Cuban and Dominican locations. Mr. Zaldívar from Fray Benito (province of Holguín) told us: *"When the majá gets tired of walking and arrives at certain age it makes itself a serpent and it goes to the sea where it turns into a fish. I do not know what the name of the fish is, but people are afraid of it. I think it might be a whale."* He confirmed that the *majá* when being in the mountains also sings as rooster.[334]

---

329 A ritual expert of Regla de Ocha from Jiguaní explained that: *"river is the life, cleanliness, tranquility, freshness, it serves to heal you, bless you, and purify you"*. The initiation of the Osha Rule is done at the river. The river is visited for cleansing, for opening you the road (positive future), for love, for health, with the help of Ochún. Different herbs (e.g. rompesaraguey) or flowers are used for removing curses or bad luck. And personally he also appreciated the sun flower as it guides your luck.

330 Interview no. 122930.

331 Interview no. 122930.

332 Simbi is also mentioned in Dominican Bánica. Note that in Palo Mayombe the *simbi* is a generic term for the forces vivifying the natural elements in the broader landscape.

333 Interview no. 112355.

334 Interview no. 122438.

One of the residents of Managuaco, Mr. Jeronimo Santana, devotee of Espiritismo del Cordón, told us about a curious encounter of one of the inhabitants of Guayacanes with a mysterious giant serpent. This serpent was said to live in the cave of Guayacán on the hill and it sung as a rooster. When this inhabitant of Guayacanes went to throw away a *guanajo* (turkey), in order to not contaminate the surroundings of the village, he saw this enormous serpent. Its appearance was interpreted as a sign of prohibition to contaminate this place. The existence of this giant serpent, said to be a guardian of the hill, was doubted by some but one contributor confirmed to have see its skeleton.[335]

The Great *Majá* also called Mother of Water personage is a quite widespread figure in Cuban oral tradition. The Mother of Water is described as an enormous *majá*, whistling, malignant and living in the rivers, wells and lakes. According to oral traditions edited by Feijoó (1996) the Mother of Water is a dangerous being that makes people disappear or drown, and sometimes may cause fever. Other narratives describe it as relatively beneficial because it preserves the water where it lives and is able to call the clouds (Feijoó 1996).

The association of the *majá* with the deities living in the Saltadero seems to be based not only on the location but also on its importance for health and wellbeing. The role of the boa as an agent in healing becomes clearer when we looking at its historical background. In order to trace this, it is vital to cite more details from regional examples, which show how the significance of this narrative seems to have shifted from that of an indigenous sacred narrative to that of "a folktale".

There are comparable Dominican examples from locations such as Bánica or Boyá. One of the residents of Bánica, Mrs. Hermania Alcántara told us about a giant serpent, which was living at the hill and when it was raining descended with the rain from the hill, it was leaving a road behind in which a river was created and then it went to the sea. It had seven heads. When it became a serpent and threw itself into the sea it cursed those who saw it and did not kill it. It sings three times at night and takes with it everything that it finds in its way: it takes away everything that it encounters.[336]

This narrative was also known in Pedro Santana (neighboring to Bánica), where Mr. De Los Santos told us: *"Before, the people used to say, there was a serpent on the top of the mountain which was singing as a rooster".* His spouse added: *"I have heard that when the water level in the river increased they said that it was a serpent descending… sometimes there are serpents that bring all this amount of the river, this is what people in the past said… In that time for crossing the river Artibonito to Haiti you would have to find a very skilled person."*[337] Later, Mr. De Los Santos linked this narrative to the destructive power of that river during the hurricane David, and suggested that the river was sometimes very dangerous and only skilled people could cross it. Similarly, in the version of Mr. León Alcántara the powerful current of the river was the serpent's body; he suggested in fact that the *"serpent is attracting the water, as his body enlarges*

335 Interview no. 152123.
336 The recorder being out of battery, this information was based on the fieldnotes.
337 Interviews no. 102432.

also the river does."[338] Another member of the founding family Alcántara, Benjamín, added: *"the serpents that were raised on this hill were jumping into the river when it was raining a lot, in this way a current was formed and it was said that it carried a thing that is called a diamond, yes a diamond. When they threw themselves into the river, when they threw themselves into the sea, when they were going there they said cursed be those who saw me and did not kill me*."[339] The narrative about the serpent was also known in Boyá. In the Boyá version, a horse stepped by accident on the diamond of the serpent and later was killed by it.[340]

As one of the residents of San Rafael from Boca de Yuma, who was initiated in Haitian 21 Division, has argued, the figure of the great serpent should not be confused with the Danbala, the creator *lwa*, who is also living in the river. In the Haitian 21 Division Danbala is the ancient omniscient Serpent, the wise Papa Danbala upon which God has bestowed the mystical priestly knowledge or profound insight about the world behind the material world. The incarnation of this *lwa* is expressed by the transformation of the healer into a serpent or an eel when trying to cross a river, after which he would mysteriously reappear again. According to this healer, Danbala is not related to the serpent that is said to sing like a rooster, because the latter was a bad creature. He further explained that when the time of this serpent has arrived, when it turns old and it sings like a rooster, it goes flying by air to the river, where it is transformed into a bad fish or serpent. When it flies and it finds something on its way it divides it in two. This serpent sometimes turns into Khon, a bird, which for the same reason people avoid to eat."[341]

The Saltadero and its meaning is situated within Cuban animated landscape wherein rivers and especially deep pools are considered dwellings of jigües. These have various physical characteristics and are mostly described as *"small boys with black or indian color"*. In the data collected at different locations their character was often described as puckish, molesting and scaring people but they also may fall in love with people and sometimes even be dangerous. They are said to appear in deep pools and rivers but also in trees (in particular the *anacagüita*) and other specific dwelling places.[342] In Barajagua this was a small well somewhere in hills.

---

338 Interview with Mr. León Alcántara, no. 170: *"After the serpents have grown up they turn into a bird (un pájaro), which was done in* (unintelligible m. 19.36) ... *sing like a rooster, and when they throw them into the river, after it has rained, they dive into the river, and create a blockade in the river like Artibonito, the Artibonito blocked, so that the water that streams grow, because this being pulls (attracts) the water together, the water raises and like this it can descend, and the river found a flat land, when the river Artibonito finds the flat part of land, it goes more than three kilometers because of this being and after that this being flows into the sea, and when this being goes to fall into the sea it gets to the hill in the sea, to this cave in the sea. As a boy I saw something from the old time because my father died at the age of 110 years."*

339 Mr. Benjamin Alcántara (no. 162) compares this further with the biblical narrative: *"This is produced like the case of the caterpillar that turns into a butterfly because of the spirit that the Scripture describes. So this is like the case of the caterpillar. What do you think about an animal that turns into another animal? It is weird but for this reason you have to read the Scripture, this says that this is like the caterpillar that transforms into the butterfly."*

340 Interview no. 043546.

341 Interview no. 4227 with a traditional healer of Haitian origin, resident of San Rafael de Yuma living more than twenty year in the Dominican Republic. I was not able to verify what bird Khon exactly is.

342 The choice of the anacagüita tree may be related to its extraordinary character because of the exploding sounds when its seeds fall on the ground.

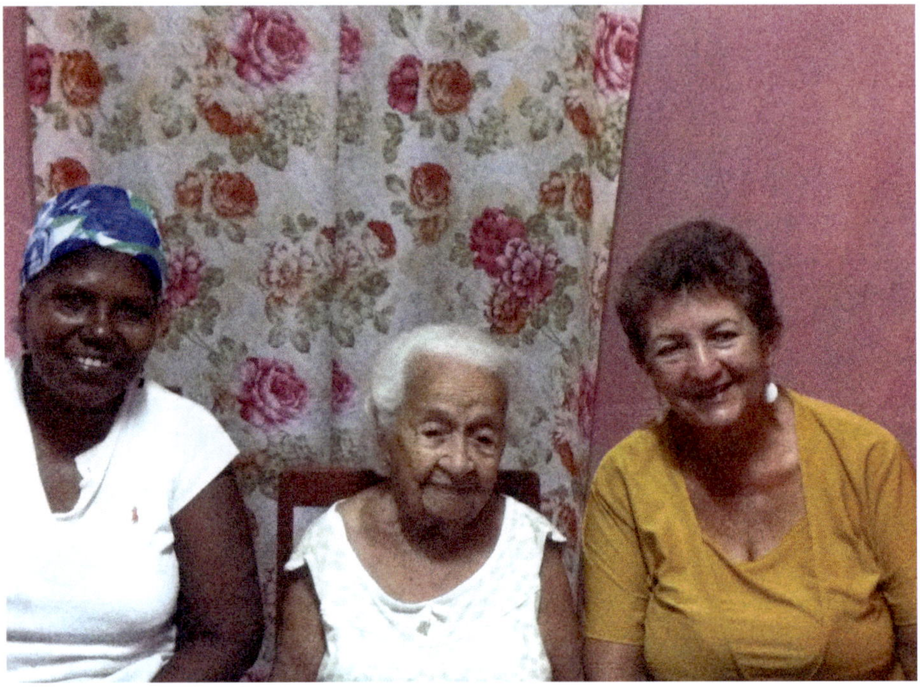

Figure 52 Celida Hernández Reyes, Mrs. Jínez Sánchez and María Palomares, inhabitants of Jiguaní, Cuba.

Mr. Alberto Pérez from Jiguaní narrated about jigüe: *"It is said that in this part of the river, where it makes a big curve, where there is an anacahüita tree, there is the well of jigüe. And they call it like this because many people say that they have seen there a jigüe emerging... They say that it had the form of a colored child and emerged in the vegetation alongside the river. So they say that there it was coming out, but I tell this to you because it is what the grandparents said and that's why they called the well like this: it was very big and had great depth... It was used for bathing... I think this was really more like a legend... I was not bathing there, not because of the jigüe but because the well was very deep."*[343] Mrs. Celida Hernández Reyes, one of the inhabitants of Jiguaní, affirmed that a *jigüe* was appearing in the river Cauto, overthrowing passersby or even making them disappear. Another Jiguanicera comments on this part that when she was a child she sometimes saw this *jigüe* at a small well and he was joshing her by sticking out his tongue (Mrs. Jínez Sánchez). During the fieldwork there were no ritual activities directed to *jigües*. Unlike what Bachiller y Morales wrote in 1883, at present in the Cuban locations *jigües* were not consulted for future telling neither were they considered to have the power to make people ill or to cure them (as suggested by Feijoó 1996).[344] Future data collections and studies on this personage should clarify the picture.

343 Jigües have figured also as a theme in oral poetry e.g. "El güije de la soledad" by Silvio Rodríguez, and even as the theme of a ballet play: El Güije by Alberto Alonso.

344 Bachiller y Morales (1883) described *jigües* as mysterious beings living in the water and presenting themselves as small "Indians" who could kill those who passed by just by looking at them. There were some in the lagoon of María Luisa in Bayamo.

The multiple meanings associated with Cuban and Dominican water sources reflect the rich cultural history of these islands. One of the cases from Managuaco illustrates how some of the attributed meanings may be based on a particular individual spiritual experience. Mr. Alcides Campo Tarragó, one of the adherents of Espiritismo Cruzado in Managuaco, explained that one night he had a revelation about a spiritual being that to my knowledge was not registered elsewhere. About this revelation in dreams he shared with me: "*This what I will tell you, I have not heard from anyone nor have I read it anywhere, this came to me in a dream, ... you are the only person that has heard this story because I have not told it to anyone (pause). She is an African lady, I know her with her name Sitochi, she is the African queen, the Queen of the Sweet Waters. This girl was carrying water in a basket, so I do not know if it was because of the droughts, but she is searching for the water and at this moment the basket breaks but there is something divine that makes the water and she turns into the Queen of Waters.*" Afterwards, he again emphasized that he had learned this through a revelation. Although he said not to make petitions for rain, he made a statue representing Sitochi which he keeps on his altar.[345]

Caribbean waterbodies as reservoirs of indigenous past

The bodies of water figure often in Caribbean cultural memory as ancestral places, as a domain of the dead, but also as a locale of renewal, of healing power and new life force. Before progressing to other features of healing landscapes, I would like to comment on the symbolic elements that are present in the narratives mentioned so far. This is will provide us with some preliminary insights into the complexity of the cultural memory connected to the water bodies. Again, following the objectives of the project, the hypothetical links with the indigenous past are highlighted.

Water sources are dwellings of different divine beings including the Divine Twins, King of Water, Simbi (D'lo) and indigenous ancestors. Occasionally they are also inhabited by *lwas* like Ogún, Santa Marta, orishas like Ochún, Catholic Saints such as Saint John or the Virgin Mary (Virgen of Charity) and other spiritual beings like the Cuban jigües.

The symbolic meaning of Twins and their relation to water sources seems to be historically related to Kongo and Dahomey beliefs. In Kongo beliefs, children with a special distinction, such as twins (*marassá*) and albinos, are associated with *simbi* (plural *bisimbi*), which are spirits of localities, inhabiting rocks, gullies, streams and pools.[346] These spirits are able to influence the fertility and wellbeing of those who live or pass nearby, and they may have a negative impact if they are not treated with respect (Macgaffey 2009). Members of lineages into which twins have been born are, therefore, in the domain of the *simbi* agency (Macgaffey 2009). At the beginning of the 20th century *bisimbi* were considered to be embodied as persons of different color (green, red, black), or as pythons, lightning, gourds, mortars or pots (Kavuna 1915 in MacGaffey 2009). Throughout West Central Africa such spirits exist under different names: they are the tutelary spirits of particular territories and the principal anima-

---

345 Interview no. 122424.

346 Breton registered various names for twins: *amayem* (sg.), *mátao* (sg.), *mataógnum* (pl.), *mónochic* (sg.), *monochicoüárium* (pl.), and *oüaríum* (pl.). De Goeje registered the word *Ibiju* for twins.

ting forces of power devices and magical objects (MacGaffey 2009). They incarnate as twins. In Kongo belief the spirit of such children born with special distinction is *nkisi Ntinu a Maza*, literally translated as "The King of the Water". This corresponds with Dahomeyan *toxosu*, which has the same literal translation. In Dahomeyan worldview, *toxosu*, those who are born with a special distinction, such as twins, become spirits of the rivers and guard the entrance to the kingdom of death. Toxosu are under the rule of the king of the children that are born with special distinction, and under that of the group of Damabala or Dambada Hwedo, powerful unknown ancestors who have entered *loko*, a silk-cotton tree or mountains (Herskovits & Herskovits 1933, p. 30).

In the Caribbean the West African concept of the King of the Water and the special importance of twins may have fused with the Arawakan figure of four divine twin brothers, who played a main role in Pané's fragmented text about the origin of the sea.[347] The sea originated as a consequence of a great flood that was caused by one of the Twins who broke the calabash wherein the remains of the son of the Creator (Yaya) were located. The motif of the great flood as origin of the sea returns also the creation narrative from St. Vincent as registered by de la Borde in 1674 (Gullick 1976). In the latter, Longuo, the great master of the Chemees (spirits) was angry with the first people because they did not offer him cassava or *ouicou* and as a punishment he sent a flood so that most of them drowned. The only ones who survived were those who fled to the hills, the peaks of which became islands. The twins are also actors in the great flood narrative that was collected in the 1940s by Lalung (1948) in Dominica. Briefly, the main plot can be summarized as follows. Jaya buried his only daughter in a calabash, which he placed at the foot of a mountain. Later he opened it and therein he found whales, manatee, sharks, and other big fish. Four twin brothers went to see the pumpkin because they wanted the fish. When the twins opened it the water gushed out, they got scared and let the pumpkin drop so that it broke. The whole plain was covered with water and only peaks of mountains remained visible above the sea. Thus the Antilles and the mainland were formed. This narrative resembles Amazon flood narratives about the destruction of ancient human life and its recreation (*e.g.* Luengo López 2009 for the Añú; Perrin 1987 for the Wayuú).

In both narratives from Hispaniola and Dominica the great transformation emerges from the fruit, the vessel in which the remains of the deceased were deposited, perhaps symbolically referring to beliefs in an afterlife, where death is followed by a new birth or by a transformation leading to a new creation. From this perspective the present-day use of calabash (higüera, güira[348], *Crescentia cujete*) for depositing offerings at pools dedicated to twins at La Descubierta, or as musical instrument (to invoke spiritual beings in Pedro Santana), can be related to the symbolism of the indigenous origin narrative. Simultaneously, its symbolic use can be related to ideas and practices in West African regions, where different types of calabashes (Lagenaria siceraria, L. breviflora and Crescentia cujete) are important elements in religious ceremonies (*e.g.* in Benin

347 The twin motif is important in many parts of the Americas. Compare the figure of Makunaima and his twin brother Pia in the Amazon or the Guayanas; as well as Tominkaru and Duid for the Wapishana. In Mesoamerica the twins (Sun and Moon) are related to "the Grandmother", the patron deity of the sweatbath (temascal). The *Popol Vuh*, a famous Maya-K'iché' sacred text, describes their descent into the Underworld and their victory over the deities of death.

348 In Kalinago: huíra (Breton 1665).

and Nigeria). They are symbols used by the Fon peoples to describe the universe, and they represent the unbroken cycle of life among Yoruba (Quiroz 2015). Among the present-day devotees of Cuban Regla the calabash belongs to Elegba and the pumpkin to Oshun and Orishaoko, and they are used in baths to attract good fortune (Quiros-Moran 2009).

The African "King of the Water" is similar to the "Master of the Water", a common figure in the Amazon cosmologies, often a boa constrictor. The serpent figure appears also in Pané´s account on two occasions. One of first possible allusion to this narrative cycle when the friar mentions briefly that the behique can be resuscitated and healed by a serpent. Secondly, when he mentions the figures of Boinaiol/Boinayel (transl. Whitehead 2011/Arrom 1974) whose representation together with another zemí (or cimimini) called Maroia/Márohu (Whitehead 2011/Arrom 1974) was found in a cavern that was hold in a great esteem, and when visited in the period of droughts it started to rain. Arrom (1974, 1975) translates this term as brown snake and adds in Amazonian worldviews this represent the mother of water. Breton registers various Kalinago´s words for a serpent, one of these *oüanáche* is described as a big serpent that turns towards the constellation called *baccámon* or Scorpion, when this raises in the morning. At last, also another element of pools as place where divine being Guahagiona bath himself in order to cure him from boils unites this text with the current meaning of pools as healing places.

This narrative seems to be related to the contemporary narratives about great boas from Cuba and Dominica, which in turn have direct parallels in the Lesser Antilles, the Guyanas and Suriname. The first historical reference to the great serpent in Lesser Antilles is from Bouton in 1640 in his description of the French establishment on Dominica: *"They say that there is a serpent in Dominica which has the power of making itself large or small and that it has a ruby or gem of the same luster in the middle of its forehead. It takes this gem off when it wants to drink and puts it back afterwards. No one may go or dares to go and see it in its cavern unless he has fasted for three days and abstains from his wife. Otherwise he should not be able to see it, or he would be in danger of being bewitched by it, that is to say, killed"* (Bouton 1640, p. 1-2).

Three centuries later, Taylor (1941) in his ethnographic study of the Caribs on Dominica registered a local narrative about a giant snake that can crow like a cock and in whose head a stone of dazzling brilliance is set. Being one of the main progenitors of humankind, Bakámo, having the body of a snake and a man's head, can transform himself into a normal man to help and counsel people. In the past, he was carried out to sea where he became the constellation of that name (in Western astronomy: Scorpio) (Taylor 1941 cited by Whitehead 1992, p. 312). Another version of this narrative mentions the two brothers as those who have received the arrowroot for charms: *"There lived in Salybia two brothers called Maruka and Siniimari, famous for the charms they made. They would go up to the House of the Master Boa … who, when all the earth was soft, made the Boa's Stairway at Sineku. He is big, big, big; has a diamond crest on his head; and he crows just like a cock. 'Well, when they had found him, they would take powdered tobacco and burn it before him on the blade of a paddle. Then that boa … vomited … boa arrowroot. After that, the boa would vanish, and in his place a naked young man would appear … and asked Maruka and Simanari what … they wanted … He explained to them how to employ the arrowroot in order to make their charms. (When) Maruka and*

Simanari ... felt old age ... they went away to 'the other country'. They reached the shores of the Orinoco and plunged into its stream ... They emerged upon the opposite bank ... (as) two young lads; and upon the water ... there floated two empty turtle shells. They never came back to Dominica; and at least one of them died, but the other, was thought to be still living" (Taylor 1952, p. 273).

Also the mainland themes of healing, Twin brothers and Divine Serpent coincide with the data from the Caribbean. To illustrate this with one example: de Goeje (1942) registered a tradition according to which the First Divine Healer, Harliwanli, from whom the other healers originate, was the older of two twin brothers. Harliwanli received from the Oriyu, the Serpent Mother (a water deity) the basic ingredients for healing and the instructions how to use them (tobacco, calabash and two white stones for the rattle).[349] Similarly, on the mainland it is said that charm plants (Calidrium bicolor) originated from the Divine Serpent (Penard 1907).[350]

The thematic coincidences between these mainland narratives and contemporary narratives about the Great Boa from Dominican Republic and Cuba provide us not only with more time depth, indicating a long continuity, but also with more details about the symbolic associations of water bodies, healing and ancestors. This fits well within the broader Amazon cosmology about the restorative and destructive powers of water. On the basis of the aforementioned comparisons, we conclude that the Great Boa narrative is part of the indigenous heritage. Most likely it was a well-known part of the pre-colonial religion and cultural memory of these islands. During the first half of 16th century it may have been communicated by the local indigenous people to the newcomers and so have become integrated into the newly formed culture. This hypothesis is plausible given the widespread dispersal of the narratives about the Great Boa in Cuba which seem to be modified versions of the Great Serpent narrative. One could argue that, given the large-scale raids and expeditions capturing indigenous people from the Lesser Antilles and the mainland, it is also possible that this motif may be indigenous heritage of non-local origin that was exchanged in the early colonial period. However, in the light of the intensive pre-colonial interactions between the islands and the mainland (as demonstrated by archaeological research) this seems less likely.

The Great Boa narrative may have provided a basis for syncretism or rather symbolic synergy with the above-mentioned beliefs from West Africa or with other water gods and beings like the *miengus*, who are said to be beautiful, mermaid-like figures with long hair that live in rivers and in the sea and bring good fortune to those who worship them. These, in turn, have parallels in European beliefs about water beings like sirens and mermaids, which may have added their part to the process of synergizing

349 In this narrative the twins are the children of the Sun and the Moon. The moon, their mother, is firstly guided in her celestial journey when following the father, but later when she got angry at them, twins take revenge by not indicating the way anymore, and therefore she is lost and later killed. In this version the twins escape the danger by using their healing art (Goeje 1942).

350 Also Okojomu is linked to Twins (see Penard 1907: 102). Curiously, the eel and firefly are seen as symbols of the force of Okojumu (Divine Beings of the Water) or the Divine Serpent. There are interesting coincides with the earlier accounts. As earlier mentioned some Dominicans and Cubans suggested that *cucuyos* are souls of deceased persons. One of the contributors from Boca de Mana declared that his uncle could transform into an eel.

worldviews, leading to the contemporary narrative about the mermaid-like indigenous woman that could be the Mother of the Water.

Again, it is highly complicated to reconstruct the exact form and meaning of the water symbolism among the indigenous peoples of the Greater Antilles. Sweet water as a source of life and death has played a prominent role in various worldviews around the world. At least, in regions historically related to the Caribbean water sources are important and empowered places. My colleague, Adrian Gomes, Wapishana PhD researcher from Guyana, after reading the previous account about the Dominican water bodies commented briefly on the importance of water resources among the Wapishana: *"...we value the water sources, springs and certain deep pools for we believe that these are sacred places with deep spiritual meanings. These sacred sites are kept by powerful spiritual beings. Therefore, every Wapishana is taught to respect these sacred places."* This respect is expressed by avoiding different activities which might disturb these sites. Mr. Gomes continues to explain that among the Wapishana: *"At certain sites, it is customary to offer tobacco or farine (a local cereal made from the cassava or manioc) to appease the spirits whilst passing the site on a journey. If no offering is made, one might become sick at a later time. We carry out our ceremonies and spiritual practices through the guidance of the marunao or the shaman who provides healing and spiritual guidance. However, persons who seek spiritual healing are not obliged to go to these spiritual places. Rather, the patient goes to the home of the marunao or the marunao comes to the home of the patient for spiritual healing. Hearing the prayer or seeing the ritual in situ is the customary law if one wants to learn about a ritual or prayer. This is how the Wapishana people pass on this particular knowledge to their fellow villagers. A person who now knows the prayer can now use it to heal others. Therefore, one should not be surprised if a Wapishana, when asked information about a ritual, he or she does not seem willing to divulge the information."*

The indigenous people of Martinique at the beginning of 17th century had a similar prohibition. An anonymous narrator visiting this island between 1618 and 1620 observed that it was prohibited to wash vessels in the currents of the river because this would bring thunder, rain and floods (Anonymous de Carpentras 1618-1620 in Petitjean Roget 1995). The narratives about indigenous spirits that are dangerous for certain persons seem to be a warning to be cautious at certain parts of the rivers which could be dangerous. Future studies should verify whether these beliefs were connected to the prohibitions to execute certain tasks like fishing or washing.

Concluding remarks

The Cuban and Dominican water sources are memory places, whose meanings are composed of sometimes fragmented past cosmologies of diverse origin situated in shared landscapes. The great sacred serpent narrative indicates an (unconscious) engagement with the indigenous past, which can be entangled into the symbolism of posterior periods. Unlike other landmarks a small water pool might not directly call our visual attention but nonetheless it may be of great importance for local history. The multiple meanings and symbolic associations of special parts of rivers, waterfalls, pools, and similar places seem to be testimonies of the universal value of certain landscape features, whose symbolism, rooted in different worldviews, converged spatially in the Caribbean context. To a certain degree this universality of landscape symbolism created the conditions for producing fusion, but also the space for masking people's own spirituality. We may compare the development of the meanings of these places with the flows of the rivers themselves. Some meanings would spread into new evolving landscapes, which themselves change, expand where possible, merge with other flows, erode on their way, dry out, submerge into subterranean and re-emerge as new small spring without seemingly apparent connections yet sometimes leaving profound imprints in these landscapes and also memories.

The next chapter focuses on another important landscape feature: the caverns, as natural sites wherein the historical memory has been inscribed and is being constantly re-inscribed through oral traditions and performances of rituals.

9

Re-membering Ancestors in Caves

Caverns are a crucial part of contemporary Caribbean healing landscapes. Caverns have been inscribed into Caribbean landscape biography as healing places, loci of (sacred) history as well as enigmatic places in oral traditions. Caverns have been a focus of, and curiosity for, narrators with divergent motives, adherents of different worldviews, archaeologists, but also looters searching for imagined treasures in these enchanted places.

Rich archeological record suggests that caverns have been loci of various human activities that in the case of Puerto Rican dates more than four millennia back (Rodríguez Ramos et al. 2018). These places served various purposes in pre-colonial era, throughout the colonial times, and during the period of the Independence War (further readings: Barnet 1987; La Rosa Corzo 1991; Ulloa Hung 2015; Pereira 2008). In oral history caverns figures as ancestral sites, places where indigenous peoples lived, as hiding places for escaped Maroons during the colonial period (see below: the caves of Gibara) and as shelters supposedly used during the Cuban revolution (*e.g.* the Santa Barbara/Chango cave known in Jiguaní but also in Niquero). Inhabitants sought refuge here during hurricanes: during David (1979) in Boca Yuma, during George (1998) in Mana, during Irma (2017) in Gibara and during Mathew (2016) in Punta de Maisí in Holguín province.[351]

Caverns on these islands have multiple meanings. Often caverns are mysterious, feared, and therefore avoided. On the other hand Cuban and Dominican devotees consider caves as places of manifestation or agency of divine beings, Saints, and remote predecessors, which can all potentially intervene in matters of human wellbeing. Adherents of Spiritism, Dominican 21 Division, Regla de Ocha, and Roman Catholicism, seek to contact and communicate with those beings, looking for improvement of their health and wellbeing in various caverns. On both islands, caverns are associated frequently with Indigenous Peoples and their past.

The following paragraphs discuss how contemporary inhabitants reinterpret and connect to their ancestral history by means of narratives and rituals. Patronal celebra-

351 For more information about how people have saved their live by hiding in caves read the news articles by Azam, A. (2016, October 17) or Romero Rodríguez (2016, October 14) or Nacher (no date). According to interview no. 152957 the Cave of Santa Bárbara was sacred and used for pilgrimages in the past.

tions and other rituals will be a point of reflection about how the indigenous ancestors are incorporated into the cultural memory. The healing function of patronal celebrations will be highlighted.

The next examples will show how ancestral commemoration is integrated within activities aimed at improvement of individual and communal wellbeing. During patronal celebrations people express their commitment and respect to Saints or *lwas* but also to indigenous ancestors, thanking them for their guidance and benefits. Like in the earlier mentioned case of La Iglesia close to La Jaiba (between Playa Ensenada and Estero Hondo), different caverns were used for ceremonial activities. During the period of fieldwork Dominican caverns that were actively used were: Cueva de La Mancha (in Boca de Mana), Cueva de San Francisco (in Bánica), Cueva del Indio (in La Hoya Grande), Cueva de Bernard, Cueva del Misterio (in Boca de Yuma)[352], and the caves of Pommier. In addition, some caverns located in the Dominican province of Mao (municipality Marmolejos, Navas) were reported as places of ritual activity in the past.

Similarly, rituals are performed in different Cuban caverns: a cavern in Gibara, a cavern near Managuaco, Cueva De Los Muertos in Guara, and in El Guafe, while in the past Cave Samuel (in Niquero) and the cavern of El Júcaro (in Antilla) were used for ceremonies of Spiritism.[353]

Mana Landscape

The Cave at La Mancha and El Hombre Parado are among the few healing places in the Mana region in the Máximo Gómez National Park. These places are related to the biography of Mrs. Viviana de La Rosa (1850?-1925), who was a healer, prophet, and founder of the Hatillo Mana community (Tejeda Ortiz in 1978). Together with Liborio Mateo she is considered the Saint and Messiah of the Dominican South. She raised the first church of the Virgen de las Mercedes and performed healings at different places in the Mana landscape.

The fame of Mrs. De La Rosa is owed to her power to divine the future and heal people. Her great-great-grandson, Mr. Julián De La Rosa, describes her as: "*an evangelizer spreading the Word of the Lord, many people were visiting her. Afterwards many ill people visited her, she prayed and cured them by the Lord's Word. Those who felt something supernatural she gave a glass of water from the jar and they were cured by faith and prayer.*"[354] Being both an evangelizer and a healer, she cured through prayers, and also

---

352 Juan Julio Castillo, guardian from the National park, who is attending Cueva Bernard, explained that occasionally traditional healers bring their patients to this cave (province La Altagracia). At one occasion he witnessed one of the ceremonies: *"they brought here a crazy women and the man said 'carry her up here' (the cave), and they carried her up, and her family together with her, and the man says 'untie her untie her' and he dressed her in black dress and when I saw her the dress disappeared and she was there naked! She was a young lady and they dressed her in white dress and she cured. And she went down and say to her mother 'I am hungry', and the black dress nobody saw it, and nobody carried it away, it just disappeared.*" (interview with Juan Julio).

353 For the details on the cavern of El Júcaro (in Antilla) see the study of Rodríguez Cullel & Peña Obregon (2000). The first studies registering ritual activities in caves are: Gleniz Tavarez (2013) on Bánica, Lopez Belando (2011) on Boca de Mana and also a brief reference by Tejeda Ortiz (1978) on Cave de La Mancha. When I use any information provided by these authors I refer to them explicitly.

354 Interview with Julián De La Rosa.

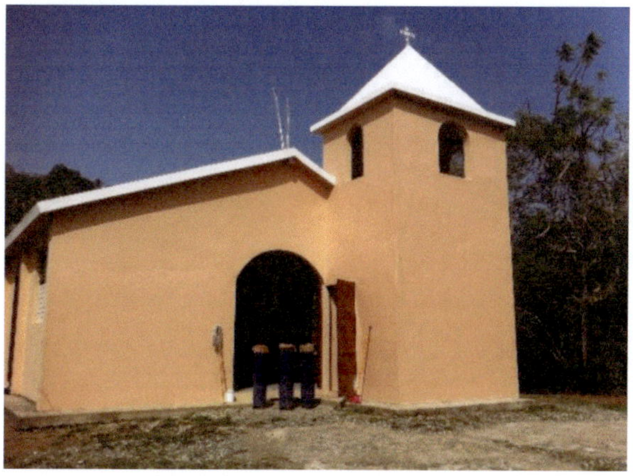

Figure 53 The church of the Virgen de las Mercedes in Hatillo Mana, Dominican Republic.

through medicinal plants. Her memory is still alive as her gift to heal and communicate with the invisible divine powers was inherited by somc family members including her great-great-grandson. On special occasions, Viviana de La Rosa incarnated into the bodies of *caballos del misterio* to help people in matters of health and wellbeing.

Among places which are connected to the biography of Mrs. De La Rosa are: the church, which is also her final resting place, and the house-temples administrated by family relatives of Mrs. Viviana, a water stream at the foot of the hill of the church, the cavern of El Conde in Monte Bonito and crosses erected by Viviana, La Mancha cavern and cavern in El Conde.

Until now, the church erected by Mrs. De La Rosa is dedicated to the Virgen de las Mercedes and is administered by her great-granddaughter Mrs. Estefanía De La Rosa and her son Mr. Julián De La Rosa. The church is visited by many pilgrims, who come especially on the day of patronal celebration. At the foot of the hill where the Church is situated some of the pilgrims purify themselves from their sins in a small water pool whose holy water is appreciated for its healing and protective powers.

Another site associated with the life of Mrs. Viviana de La Rosa is El Conde (abbreviation of El Escondito), with a nearby cave from which she was transporting herself to the cave of La Mancha (spiritually, in her state of grace). The path to the cave is marked by a massive natural rock arch, which forms a physical transit zone from the profane to the sacred. Here, first offerings are brought in the form of candles, and also ritual bathing takes place as one can see from the remains of plants and tobacco. The path to the cave is further delimitated by one *calvario*, dressed in yellow, red, and blue colored papers.[355] Near this *calvario* visitors make their first prayers and light candles. Inside the cave there are small altars with images of Virgins (Altagracia/ Mercedes), Belie Becán/San Miguel (the popular patron of Dominican healers), Sacred Heart of Jesus, the All-Powefull Hand. In front of some small altars there were still *Véves* visible, secret symbols that serve as signs for *lwas* to descend on this specific site. Also, on one altar, a candle was burning with some fresh food offerings of calabash, deposited with older

355 All colors have meaning in Dominican 21 Division. The blue can symbolize Ogún Balenyó/ Santiago, or in this case maybe Saint John, Yellow Anaisa Pié/Santa Ana. Red stands normally for Papa Candelo/ San Carlos Borromeo but if it is in combination with green it symbolizes Belién Belcán/San Miguel.

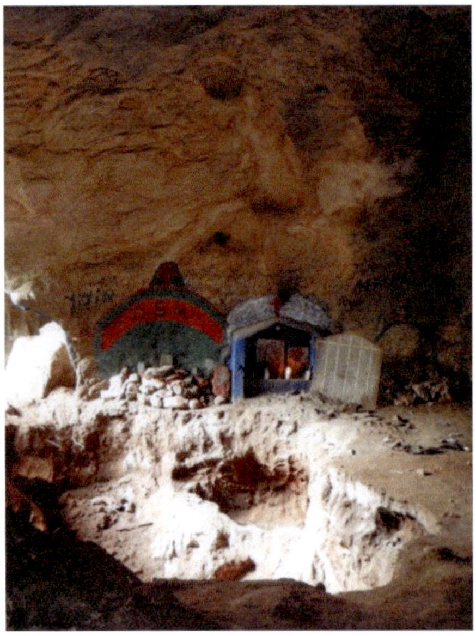

Figure 54 One of the altars in a cavern near El Conde, closeby to Boca de Mana.

empty bottles of alcohol and flowers in water. Although it was not possible to interview a healer about the practices in this particular cavern, the material evidence encountered here suggests that the place is of profound religious significance. Unfortunately, this cavern has been affected by the excavation of *guano* that is used as a fertilizer for agriculture: one of the altars has been demolished together with possible archaeological evidence.

Cave of La Mancha: Healing with Indigenous Lwas

A cave situated in the community La Mancha is one of the places used for healing in the Mana landscape.[356] La Mancha is an abandoned settlement, which is accessible only by foot – it takes approximately forty minutes from Boca de Mana in the municipality El Yaguate in the southern Dominican province San Cristóbal. The oral history of this cavern is closely related to the biography of a specific traditional healer: Mrs. Viviana de la Rosa.

One of the places utilized in the past by Mrs. De La Rosa for healing is the cave at La Mancha. Juan Pablo Rosario Araujó described Mrs. De La Rosa's first encounter with this cavern: *"According to the predecessors, Viviana discovered this cave, being a daughter of Indians, and those living in the cave were Indians and she fought with Indians*

356 The information from this case study is based on personal participation in the rituals and interviews with different contributors including the family of Viviana De La Rosa, inhabitants of Hatillo Mana, Boca de Mana, Mancha, as well as traditional healer Giovanni Guzmán, who is still coming regularly to the cave. For specific details see my interviews in the Leiden depository. The contact with Giovanni Guzmán was kindly facilitated by José Antonio (Toño) Arías Peláez, a student of Anthropology at the Universidad Autónoma de Santo Domingo, who is planning to publish a thesis on the community of Hatillo Mana. He has visually documented many of the ceremonies that take place in the cavern and also interviewed many members of the Mana community throughout the years. In his presentation in Museo del Hombre Dominicano in 2016, called 'Cueva Mana, entre la memoria exigua y el olvido', he referred to the rapid changes of altars taking place in this cavern.

under the (influence of) rum, with a cavalry of people, she discovered the entrance of the cave and under the (influence of) rum she drove them out, and separated them, to take her place in the cave (while) giving rum to people of the group in the cavalry with a lot of rum, food and things".[357] In brief, this fragment could be interpreted as: Viviana de La Rosa, a person with a gift to heal and to communicate with indigenous *misterios*, discovered this cavern wherein she performed rituals (including a trance, or a dream) that enabled her to gain her own space at this cavern, which was previously governed by indigenous ancestors. Afterwards Viviana de La Rosa performed some of her healing in this cavern as well as in other places of the Mana landscape.

Mrs. De La Rosa was considered by various inhabitants "*a daughter of an Indian man*". Also one of the evangelist neighbors, who condemned the healing rituals in caverns as witchcraft, confirmed the well-known narrative about how Mrs. Viviana's mother was lost in the water pool. This family history should be seen in the broader cultural context in which healers are said to be taken away by "Indians" (*i.e. misterios*) and so develop an ability to communicate with the invisible and to cure. In my view, this narrative illustrates a deep spiritual identification of this healer with indigenous ancestors, which gave her more social recognition as a powerful healer.

Until today the cave of La Mancha is a spiritual and sacred place where different *misterios* can manifest themselves and provide advice in matters of wellbeing and health. Devotees have been coming here from Baní, Hatillo Mana, Bajo de Haina, Yaguate, Altagracia, and in the past also from Bánica (on the Dominican-Haitian border). Some 11 traditional healers visit this cavern regularly as part of initiations, healing rituals, peregrination, and during the feast of Saint John. One of them is Giovanni Guzmán, *caballo del misterio* of 21 Division. Mr. Guzmán has been going to pilgrimages to this place for approximately 30 years already. As a child he used to walk to this cavern from Bajos de Haina (30-35 km) together with his mother, grandmother and groups of pilgrims. The first stop of his pilgrimage in the Mana landscape is a part of the Mana river called *El Hombre Parado* (The Standing Man): *"Every time they were first bathing in the river and then they went up to the cave* [...] *A lot of people were lighting candles, many went to bath to ward off the negative"* (interview with Mr. Guzmán 2014).

Following this tradition Mr. Guzmán brought me to El Hombre Parado, which is a water pool roofed by an extraordinary rock positioned at the upper part of the Mana River, about a thirty minutes' walk from the community Boca de Mana. *El Hombre Parado* represents an important site in the local healing landscape. Mr. Julián De La Rosa confirmed that this place is very spiritual; it is a popular place where people with certain health problems come to ask for favors and health. Together with the Cueva de La Mancha it is an important place in the initiation of healers who are being prepared to work with indigenous *lwas*. This site is also a place where the indigenous past is remembered through ritual engagement with indigenous *misterios*.

During the first visit with Mr. Guzmán in 2014 bathing started with a prayer to the Indigenous Division, followed by smoking tobacco and offering a candle; the subsequent submersion into the pool should ward off all negative energies. On occasions, more elaborate baths are organized here. During these activities the *indigenous misterios* and Saint John are asked to attract the positive (like health, good luck in love or bu-

357 Interview with Rosario Araujó.

siness) while taking sweet baths or to ward off the negative (*e.g.* harmful spells) while taking bitter baths. For the cure to be effective the belief in the *misterios* of the stream is essential. Depending on the exact problem of the person various ingredients may be used. Mr. Guzmán uses frequently: flowery waters (one can buy these in botanic shops), water from coconuts, red wine, beer, teas of *manzanilla, canelilla* and *mejorana.* Also fruits (watermelon, papaya, *guineo*) and flowers of different colors are dedicated to the Indian Division in order to receive good luck.[358]

After the spiritual cleansing at El Hombre Parado, pilgrims continue their journey to the cavern La Mancha. Mr. Guzmán narrated: *"I have started to bring pilgrims there since I am 14 years old. I started to bring people there for a bath to ward off the negative, in quest for a blessing, we were going to the cave and to the spring so that people receive force, the Light, spiritual cleaning of their body, because the cave is a place of healing, a place of spiritual material healing, of inner and outer corporal healing."* Cueva De La Mancha is a site of therapeutic consult with *misterios* throughout the whole year. Healers and their followers come from different locations for individual healing rituals and also to express their gratitude after successful renewal during the celebration of Saint John, the patronal saint of this cavern.

The feast of Saint John is celebrated on June 23rd, around the time of the summer solstice, for which healers, their followers and pilgrims from different communities (including Mana, Baní, San Cristobal, Bajo de Haina) come together in Cueva de Mana in La Mancha. The participants state explicitly that for them the main goal of this celebration is to fulfill their vows to St. John and other Saints, *lwas* and spirits that enable them to cure illnesses and overcome other obstacles in their lives.

I have participated in the St. John celebration in the Cueva de Mana in 2015. This celebration was marked by extraordinary circumstances because a close friend of the administrator of St. John's house-temple (a small chapel which was not consecrated by The Church) had suddenly died. This death and also her own health condition impeded the organizer, Mrs. Candelaria Bautista De La Rosas, who is Mrs. Viviana's great-granddaughter, to attend the traditional mass at her house-temple. In addition, due to the severe droughts of that year pilgrims did not perform the ritual cleansing at El Hombre Parado before continuing their peregrination to the cave, as is the custom, because the stream had nearly dried up. Both events downsized the number of participants of the feast of that year. The droughts clearly formed also an economic obstacle for those living from agriculture.

Many days before the feast begins, the participants prepare themselves individually. This preparation starts with a personal sacrifice, *i.e.* saving enough money to be able to afford the journey. For the organizing healer this means that she must arrive earlier with her family, friends, and followers to prepare the ceremonial meal and organize the drummers to make offerings to the *misterios.* This self-sacrifice is to a certain extent also physical. Some pilgrims carry a lot of belongings, following a steep path to the cave where they have to circumnavigate crosses. There candles are lit and stones deposited. The last stop is made at a third cross where devotees ask permission of El Dueño de la Cueva (The Owner/Master of the Cave) to enter the cave, by ringing an iron object (in the past a bell) to make the *misterios* aware that people are coming.

---

358 Interview no. 95 and 96.

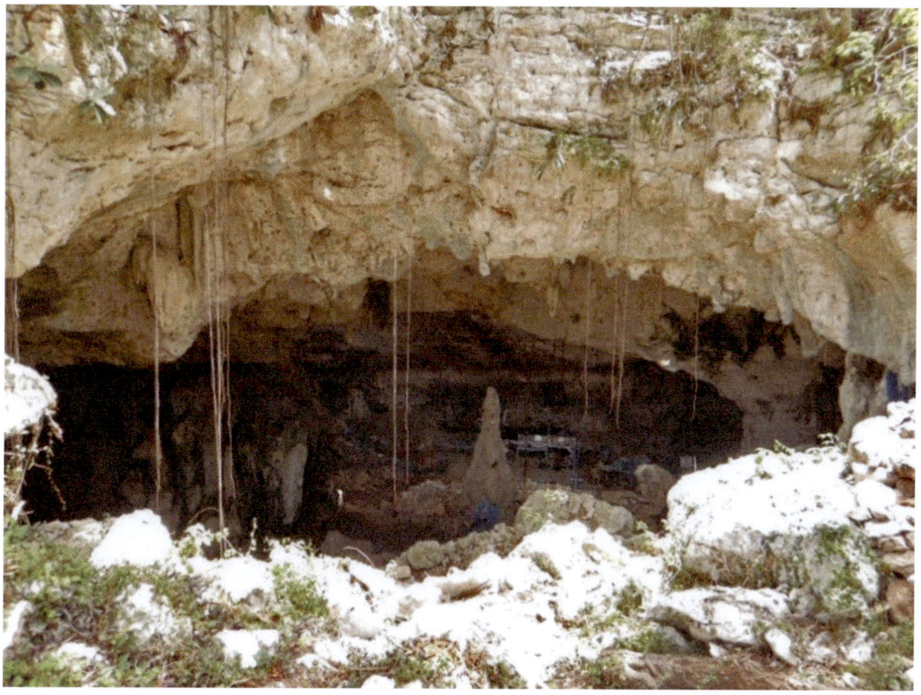

Figure 55 The entrance to the Cueva de la Mancha with the stalagmite that represents Saint John, Dominican Republic.

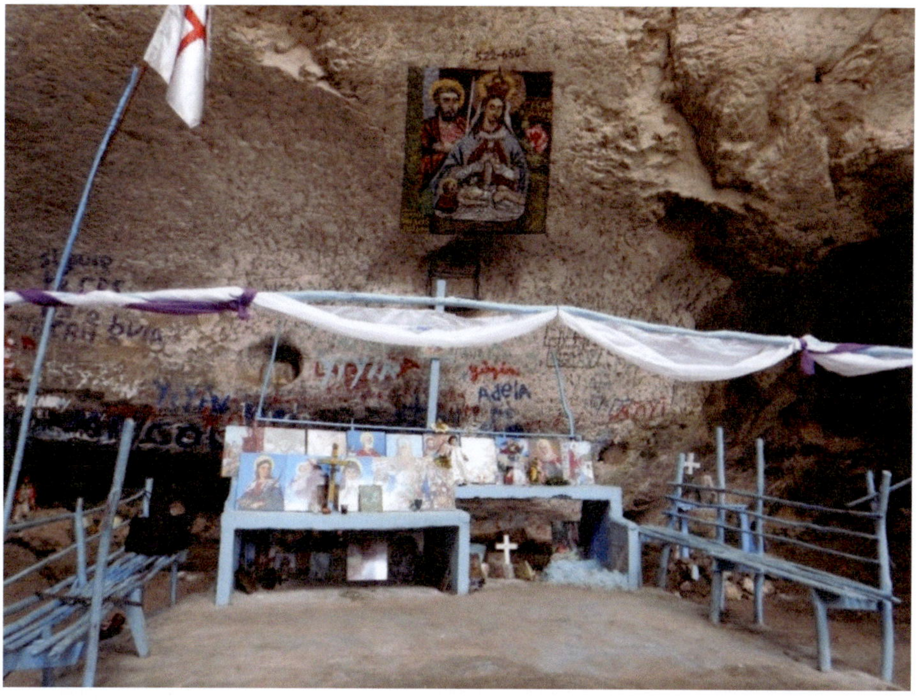

Figure 56 The main altar during the feast of Saint John.

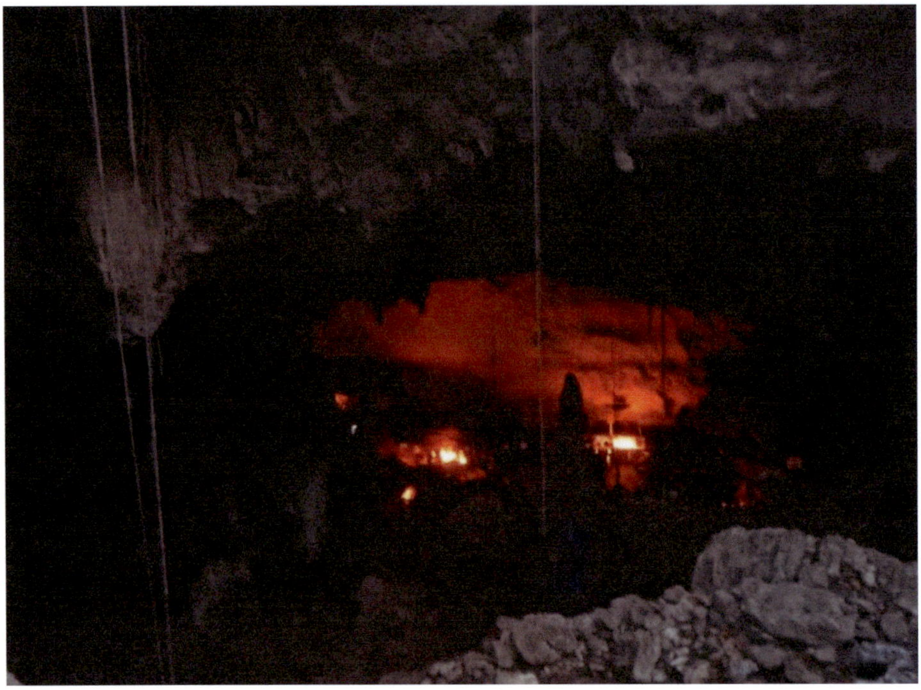

Figure 57 The entrance of Cueva de La Mancha at the night of Saint John.

From this point, visitors proceed to an altar of Saint John, carved in a large stalagmite in front of which devotees wait until holy water drops on their head from the ceiling of the cave. Then they light a candle and proceed to chambers with smaller energy points of Papa Legba, Belié Belcán, and *lwas* of the Ogún division, such as Ogún Balenyó and his spouse Ofelia Balenyó (Virgen de las Mercedes). Further in the cave are Los Petroses (earth lwas) of Santa Marta La Dominadora, Barón del Cementerio (San Elías), Yemayá, Alailá (Virgen de Altagracia, the Dominican patron), and the chamber of indigenous ancestors. The pilgrims encircle the main altar of 21 divisions with Saint John. Mr. José De Los Santos one of the last inhabitants of the small settlement La Mancha, brings the small statue of Saint John from De La Rosas´ the house-temple. The statue of St. John stays at the main altar for the day and the whole night; later it is returned to his house-temple.

Participants of the celebration deposit at the main altar their votive offerings symbolizing their prayers, gratitude, and commitments to the Saint(s) and/or lwa(s). At the main altars as well as at small points for specific lwas we find candles, cigars, flowers, food (fruits, peanuts, corn, bread) and beverages (coffee and/or alcohol). Yenni, a traditional healer originally from La Mancha, offers to the *misterios* and participants a dish of Chicken with Moro (rice & black beans), and arrange the music as part of her vow. Musicians invoke misterios by singing, playing of drums and güiras (metal scraper instruments). The prayers are sung and are dedicated to different *misterios* starting with Papa Legba, Bon Dieus/Gran Dios, Santa Marta, Barón del cementerio/San Elías and the indigenous *misterios*. Together with the music (while the drums crucial), tobacco, and alcohol are important means to make misterio arrive. Following the drums, echoing powerfully throughout the cavern, the *misterios* manifest themselves through the bodies of *Caballos del Misterio*.

The celebration culminates with the arrival of the *misterios*, when these descend into the heads of those initiated or gifted and through them participate in the celebration by dancing, drinking, and eating. The representations of the incorporeal mysterious agency become substantial in clothes and behavior, which are characteristic of the personage of the *misterio*.

Engaging with Misterios of Indigenous Peoples at La Mancha

The Saint John cavern is a place where different *misterios* including indigenous ancestors can be consulted with regard to matters of health and wellbeing. Like other *misterios* indigenous ancestors are called upon with offerings and music to descend. The lyrics dedicated to the indigenous *lwas* could be translated as: *"The Indian woman is, the Indian woman goes, the Indian woman lives under the water, the Indian woman arrived from under the water"*. This song was played at the beginning of the feast. During my presence, *indigenous misterios* did not enter into the head of (initiated) healers, ritual specialist or of other believers. This could be explained by the circumstance that at the moment there were no healers present who had an indigenous *misterio* as their main protector. There were other healers, however, *e.g.* Mr. Guzmán, who had been initiated to work also with indigenous *misterios*. This indicates that indigenous ancestors were part of the celebration and were honored though offerings and prayers but not the most important force to be recognized that night.

Among the offerings dedicated to indigenous ancestors were: tobacco, candles, fruits (*e.g.* watermelon, mango), flowers, maní, and maize. These offering were placed under the main altar at the man-made pool, at the personal altars of the healers, at places where the water from stalactites concentrate and at a specific section of the cave called the "Indian chamber". According to Mr. José Isabel Jiménez de los Santos this part distinguishes itself from the rest of the cave by its hollow bottom, which is indicative that underneath there could be water, a small pool where "Indians" live. In the altar setting they are represented by icons of indigenous national heroes and historical personages, such as Enriquillo, Caonabo, Anacaona or similar figures from abroad, such as the Venezuelan Trinity (Maria Lionza, Guaicaipuro, Negro Felipe) and by manmade small pools of water.

As in the case of other altars of 21 Division specialists, these images of indigenous heroes were accompanied by Yemayá, the sea goddess. Her blue color and water symbolism link her to the "Indian division".[359] The Indigenous division is not considered to be one of the many representations of Yemayá. There seem to be generally related through water element and through landscape as Yemayá guards the mouth of the river and the sea. Similarly, there is a close relationship (parallel) between the Indigenous *lwas* and Saint John. More specifically, they share the blue color and elements (sweet water), as well as particular places of worship such as this cavern or El Hombre Parado and both share the aspect of having purifying powers to ward off all sins and spells. Mr. Guzmán clarified that although both share the water symbolism, according to him

359 In Cuban Palo Monte she is often not the Mother of the Sea but Mother of the Waters including sweet water.

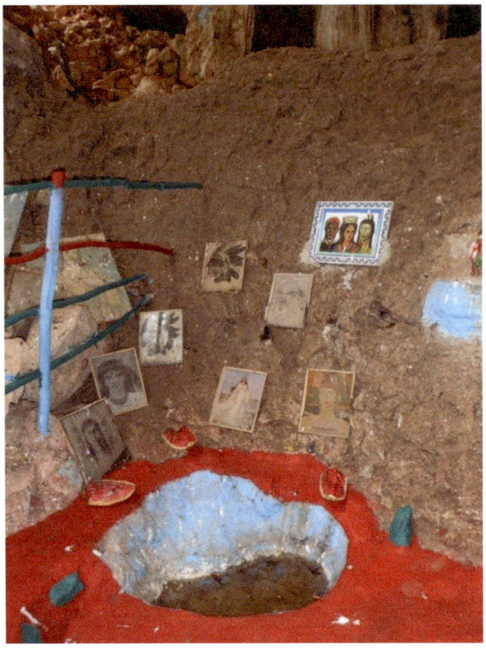

Figure 58 A part of an altar in the Cave of Saint John in Mana. Observe the stereotypical representation of indigenous heroes such as Coanabo with the feather headdress, on the left.

Saint John is *not a* patron of the "Indigenous division". He assumed that Saint John has been chosen as patron of this particular cave because Mrs. Viviana came from Baní where he is patronal saint of the city. According to the literature (Lundahl & Lundius 2012) several devotees of Indigenous Division from Baní do consider that this division can be represented by the image of Saint John.

Mr. Guzmán considered Tindjo to belong to the Indigenous division. Tindjo is associated with the Catholic Saint San Rafael, considered to be a divine healer, who has water and fish as his attributes. Mr Guzmán described in general terms his consults with Tindjo, which took place throughout the year in the cavern La Mancha: *"Tindjo emerged, went and took the water, purified and blessed the whole world* [...] *This was inside of the cave because the cave contained a lot of water pools and before there were water and lagoons everywhere. Now not anymore because of* [the lack of] *the rain, because people made a lot of stuff. So there the misterio was manifesting and bringing devotees, cleansing, healing them and giving them the water to drink and you could feel that you were healing from inside because you got diarrhea and this was cleansing you from inside."*[360]

Also initiations of *caballo del misterio* take place at this cavern throughout the year. For these the initiates come from remote places. One of the healers from Monte Plata declared that approximately 30 years ago she came to this cavern as part of her initiation, which now enables her to work with indigenous *lwas*. The indigenous past is not only remembered in the cavern at La Mancha but also in other sites of the Mana landscape.

In recalling childhood memories Mr. Guzmán associates this cavern further with indigenous predecessors: *"We were climbing there with a candle, food, and all people were very organized. If it was said you leave there, fruits, mapuey, ñame, yautía, cassave, big*

360 Interview no. 130615.

dishes in higüero they went and left it there. And there were not so many altars as now, there were crosses, neither Saint John, there was nothing. Up there was an altar and a hermitage, where people were resting and were going down to the cave and were communicating with the Indian Division. They were every time bathing there. There was some water that was used to cure you from inside, from everything, if you got diarrhea even better because this was a sign that you were cleaning. And the objective was to collect water here, there existed seven spaces of cavern to search seven drops of water. Similarly, you had to make seven circles before entering the cavern." He elaborated on the changes within the Saint John cavern: *"Before, it was not the same as it is now. Before, one did not find Saints there as quickly as it is now. The Saints were from the Catholic Church, there were not so many botanic shops. Before, in the cave there was no altar. There was the Virgen de Altagracia, small images, and a wooden cross... The first Saints that were there belonged to persons who did not want to have an altar any more so they were depositing their Saints in the cave, to not throw it away (because this could have negative consequences). Since then it is that all these things were constructed. Without this it would remain with the belief in Indians because this was what was there in the past. People were coming to the cave because it was a sacred indigenous Taíno point where you make contact with Taíno gods of nature. Now all Caballos de los Misterios who went there put their candle and all other divisions but in reality this cave is a sacred space and point of the Indian Division."*

Also in another part of his reflection about past pilgrimages Mr. Guzmán linked this place to the indigenous past. When asking permission of the Owner of the Cave before entering the cavern, he recalled that his grandmother used to hit the rock in front of the cave with a stone, and continued: *"I think she was doing it because of having fear of the Indians so it was a sign for them to hide, I am thinking it could be this because I have kept the tradition. Before, they were doing it with a stone, you know it was a signal that they arrived. Because every time it was said there was an Indian, if you have left there something, some rubbish, in the morning it was cleaned, it were the Indians who were cleaning it".*

Multiple sites of the Mana landscape, narratives and practices have explicit connections to the indigenous ancestors. The memory of the indigenous past is interlinked with the cavern, particularly through the feast of Saint John, which includes explicit indices to their commemoration. This memory is also integrated in therapeutic sessions wherein the ancestral forces are invoked, with testimonies of their agency and initiations. Specific sites such as Hombre Parado, Cueva de La Mancha are not only places of healing but also ancestral places where that memory is kept alive.

Conflicts in Mana landscapes

As in other regions, also in Mana there seem to exist religious tensions about the value of ritual activities at diverse healing places including the La Mancha and El Conde caverns. These were also displayed during the feast: the celebration was briefly interrupted by members of the evangelical church, who started to offend participants and play loud music to drown out the drums. This incident was preceded already by other examples of tension, which resulted in the destruction of *calvarios* or painted rocks. During illegal road construction in 2018 the path towards the cave of la Mancha including calvarios have been destroyed (Arías Peláez, personal communication). The damage of the archaeological sites in the surroundings of this cavern is yet to be assessed.

These incidents raise concerns about the protection of sacred sites like this place in the Dominican context wherein devotees of 21 Division are attacked for their beliefs. In the case of La Mancha local authorities were mobilized to stop the destruction of the path of the pilgrimage, not because it was recognized as sacred place but because the cavern is situated in a nationally protected area. In other cases like the pool of Tamare in La Jaiba the destruction of this places is difficult to prevent legally. According to the law no. 391 devotees of Vudú can be sentenced to a fine, even to days in prison for organizing their festivities. Likewise those who provide their houses for these ceremonies can be officially persecuted. This law was criticized for being against the own Dominican constitution, and as openly discriminative and racist (Tejeda Ortiz 2013)

The Cave of Saint Francis as a Healing and Memory Place of Bánica

Cueva de San Francisco in Bánica (province Elías Piña) is located at the top of Saint Francis Hill, a walk of approximately half an hour from the municipality. The Sacred Mountain is a protected natural monument because of an endemic cactus, Rosa de Bánica, and the presence of petroglyphs with stylistic features of the pre-colonial period (Puello Nina & Tavarez 2014). The Saint Francis cavern is one of two caverns in this mountain. The second cave is situated at the northern side of the mountain facing Pedro Santana, well known for the La Zurza sulfur spring. The Cavern of Saint Francis is a sanctuary of regional importance. Each year, this sanctuary is visited by thousands of pilgrims (approximately 25,000) from different regions including the provinces of San Juan, Azua, even San Cristóbal. The Cavern of Saint Francis is a focal point of the patronal celebration during which people come from far and wide to pray for their health and wellbeing. The subsequent paragraphs will address its relation with healing during the time of the patronal celebration, which is intertwined with the commemoration of the spirits of indigenous peoples.

The cave and hill of Saint Francis are sacred locations because Saint Francis has manifested himself there. Different accounts of his appearance have been preserved in oral history. Mr. Lionicio De La Rosa Alcántara, told how this event was described to him.[361] A man named Godo was searching for bees on the hill when he suddenly heard hammering sounds; following the noise he arrived at a huge cave where he did not find anyone, only an image, so he went and announced his discovery to the church whose administrators returned to the cave and saw that the image was that of Saint Francis. They brought the image to the church where it was hung but later the image disappeared. Saint Francis returned back to the cave. After being forcibly displaced a third time he never appeared again. In another version by Xavier De Los Santos Saint Francis first manifested himself as a person in the church of Bánica and afterwards he disappeared. People were searching for him everywhere and found him in the cave. They brought him back to the church down town. But he escaped back to the cave

361 All further discussed contributors of this section are inhabitants of Bánica who regularly participate in the celebration of Saint Francis.

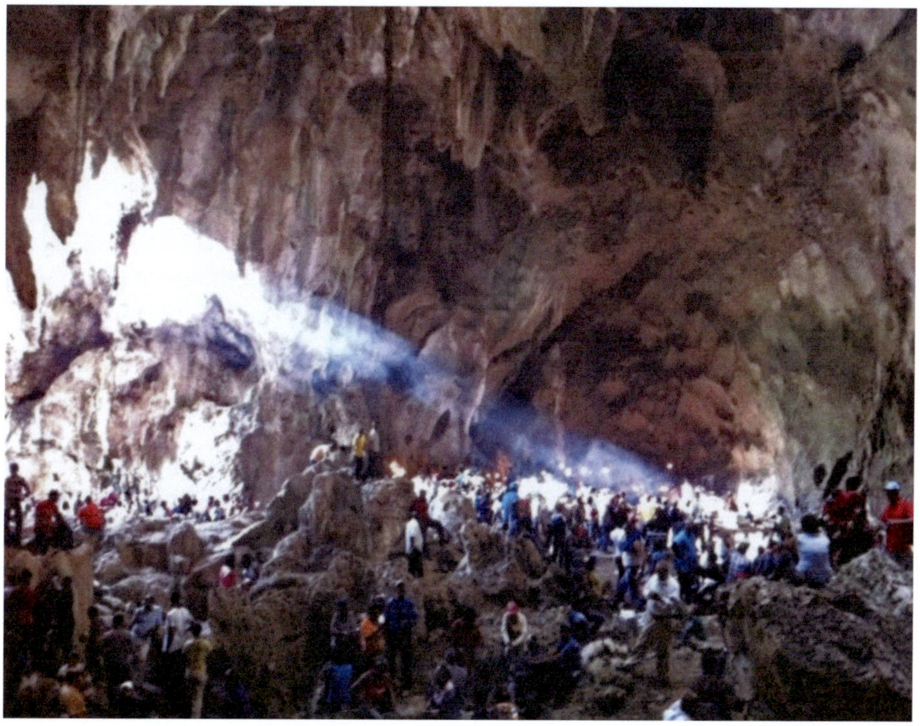

Figure 59 The view of the Saint Francis Cavern on the 4th October, a beam of sunlight hits the Saint's altar, Bánica, Dominican Republic.

because that was his home. This sequence of events repeated itself several times until Saint Francis disappeared forever.[362]

There is no consensus as to when exactly the celebration of Saint Francis started to be celebrated in the cavern. For some this should be the date of the foundation of the city, for others it goes further back. Mr. Xavier de Los Santos asserted that since the time when God created the world the cavern was visited. According to him, it was visited by the predecessors, "*the first people that were here in the world*", from those days onwards people have been visiting the hill, but then, after Trujillo, people started to make vows.[363] Other statements that this celebration has always existed show that it goes further back than the collective memory.[364] Another spiritual leader of Bánica, Mr. Hecfredes Gómez, described the cavern of Saint Francis as a holy place, comparable to a church, which in his words is a center of indigenous peregrinations since the time that indigenous people lived here.[365] Another Baniquera, Ms. Flor Celeste, from the Oviedo family (according to oral tradition one of the founding families of the town),

362 Interview no. 073947.

363 Interview no. 170.

364 Interview with Mr. Manuel María Moreta De Los Santos (no. 160957).

365 Mr. Hecfredes Gómez's view of this cavern as an indigenous pilgrimage site is rather unique but he is an important spiritual and influential leader so it has to be considered. His interpretation can be explained by his own deep spiritual link to this place as well as his contacts with an archaeologist from the Museo del Hombre.

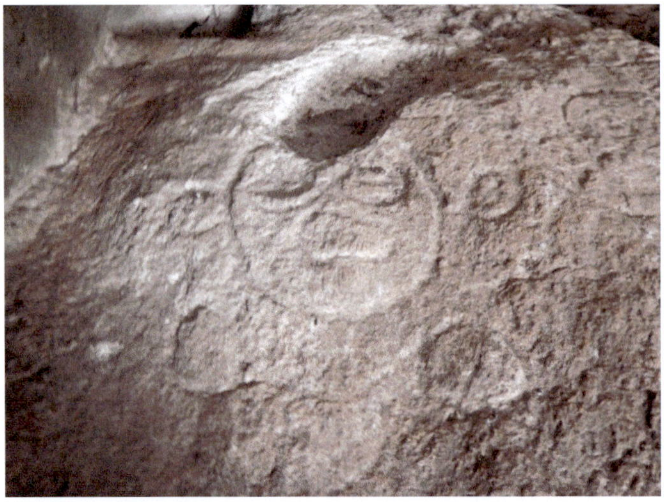

Figure 60 One of the petroglyphs in the cavern of Saint Francis.

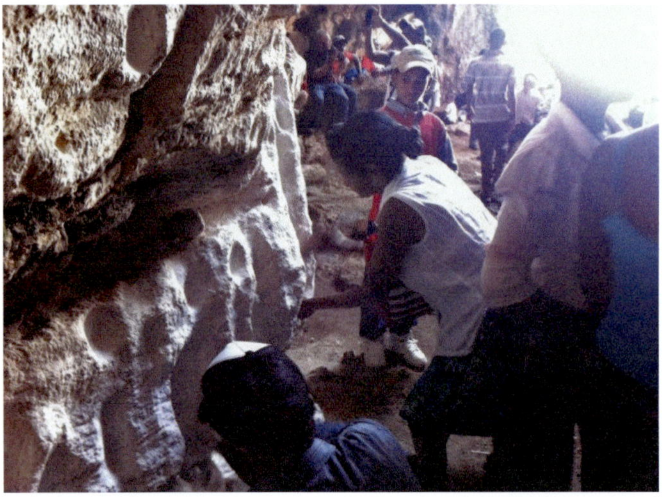

Figure 61 Pilgrims collecting a calcic powder in the Saint Francis' cavern.

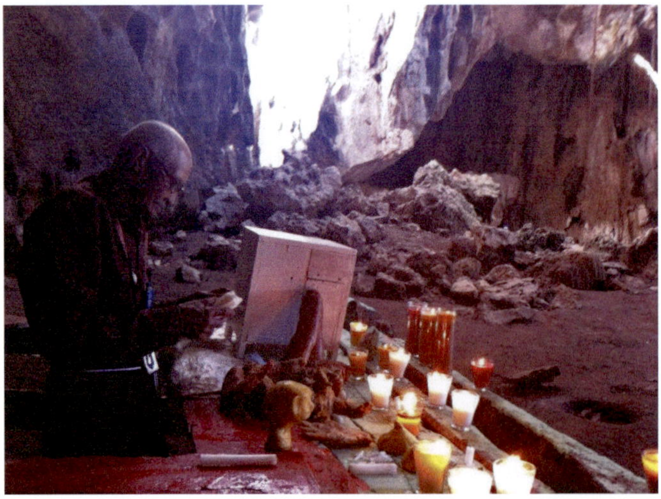

Figure 62 Mr. León Alcantára collecting offerings from pilgrims, Saint Francis cavern.

proposed that the feast started after the villa Bánica was founded in 1506 because the cave in her view belongs to the church, and the church dominates it.[366]

A Journey for Spiritual and Physical Wellbeing during the Celebration of Saint Francis

As a usual patronal feast, the Saint Francis celebration lasts nine days (a Catholic novena). A mass for Saint Francis is organized each night in the church, while on the last day, the 4th October, there is also an official Catholic mass in the cavern. The major flux of pilgrims towards the sacred shrines dedicated to Saint Francis, the local church and the cavern, starts on the 2nd of October and intensifies during the following two days. The actual celebration in the cave is on the third night when many pilgrims stay overnight and attend a morning mass in the cave. The last day pilgrims arrive predominantly from further away, from the province of Elías Piña but also from other provinces, such as Dajabón, San Juan, Azua, or Bahoruco.

During these days thousands of pilgrims of different social classes climb the steep mountain in order to express their faith and devotion, and to fulfill their vows or show their gratitude. On their way the pilgrims encircle crosses (four in total but three of these are the more frequently used) and light candles, deposit stones (representing wishes, sacrifices or sins), and pray. According to the nature of their vows the pilgrims are dressed in brown henequen clothes, sing liturgical chants (*plegarias, salves*) climbing the steep hill individually or in a group. Their journey is physically demanding due to its length, the steep elevation to overcome, and the necessity to carry heavy equipment for the nightly feast. The commitment to maintain a good relationship with this Saint and his sanctuary is expressed in the invested time and effort as well as in the offerings.

From the last stop at the cross at the entrance of the cave, pilgrims continue to the altar in order to deposit offerings and to receive the blessing from Saint Francis. Many people before approaching the altar sanctify themselves with the holy water from stalactites and calcic powder from the cave walls. Sometimes they collect water and powder to take them back home and use them as remedies. Afterwards, the pilgrims approach the main altar, where a church assistant receives their offerings and places the image of Saint Francis for a short moment on their head, so that it may communicate his blessing to them. When going around the last cross, pilgrims touch the surrounding walls of the cave.[367]

Offerings brought during this event should be seen as fulfillment of a vow after having been cured or as an invocation and appeal in order to be alleviated from illness or economic problems.[368] The typical offerings brought to Saint Francis are candles, animals, objects made of wax, food, and money. The animals (cattle, goat, and chicken) are received by the church officials who are in charge of the event and are deposited

---

366 Interview no. 160957.

367 Note that people experience the physical link with this sacred places also through direct contact with the earth by being without footwear: this feeling to communicate with the invisible contributes to the state of grace of the participants.

368 León Alcantara explained: *"When you are sick you make a vow to Saint Francis asking him to cure you. And you told him: Saint Francis I would like to that you cure me from this illness I will give you as a present a cow. And at the Saint's Day you will bring it. And it is like this. When you cure yourself, the day of the feast, you will take and bring this cow to the mountain, and there you will give it to one young man, called Hecfredes, and after you have carried out this vow your body starts to feel well and you recover."*

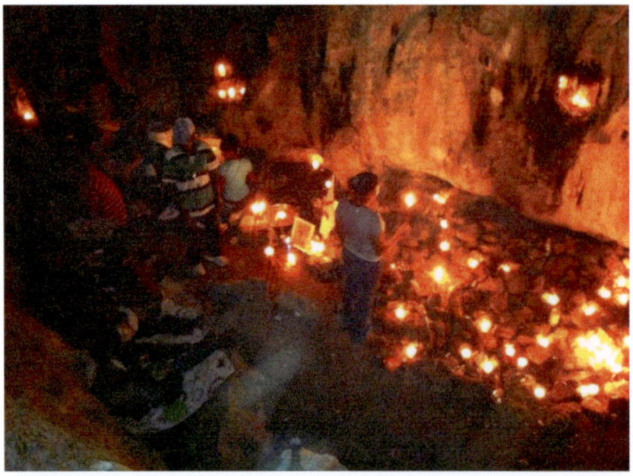

Figure 63 Devotees making their vows.

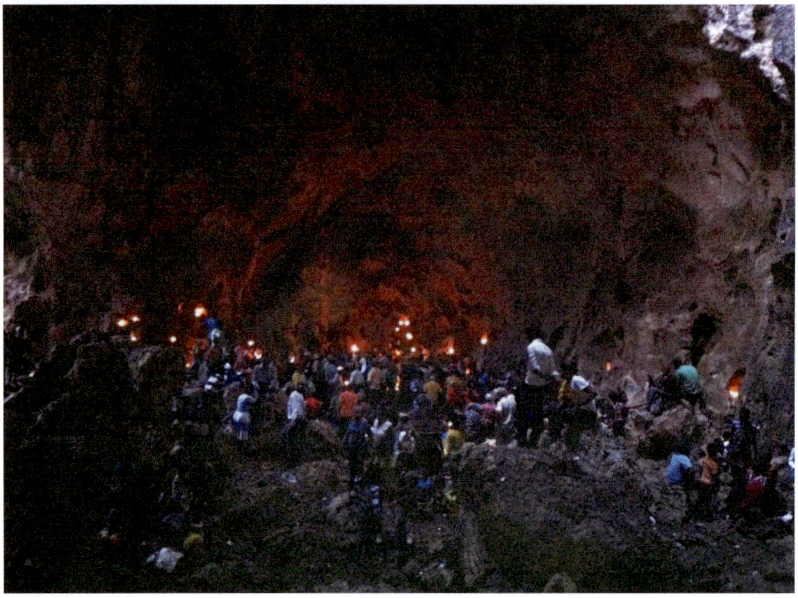

Figure 64 Celebration of Saint Francis at night of 3rd October.

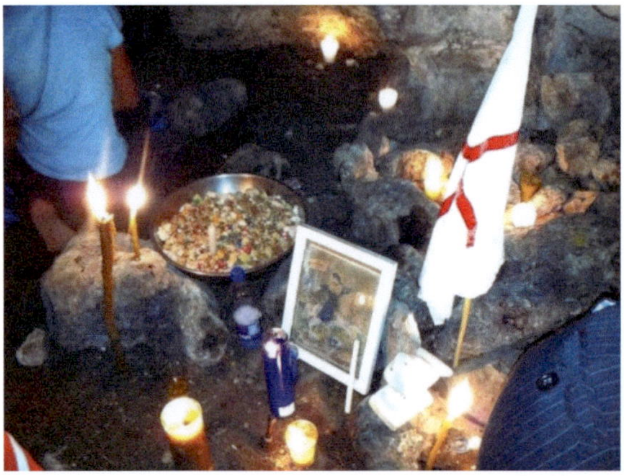

Figure 65 The image of Ogún Balenyó/San Santiago at night on the 3rd of October.

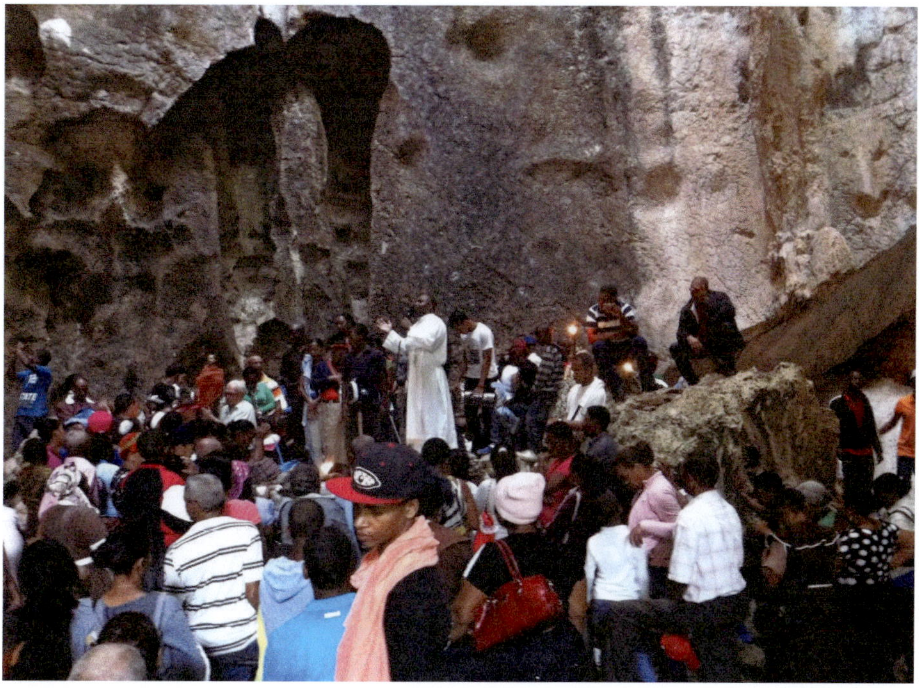

Figure 66 The Mass in the Saint Francis cavern at morning 4th October.

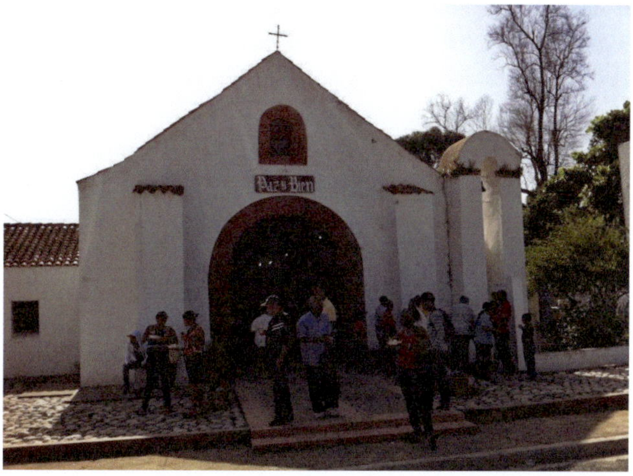

Figure 67 The church of Saint Francis on the 4th of October 2014.

somewhere else until they are sold.[369] According to Mr. León Alcántara, a church assistant during the celebration, the ex-votos of wax that represent requests to the Saint for healing specific illnesses take the material form of affected body parts. Other offerings in the form of small houses, animals, and other things are materialized requests for economic wealth.

Some participants of the feast also offer peanuts and bread crumbs to the "Indios", the spirits, or, as one of the contributors said, to the *marasás* (the divine twins).[370] These

369 Interview no. 158.
370 Interview no. 170.

are deposited in the area of the petroglyphs (possibly pre-colonial because of their Indigenous style, see Fig. 60), which are mostly located on the left wall in front of an altar, while some are just put on the ground near the cross and altar. Moreover, a huge rock near the altar is considered by some to be an indigenous altar.

As a sacred place the Cave of Saint Francis is often referred to as a church and it is, obviously, consecrated to Saint Francis. Unlike in the case of La Mancha there were nearly no images of any other Saint. In person, I have seen only two images of Ogún Balenyó (San Santiago), which were carried as personal protecting *lwas* at the night celebration.

The night of 3 October is an important part of Saint Francis' feast. Prayers accompanied by the music of *palos* intensify through the night. The *palo* is a type of a long drum, seen as the main sacred instrument. The *palo* musical groups are comprised of a person playing *güira* (a local metallic percussion instrument) and three drummers. Devotees are celebrating by dancing, eating, and waiting for the sacred to manifest itself through the bodies of the *Caballos del Misterio*. Like in other patronal celebrations the *güira* and *palo* are indispensable to invoke *misterios* and to bring them to incarnate into the bodies of those with "the grace". One drummer is typically a leading singer who directs his verses towards the Saint and the *misterios*, while a chorus of other *paleros* and attendees repeat the refrains. In this case the music was also accompanied by the ringing of a small iron bell.

During the feast of 2014, an Indigenous *Misterio* materialized through a young man "with grace" from San Juan de Maguana, who reached a state of trance by dancing to the rhythm of the *palos* in front of the altar. As their identities merged, the young man in a state of grace fell on the ground without any movement, remaining in this state for about ten minutes, protected by his company from the crowd that continued to dance and sing. During this time the music intensified. After the trance, the young healer did not remember anything of what just had happened. Like Mrs. Viviana De La Rosa he seemed to communicate with the spirit world through the earth. The feast continued into the late hours, many of the participants slept overnight there to attend the next day's mass.

On the day of the Saint, the 4th of October, an early morning mass was organized by the priest and other representatives of the church. At this point, the only image present was the one of Saint Francis and the music was played only by the priest's assistants. While pilgrims continued to attend this sacred place throughout the entire day, those who had come the day before descended towards the church to participate in the mass that was held there. Again, many repeated the circle to greet and touch all Saints of the walls in order to receive blessings at the major altar of the Bánica church. Mass started with singing *salves* and after that was finished, the attendants received hot chocolate and bread. Then a procession followed in which selected men carried the Saint on their shoulder through the village, accompanied by singing and bell ringing, and finally returned with the Saint to the church.[371]

---

371 The images are not identical. The smaller is used for ceremonies in the cavern and the original is kept in the church and only taken out during the procession in the village.

Forgetting and Remembering Indigenous Past in the Bánica Landscape

At present people are generally not aware of the fact that Bánica once had indigenous inhabitants. Many agreed that the above-described feast was certainly celebrated by their great-grandfathers, who are considered to have been of Spanish origin.[372] According to the contributors there are some people who might be considered descendants of the indigenous population, but this is because of their appearance rather than self-identification or genetic evidence.[373] There is, however, a strong spiritual connection to the spirits of the Indigenous People. The Indigenous *lwas* are often called Saints.

In Bánica there are various narratives about indigenous *misterios*. These were related to people "with grace", who were said to have been taken away but who returned with the grace or gift to heal.[374] In the past, there were more healers who had gained their grace as a consequence of having been taken away by indigenous *misterios*. One of the local examples was a healer, Kusha, who went to their place and when she returned she told that she was another person. In her house there was even a stone from which water was streaming. Mrs. Carmela Alcántara (78 years old) told us about her grandfather who gained his healing grace by living under water for seven years, after which he re-emerged with *Misterio* and the power to cure. At present there is one person who has developed this grace to heal. As part of another Saint´s celebration this person and his followers, but also Baniqueros in general, bring offerings to the river for Indigenous *lwas*.[375]

Mr. Alcántara distinguished between two categories of indigenous *misterios*. The first had positive effects and was playful, but the second consisted of "Caribs", which if they arrive to the mind of persons in trance, are very violent: they *"throw them to the ground"*, *"harm them"*, and *"massacred them"*. When one receives *"a Carib Indian"*, it is always hurtful, because these can even *"eat people from inside"*. And he explained further "*a Misterio that throws you on the ground is good but only if you have one that speaks normally peacefully to you, like a good Misterio, he knows the reason of your visit. And if you think of lighting a candle for him, it is not your own idea, it comes from the mind of the Misterio.*"[376]

These two witness accounts are illustrative examples of how oral traditions keep the spiritual link with *indigenous misterios* alive from one generation to the next. This confirms the existence of an encompassing structure of participating in cultural memory, which is refreshed on various occasions. The memory of the indigenous ancestors is embedded in the landscape. Different places in the Bánica landscape, like the Cave of

372 See also the historical overview. Although it is not clear when patronal feast was for first time celebrated in the cavern, it is at least since the 18th century that Saint Francis de Paula is the patron Saint of Bánica; the first references to the church we have are from the 17th century.

373 One of them was the aunt of Manuel María Morela de Los Santos, Ms. Binda de Los Santos Valenzuela.

374 *Se lo/la llevaron*, they took him/her away, was understood as soul loss because the body could be present but without consciousness.

375 Among Baniqueros Saint Francis is not a patron of any *lwa*. In Haitian Vudu he is the patron of Loko. According to Tejeda Ortíz (2013) Virgen del Carmen stands for "Indio Carmelo" but this author does not elaborate further on the symbolism of these figures. In Haiti Our Lady of Mount Carmel is associated with Ezili Dantó and has dedicated a popular pilgrimage place at Sodo (Saut d´Eau) (Ramsey 2011).

376 See the interview with Doña Carmela.

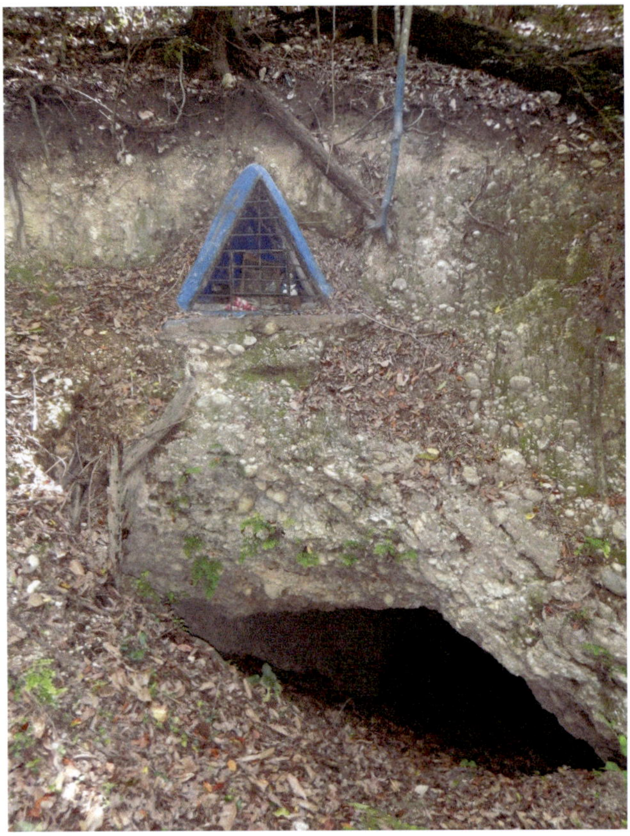

Figure 68 A shrine dedicated to Virgen of Altagracia, Bánica region.

Saint Francis, the springs La Zurza, La Descubierta, Las Tres Piedras and La Chorrera, at Río Artibonito, in the cavern at Sabana Mula and in the church of Saint Francis are associated with ancestral agency. Baniqueros refer to the Cave of Saint Francis as a church, just like the church in the town.[377] Both places are connected by the pilgrimage but also by associations with the indigenous *misterios*. Similar to the cavern, the church is said to have an Indigenous *Misterio*. As Mr. Benjamin Alcántara explained, in the past people could hear Indigenous People hammering and making other sounds of construction in the church at night. When asked why he thought that the sound was made by indigenous workers, he answered: "*because they make marvelous things*". The sound of hammering is also associated with the manifestation of Saint Francis. The cavern connects to the indigenous ancestors through the elements of sweet water (from the stalactites) and earth. These elements also play a role when people share with the Indigenous *Misterio* the first crops or ceremonial meals after the patronal feast, as they bring these offerings to a specific part of the river, *e.g.* the whirlpools Las Tres Piedras and La Chorrera or springs such as La Descubierta.[378] According to Mrs. María García Alcántara, Saint Francis lives in the La Cidra Cave, which is connected by a subter-

377 The same statement was made by an elderly woman from Fermíz Beato in Piraguas Arriva (interview no. 201430) when speaking about the sacredness of the cavern. On my question why she thought this cavern is sacred she answered: because it is there were Indians live.

378 See also Interview no. 105416.

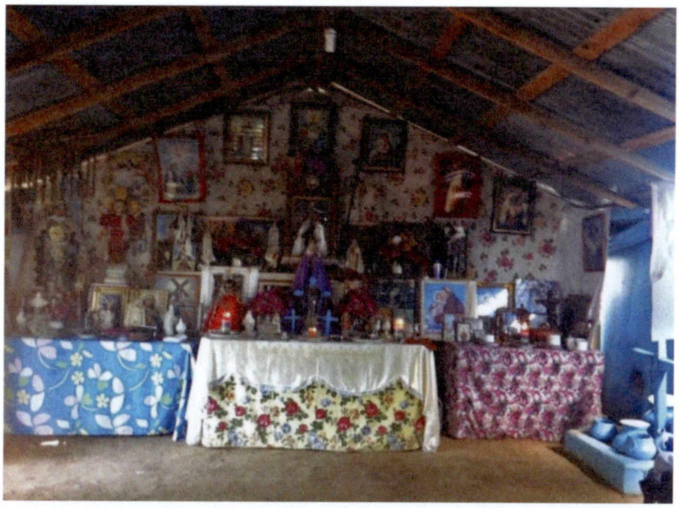

Figure 69 The altar at the day of celebration of the Virgen de las Mercedes, Bánica.

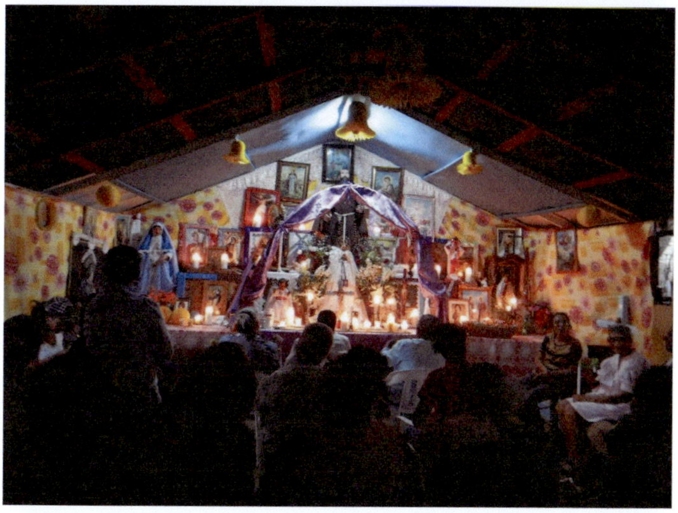

Figure 70 A Mass in house-temple on the day of Virgen Carmen.

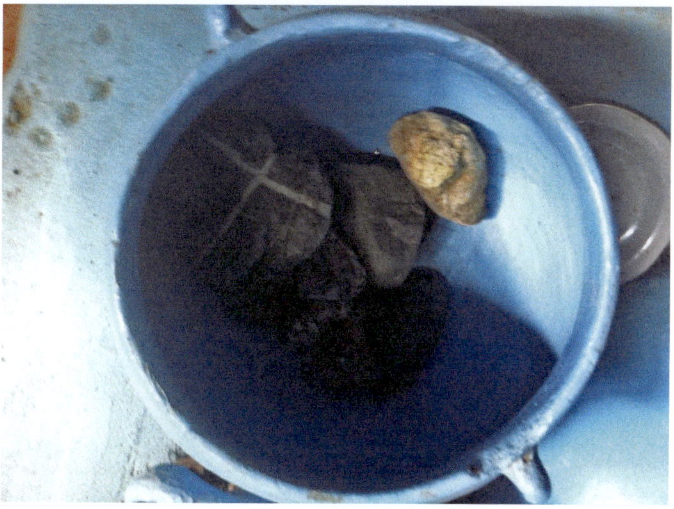

Figure 71 A Vessel for indigenous misterios house-altar Bánica.

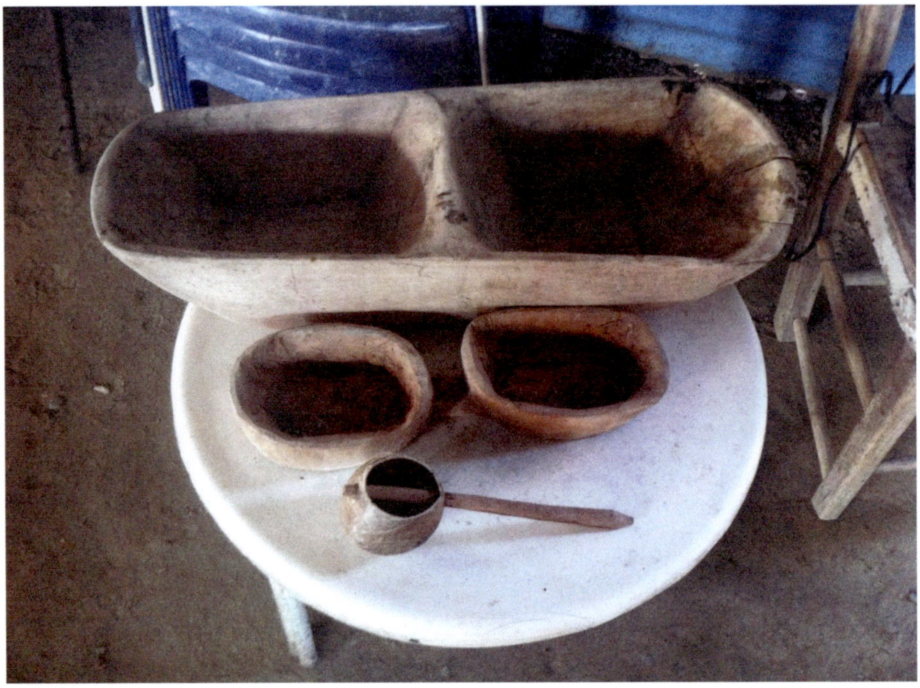

Figure 72 A batea for offerings for the twins from Bánica.

ranean river to the cavern in Bánica.[379] Saint Francis was not even once associated with another *lwa* or indigenous *misterio*.

The Saint Francis cavern is not the only cavern were ceremonies are organized in the Bánica landscape. Next to the afore-mentioned springs and part of rivers, ceremonies were in the past also organized in another cavern consecrated to the Virgen de Altagracia at Sabana La Mula (approx. 10 km from Bánica). Some details about how this place was consecrated are considered complementary to the changing meaning of the Bánica landscape. Mrs. Carmelita de La Rosa Oro, one of the traditional healers from Bánica, devotee of God and Saints (*lwas*), explained how she started to celebrate Altagracia in this cavern. It was because the Lord had sent her to this place to organize the celebration requested by the Saints. Next to the cavern she built a small altar, dedicated to the Virgen de Altagracia and a small wooden house next to it. She offered these as an expression of her penance. After the death of her husband she did not continue the celebration. This healer asserted: it does not matter what you pray for, as long as your request is made "with a clean hearth". She explained also that, because the cavern is a sacred place, different Saints can manifest themselves there – in her words "*where there is one, there are many Saints*" – and therefore one should also pray to the Indigenous Saints.

The celebration of the Virgen de Altagracia drew on previous traditions of local inhabitants, which were bringing offerings to the "Indians" long before Mrs. Carmelita de

379 I have not visited La Cidra; it is to be verified in the future whether this is the same as the La Cidra Cave that is known as an archaeological site in the same province.

La Rosa started her celebrations. One of the residents of the location Patricio Luciano confirmed that after Mrs. De La Rosa stopped with the celebration, only very few persons continue to visit the cavern. He considered such visits as a custom stemming from the generation of his parents and grandparents. In addition, he explained that in front of the cavern there is a *higo*, a fig tree (*Ficus genus*), which is very much respected because "the *Misterio* enters your body there" ...and continued: *"They say that indigenous peoples were coming out, they guarded themselves in the cave; to my mother appeared a marked goat, with combed hair."* The last remarks refer to a belief that we encounter also in the northern region of the Dominican Republic, namely that braided hair can be sign of indigenous agency. This account illustrates that even if in this account it is easy to date the beginning of the celebration started by Mrs. Del Oro, according to Luciano this tradition was preceded by older traditions conducted by his parents and grandparents in which he did not participate so he could not give us more details.

Ritual activities and healing practices in caverns at La Mancha and in Bánica are just two examples of how people engage spiritually with places that are associated with the indigenous past.[380] The next section will illustrate how some Cuban caverns connect present-day people with the indigenous past.

Healing among Spiritists, Managuaco cavern, Holguín, Cuba

Cuban caverns are also accompanied by narratives about and rituals dedicated to indigenous spirits. Narratives about how trash that was left behind mysteriously disappeared and was apparently consumed by "Indios" – are told in the different Dominican and Cuban places that I visited during fieldwork. In general, these are considered "tales of old people". However, devotees of Regla de Ocha and Cuban Spritism believed in the agency of the indigenous spirits in daily life. Devotees of Espiritismo del Cordón perform ceremonies in which these spirits are regarded with great respect. They do so in Managuaco, and, in the past, performed these also in Niquero. In Managuaco I got the chance to collect more information on these practices.

Managuaco is a small settlement in the province Holguín and has been previously discussed as one of first small farms in this region, and the first Catholic hermitage in Holguín province built at the end of XVII century. Currently there is only a small altar outside for the Virgen of Charity and many inhabitants are devotees of Espiritismo del Cordón.

One of the *cabeceros* (Head Medium) of the Espiritismo del Cordón, Mr. Jerónimo Santana felt a spiritual link to indigenous forefathers that he believed was inherited through the mother side of the family. The spiritual connection with the indigenous past may be reinforced by invoking the *"Indian commission"*. This is a group of spiritual entities, summoned with the objective to achieve their help and protection. The devotees seek communication with those spirits in their dreams and most often in cord ceremonies at a house-temple.

The ancestral agency is also connected to specific places and features in surrounding landscapes. Mr. Jerónimo Santana described places that are used for healing practices

380 The cavern is sometimes also used for other types of ceremonies like ritual cleansing. The description of these is left out in accordance with the wishes of the local spiritual leader.

according to domains of two major commissions: the "African" and "Indian" commissions.[381] Each commission has its own specialization as to curing, remedies and places that are especially apt for communicating with the respective spirits of each. The domain of the "African" commission consists of mountains with trees of hard wood such as *yaya, ciguaraya, or quebracho*. Like in Regla de Ocha, Palo de Monte and Mixed Spiritism, the head medium asks permission before entering "*el monte*".[382] The Indigenous commission works with plants like *yerba mora* and *romerillo*. In the contributor's opinion even if the plant is sent by an "African spirit" the botanical knowledge is the domain of "Indian spirits". The curing receipt is passed down from spirits via mediums to their patients.

Rituals for spiritual cleaning and empowerment are performed at the banks of rivers where prayers are dedicated to the Mother of All Waters (here: Yemayá) and Oshún (the river flow). As we mentioned earlier, Mr. Alcides Campo Tarragó, another medium, from the same house-temple, considered the water bodies in the same location to be the domain of Sitochi, The Queen of the Water, as she revealed this to him in a dream. Like Sitochi, also other beings or spiritual entities of other commissions can reveal themselves to the people in dreams or during the cord ceremony.

The contact with this *"Indian commission"* can indeed be facilitated through dreaming and it can take place in house-temples. For Mr. Jerónimo Santana from Managuaco this communication is also established at places *"where there have been communities in the past, where they (indigenous spiritual entities) can feel well, where there is a better fluidity, such as temples, mountains, caves, and rivers"*. One of the places where a mass is organized is a cavern near Managuaco. Mr. Santana explained the motive for selecting the cavern as a place to celebrate mass: *"in their world they have lived there, they have their own forms, for example when you are going to communicate, the caciques who were living there with others, did not go away; their spirit remains there, it does not leave the place, if you want to communicate directly with it you have to go there."*

The mass takes a place in the cavern approximately every four months or when a special necessary presents itself, *e.g.* in the case of an illness. Not everyone who participates in the mass in a "house-temple" is selected to join for the ritual in the cavern.[383] People with health problems are more likely to be designated by the guide spirit to receive advice. Before entering the cavern, permission is asked to form a circle and through dance and singing of hymns communicate with the spirit.[384] The ultimate goal of the ceremonies organized for the indigenous commission is the spiritual development of the practitioners and a means of recovering health and of obtaining spiritual protection.

The cultural memory of the indigenous past does in this context not rely on only one individual to transmit the values and meanings of rituals. The collective nature of the *cordón* also broadens the participatory structure of the cultural memory. The

381 Interview no. 103025.

382 The word 'monte' may have different meanings: hill, or uncultivated land covered with trees, shrubs, bushes or grass.

383 The reason for the selection may be the spatial limitation of the place: this cavern is rather small and not many persons fit in.

384 *Pleiada* is a type of song in which the spirits are mentioned and called to descend to the place where the mass is held.

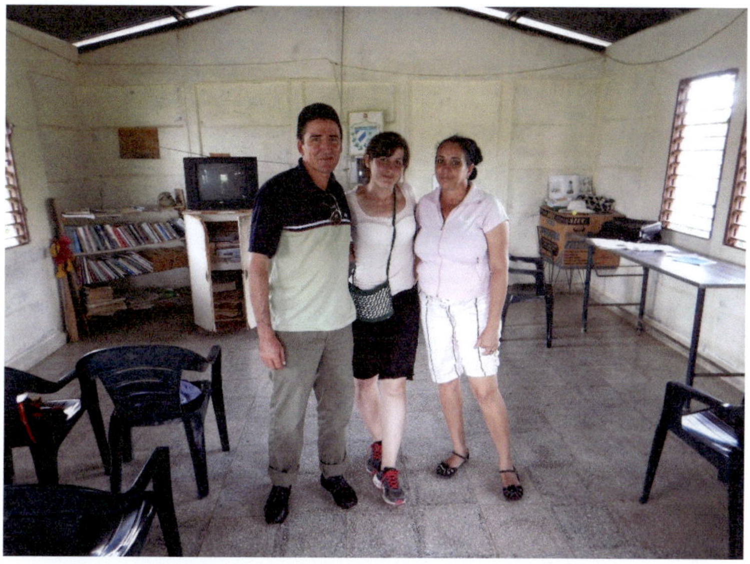

Figure 73 Mr. Jerónimo Santana in Managuaco, Cuba.

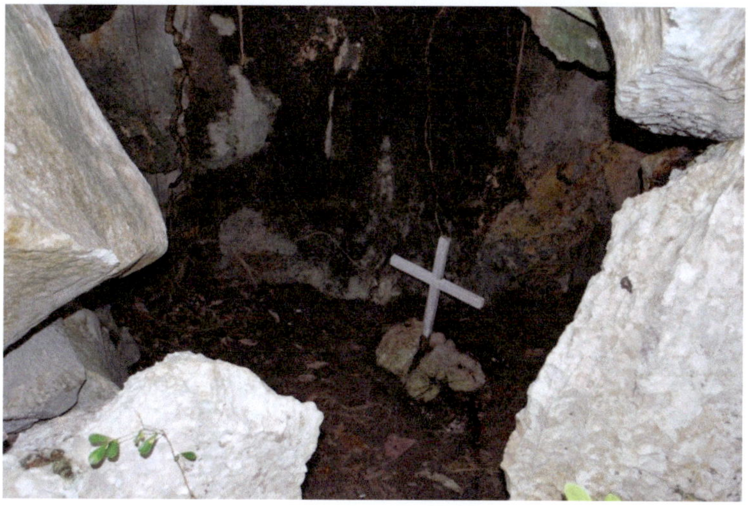

Figure 74 Cavern used by Spritism´s devotees from Managuaco. Photo Courtesy Dr. Roberto Válcarcel Rojas.

continuity of Spiritism in this location can be explained by the meaningfulness of these practices to the people, especially to those who have been cured in this manner: the therapeutic function of religion is in general a binding element for the community. Broader societal contexts, however, such as the aging of the rural population and the limited job opportunities in these areas, are important factors that may interrupt the further transmission and local expression of collective memory about the indigenous past.

The spiritual link that is felt by some of the Managuaco inhabitants should be contextualized within the broader region where the commission of indigenous spirits is also recognized by other centers of Spiritism in nearby Guayacanes, in more remote

Jiguaní or in Cienfuegos.[385] These particular expressions of the cultural memory take also place in a landscape with rich material imprints of the indigenous predecessors. While Managuaco´s contributors did not if indigenous ancestors resided here during the colonial period or that some of the present-day families might have genealogical link with the past indigenous population, they were well aware of the historical link that – in conjunction with formal education – was situated in the pre-colonial period. The recent excavations by the CITMA institute of Holguín is likely to reinforce the awareness of a historical link with the indigenous predecessors.

Cueva De los Santos Gibara, Cuba

Not all Cuban caverns are associated with indigenous spirits. The reflection of Mr. Torre Anguilera about his past spiritual works at Cueva de Los Santos is one of the testimonies about the spiritual value of these places for the Cuban population at large. Mr. Torre, as *taita*[386] of *Regla de Ocha,* founded his altar in one of the Gibara caverns approximately 17 years ago. Like in the case of Mrs. Del Oro´s from Bánica he decided to construct this altar after a revelation. In this revelation a spirit of a dead indicated this site to him as a powerful place where he had been spiritually working before. While this *taita* did not share many details about the biography of this dead he remarked that he was was living in *el monte.*

The cavern was consecrated to Chango/Santa Barbara and Oya/Santa Teresa de Jesús, who dominates the tomb/the world of the dead. The main guardian of the cavern is *Oggun guerrero,* who together with Ochosi is considered to be the owner of *el monte* or to be *el monte.* Oggun gives followers of *Regla de Ocha* the authority to enter this place and work there. Like in the La Mancha case, before entering the cave a bell is rang to announce that people are arriving.

Mr. Torres explained that the altar at the Cueva De los Santos, Gibara, was founded with the aim to heal and develop strong spiritual links with the dead.[387] The cavern was designated to that effect by a muerto, *i.e.* the spirit of a deceased person, and therefore the presence of other remaining dead could be felt better at this place. According to Mr. Torres, the spirits of the dead are most likely "Afrocubans", and on the basis of their form of speech most certainly are Cubans. Although he does not personally work with the spirits of indigenous people, these are considered one of many agencies dwelling in the landscape. They are not associated with this particular cavern, however.

The ceremonies that took place here were organized in groups of seven different priests (for whom the Spanish word *sacerdote* is used). Each priest has his own group of dead to work with. Like in the Dominican cases explained earlier, the

---

385 In the nearby settlement Guyacanes the adherents of Cord Spiritism also organized their mass in home temples to the commission of indigenous spirits. The lyrics were composed by one of the devotees who was always searching for inspiration at the rock wall where he felt he had a better connection. An example of such lyrics: *"Que lleguen los indios buenos, porque yo les estoy llamando, yo le hago un llamamiento pa' que vengan labrando."* Another *pleiada*, called The Drum, sounds: *"Llegan indios misioneros hoy llegan con su tambor para que quiten el dolor a todo el mundo entero."* These texts illustrate how the indigenous past is actively engaged with in the context of the healing practices.

386 *Taita* is an initiated ritual specialist who can train novices.

387 For more on the role of dead in Regla de Ocha see Rodríguez Reyes (1993) and González Peréz (1997) or those of Yoruba Vidal (1993).

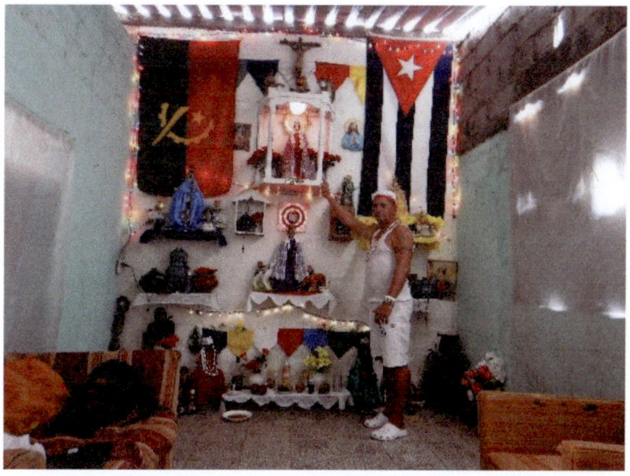

Figure 75 Altar of Mr. Torres, Gibara, Cuba.

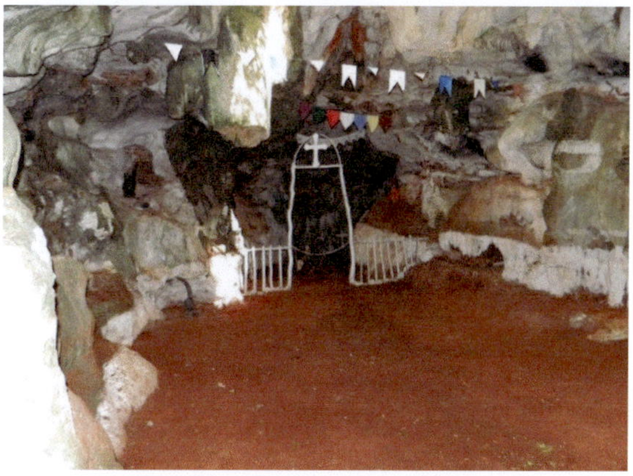

Figure 76 Cueva De Los Santos, Gibara. Photo Courtesy J. J. Guarch Rodríguez.

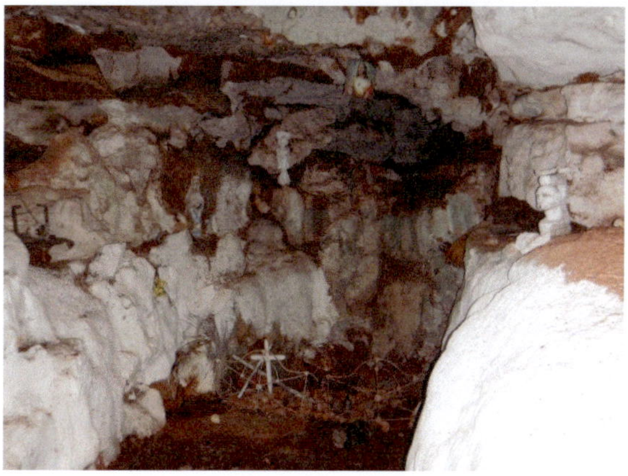

Figure 77 Cueva de Los Santos, Gibara, after its altar has been demolished.

ceremony culminates when the spirit of a dead person is reached through trance elicited by drum music, chanting, and stimulants like tobacco and alcohol. One of the priests asks in trance to receive a recipe for medicinal plants, and an assistant (*perro de prenda*) goes to search for the plants in *el monte*. Almost always medicinal plants that were used by "*los muertos*" are applied. Among them are: *Zazafaraparilla, Rompezaraüey* and *Pederaja macho*.

Different testimonies speak about cures of illnesses (psychological and physical ailments), which were made possible through the agency of the *muertos* (the dead) from this cavern. In addition, if there is a type of problem that is considered to be the domain of another deity, this other deity can also be invoked here. This was also the case of a newborn of one of the members, which was saved through the help of San Rafael (Inle, *orisha* of all medicinal healing) invoked in this place.

Also Cueva de los Santos did not escape the above-mentioned disputes and the altar was destroyed. The vandals, it is said, will be punished by the dead; in the meantime there are already plans to reestablish a new altar there and to continue the ceremonies.

Although these ritual activities seem to have been entirely initiated rather recently, there are some precedents of ritual cavern use in the same town. Mr. José Corella Varona, cultural promoter and speleologist from Gibara, tells us that at the beginning of the 20th century peregrinations were organized to the so-called Cueva de la Virgen, now known as Los Panaderos. This cavern was named after a rock formation associated with the mantle of the Virgin, where flowers were brought as offerings. The exact details are not known. Today, this cavern is known as an archaeological site and by some related through a narrative with the cacique Catuco. Mr. José Corella described how according to this local narrative cacique Catuco and his daughter, when fleeing from the Spanish invaders, could escape because a deity, Granma (Bayograma), transformed them into a rock formation inside this cavern. This rock formation is more distant from the cave opening than the altar of the Virgin.[388]

According to oral history, the Gibara landscape is entangled with the lives of escaped enslaved people. In the context of explaining sacred places related to the ancestors, Mr. Tomás Rodríguez Gonzales from Holguín also mentioned Palenque de Gibara. After describing *el monte* as a place related to ancestors *"because it was there where enslaved Africans where cutting the sugar cane, collecting the coffee, and therefore there developed also more their religion"*, he gave as an example *"Palenque in Gibara, where there are some caves that everyone knows."*[389] These caves are situated near an old sugar mill. Being very conscious about his West African heritage from his mother's side (Angolan) and from his father's side (Cuban), Mr. Rodríguez added a popular Cuban proverb saying: *"who does not have something from Congo has from Carabalí"*. He clarified that when talking about sites of the ancestors he referred to places related to the enslaved Africans, but added that he honored also an indigenous man ("Indian"), whom his grandmother and

388 Likely the opinion of José Corella from Gibara was somewhat influenced by his role as a local historian and cultural promoter: *"In Catuco there is a site of cultural encounter. There lived a cacique with his daughter who was very beautiful. When the Spanish conquerors arrived and started to attack the village they flee to the mountain. Catuco and his daughter with a child in arm fled to the mountain and four Spaniards with dogs chased them. When they arrive at the cave of Los Panaderos they invoke the god Bayograma to help them hide and then Bayograma magically illuminates the path of these Indians who are running away while the Spaniards lost their time to light their torches to enter the cave and then they got advantage over them and the Spanish keep up with them and when they almost can reach them and let's say that by the same intervention of Granma these Indians are turned into stone. There are two rock formations that are identical and one is like an Indian in the position of a cuckoo with a spear and the other is an Indian with a child on her arm and when you look at them they are identical and they say that these are the stone statues of Catuco and his daughter."*

389 Interivew no. 150617.

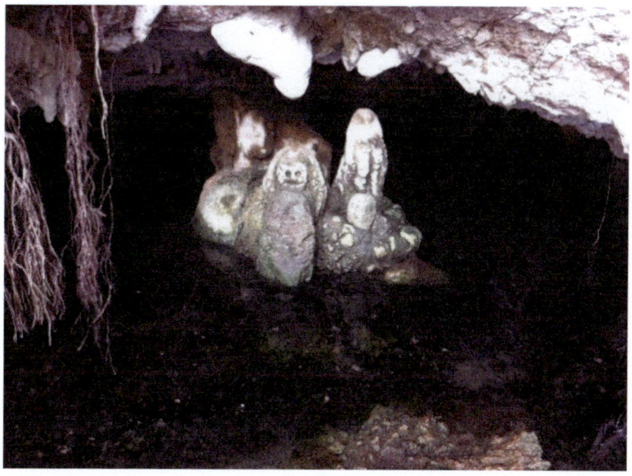

Figure 78 The Cavern in El Guafe where Neo-Taíno activists and adherents of Espiritismo have organized a ceremony, Cuba.

mother knew, and to whom they were praying, and to whom he sometimes is praying too. In Mr. Rodríguez' view, this docs not mean that he is indigenous descendant.

More caverns figure in Cuban collective memory and sacred history. In many the religious practices have by now been abandoned, like in the case of the Cavern of the Virgin. Another example of a cavern where the use for spiritual aims has been discontinued is the Cave of Samuel in Niquero. This cavern was valorized for its huge concentration of spiritual energies by past *Espiritistas* from Niquero.[390] This special character was revealed to one *Espiritista* approximately 40 years ago in a dream. The use of the cave ceased after the death of the spiritual leader but some people still remember the ritual experience and *plenas* song in the cavern. *Espiritismo* has a strong tradition in Niquero, and until the present day it is estimated that there are nearly three hundred different house-temples. This spirituality is sometimes translated into occasional visits of the caverns of El Guafe, which are situated in the national park neighboring to Niquero. In the recent past, an investigator from the Smithsonian, and young *Espiritistas* from Niquero organized a ceremony in the cavern of El Guafe. The role of the investigator in dealing with the collective and cultural memory of the indigenous past is often much more subtle but may trigger its preservation, modification or even discontinuity. Personal observations at the caverns and the testimonies of park rangers, suggest that the caverns of Guafe are sometimes visited for spiritual purposes by "people from Habana". One of the constraints for the renewal of traditions by inhabitants of Niquero is the general poor state of transportation in Cuba.

Cuban and Dominican caverns as memory places of indigenous past

Caverns are sacred and empowered natural sites, loci of history, and settings for oral traditions. In describing a few examples I have highlighted some of their rich symbolism on the basis of discussions with devotees of Roman Catholicism, 21 Division, Spiritism and Regla de Ocha. Within these plural meanings I have emphasized the role of caverns in healing from a cultural memory perspective. Regardless of their re-

390 Interview no. 152957.

ligious affiliation, and their specific invocation of divine beings and spiritual entities, the visitors undertake their journey in order to improve their health, wellbeing, and protection (spiritual and physical, also for example in the hurricane period). Being physical, natural features of an extraordinary characteristics, caverns create easily a bridge towards invisible worlds and, as we have seen, also across generations.

This chapter elaborated on the meanings of these heritage sites in contemporary societies. The connection with the past is made across different religious affiliations and according to people's own perception of history. More specifically, I have focused on cases where the commemoration of the indigenous ancestors has been integrated in the patronal celebration of Saint John and Saint Francis. These data were complemented by the information on the significance of the cavern during the Spiritism ceremonies in Managuaco and by accounts of the agency of the dead in healing ceremonies in Gibara.

While during the patronal celebrations it was possible to communicate with *lwas*, and consult them about different cures, the emphasis at these moments seem to have been on the attendance of celebration. People's own participation can be conceived a way to express one's commitment with the *Misterios* or the Saints who will be of benefit for one's life. From this viewpoint the commemoration of indigenous ancestors within these celebrations seems to be a confirmation of a mutual caring relationship, by looking after, honoring and keeping the memory alive of those who passed away. In a symbolic way, it is at the same time a recognition of those predecessors who passed on their knowledge of what to do in time of illness, who warn and protect us with their previous experience and accumulated knowledge.

People's inclusion of indigenous ancestors into their own pantheon in landscapes that are scattered with historical imprints provides them also with a sense of belonging, as it positions the devotees in time and space. Personal participation in feasts or listening to elders creates a shared cultural background; shared experiences and as such it promotes a community identity and fosters group cohesion.[391] According to social psychology social inclusion contributes positively to mental health as it fulfills the basic human need to belong (Baumeister & Leary 1995; Walton & Cohen 2011).

Devotees of 21 Division, Spiritism, and Catholicism commemorated Indigenous *lwas* and spirits in cavern settings. Similarly, indigenous ancestors are also recognized as important forces in Haitian Vodou Brazilian Candomblé, and Surinamese Winti (Stephen 2002; personal communication Sony Jean 2015). As earlier suggested, from the viewpoint of popular Catholicism a cavern can be a place where the indigenous spirits dwell because their souls are in penance. Being historical places with rich material imprints of the indigenous predecessors, these sites are likely to be situated in locations where the communication with the ancestral world may take place. This seems to be a shared belief among Spiritism, Regla de Ocha and 21 Division.

The altars dedicated to Barón del Cementerio/San Elías, the head of the *guedes,* in Cueva de La Mancha or those for the dead Maroon in Gibara indicate that these caverns are – together with cemeteries – gateways to the world of deceased ancestors in general. This view overlaps with archaeological records about the rich funerary practices from the pre-colonial period (*e.g.* Vácarcel Rojas et al. 2003) and with information that suggests that these sites were used by Maroons (*e.g.* Pereira Pereira 2008). The accounts

391 The community identity is comparable to the Turner's communitas as referred by Rappaport (1999).

about spiritual entities residing in specific places may sometimes have historical value as it is bounded to local histories. The testimony about the agency of the dead from the cavern of Gibara, for example, is connected to the oral history about Maroons in this particular place, an information that is open to verification by future historical and archaeological studies.

One of the crucial questions concerning these ritual places, which have been the focus of attention for Caribbean residents during centuries (and in some cases even during millennia) is whether and to what extent the present-day meanings and practices can be considered a continuation or reinterpretation of previous traditions. Within the framework of the Nexus project one of objectives of this study was to examine the possible link between the ancient indigenous population and contemporary traditions. One of few accounts that we have about indigenous worldviews concerning the caverns in the Caribbean is that of Friar Pané (ca. 1498/2011). This source depicts caverns as sites where the ancestors had originated and where Sun and Moon had emerged. It suggests that one of the caverns was held in great esteem as a place to celebrate religious ceremonies. It is plausible, therefore, that the present-day association of caves with indigenous ancestors and their ritual use echo – at least in a partial and transformed manner – pre-colonial ideas about the landscape.

Another (possibly unconscious) continuity of ancestral practices may be the selection of maize, beans and possibly also maní as ritual offerings. Maize and beans have been found in pre-colonial cavern sites (Pagán Jiménez 2008) and maní at one Cuban site (Birama, Trinidad), dated to the beginnings of the 12th century (Angel Bello et al. 2002).[392] As earlier suggested, corn and beans, however, may have been recognized by the African ancestors upon their arrival to these islands since the second half of 16th century: they continued to be important components of the diet during colonial times.

The indigenous conviction that these places were connected to miraculous ancestral forces would have been easily incorporated in popular Catholicism and West African beliefs. The development of these traditions cannot be divorced from the specific historical context. Caverns were centers of both Catholic and non-Catholic beliefs for many centuries in Europe, and also Spain they were popular for ascetic practices, sites of pilgrimages, and healing in for centuries.[393] From this perspective, Spaniards observing the indigenous rituals in local caverns were also able to understand its symbolism according to both Catholic and non-Catholic European reference

---

392 The analysis of the starch residues in the cavern site Cueva de los Muertos in Puerto Rico (Pagán Jiménez 2008) identified guáyiga, maize, sweet potatoes, batata, yams, lerén (Calathea allouia), yautía, corozo palm seeds (*Acrocomia media*); beans (*Phaseolus vulgaris*); arrowroot (*Maranta arundinacea*); manioc; and the seeds of *achiote, bija* (*Bixa orellana*). The presence of these plants in a non-residential context, whose functions relate to religious activities (based on the archaeological record identified as burial, postmortem rituals and/ or ceremonies related to the numinous petroglyphs), was interpreted as having dietary (e.g. as preparation meals for attendants of commemorative ceremonies) and religious significance (e.g. as offerings).

393 Among the sacred cavern in Spain are e.g. Cueva Santa, Virgen de Montserrat, Virgen de Covadonga, Cueva de Santo Domingo de Guzmán in Segovia, Cueva Sacra San Miguel, Virgen de la Peña in Mijes.

(Pané as a Catalan had to sacred cavern of Monserrat, see the previous D'Aghieri's comparison to Greek beliefs).[394]

Spanish caverns have been sites of pilgrimages and sites of healing prior to and after the conquest of the Americas.[395] One of many examples is Virgen Candelaria which had her shrine also in a cave in Tenerife. The same Virgen became a popular in both Cuba and the Dominican Republic.[396] The Marian manifestation in both islands registered also historically (Tricando 1997; Portuondo 2016), during this study in the form of ascetic use of caverns in this study (Evangelist in La Jaiba and Boca de Yuma) should be seen in the light earlier miracles which occurred in the caverns.

The insertion of markings of crosses, biblical phrases, Spanish names, and dates in Mona caverns reveal that these places were visited by Europeans throughout the colonial period (Samson et al. 2016; Samson 2017). The insertion of Catholic symbols can be explained in various ways, including their utilitarian use (if as in this case the only sources of permanent drink water), a contestation of signs of indigenous worldviews depicted on the walls, but also as an evidence of evangelization efforts, and an engagement of Christian individuals with places with indigenous rock art. The Baniqueros, who are also European descendants called the rock art in the cavern of Saint Francis, "Indian altar" and it was one of places were the offerings were deposited.

The meanings attributed to caverns, even by atheists, are interwoven with socio-political relations, which sometimes have conflictive historical backgrounds. Although caverns were once sacred natural shrines in Spain as well, the Spanish ruling orthodox policies in the 16th century aimed at demonizing caves in the colonies. Already during the early colonial period, this official discourse was contested by local spiritual practices. From different accounts, it is clear that Caribbean caverns raised fear and curiosity among Europeans. D'Anghiera describes how one of the colonizers, Morales, was scared to enter a cave in the province of Caizcimú in Hispaniola because his crew

394 Caverns have been important, religiously charged places in many other worldviews. Petrus Martyr D'Anghiera compared "the superstition" of the indigenous peoples of the Caribbean with ancient ("pagan") Greek beliefs about the caves of Corinth, of Cyrrha, and Nissa, and also compared the indigenous cult to his own belief system saying that: "*They go on pilgrimages to that cavern just as we go to Rome, or to the Vatican, Compostela, or the Holy Sepulchre at Jerusalem*" (1492 -1526, First Decade, Book IX).

395 Examples of some of the holy caverns in Spain are e.g.: Cueva Santa, Virgen de Montserrat, Virgen de Covadonga, Cueva de Santo Domingo de Guzmán in Segovia, Cueva Sacra San Miguel, Virgen de la Peña in Mijes). In addition, official Catholic teachings (e.g. the hagiography of Saint Francis) also confirm that caverns were utilized for ascetic practices in Europe (for the late medieval age see Fernández Conde 2000).

Diverse European worldviews related to caverns should be taken into account when reading for example Gómara's narrative about a group of indigenous men who were hiding in a cave for a storm. Those who had derided God's name were struck by lightning. The only man who prayed to the Virgin Mary survived (López de Gómara 1922 [1551-1552], Chapter XXXIV, p. 79). *"[...] el uno se encomendó a Santa María, con temor e rayo, los otors hicieron burla de tal Dios y oración, y los mató un rayo, no haciéndoles mal al devoto"* (López de Gomara (1551-1552), 1922, Tomo 1, Cap. XXXIV, p. 79). Without doubt, Gómara aimed to exalt the success of the Catholic missionary activity in rescuing indigenous souls through their conversion, but at the same time his text is evidence of the widespread belief that a manifestation of the Virgin Mary could take place anywhere, including in caves, because the divine power was omnipresent.

396 This Virgen is patron of Tenerife and now is also patron of following locations San Fernando de Camarones, Camagüey, and Sabana Grande de Boyá. One of first brotherhoods from Santo Domingo composed of "Biafaras and Mandingas" had her as a patron. In Dominican 21 Division she represents Candelina Sedifé and in Regla de Ocha her image represents also Oyá.

"was terrified of hell" (D'Anghiera 2002 [1494-1526]). The fear of the unknown is also present when these dark caverns were described as gates to hell or as hiding places of Amazons as in the case of Madanina or Matinino (possibly Martinique) or loci of human sacrifices in Venezuela (D'Anghiera 2002 [1494-1526], First Decade: Book II & VII; Lopez Gómara, as cited in Urbani & Urbani 2011).

Even if Caribbean caverns raised fears of gates to hell and the unknown, in exceptional cases this did not impede for Spaniards to consult piaches in Venezuela about their future, the same persons who were known to be initiated and perform ceremonies in these places in Venezuela (López de Gómara 1551). News about indigenous treasure hidden in caverns from the mainland (Mexico, Peru, Brazil) arouse enough curiosity. The long-term piracy and privateering in the Caribbean regions contributed even more to expectations about the findings in these places. One of account about treasure hunting from the second half of 18th century Cuba illustrates how one of caverns close by to Bayamo was a mysterious place where indigenous spirits revealed and where the Virgen of Charity miraculously rescued her devotees (Portuondo Zúñiga 2016).[397]

As today the past early diasporic communities were likely attributed to cavern various, sometimes contested meanings. Contemporary religious disputes often follow the argumentation of colonial discourse, in which the religions of the colonized are stigmatized and considered to be witchcraft. The recognition of some of these places, like Saint Francis' cavern, by the Church authorities is clearly reflected in the number of pilgrims that come to visit them. The great popularity of Saint Francis' cavern in Bánica has parallels in other pilgrimage sites in sacred landscapes elsewhere, for example Monserrat in Spain, the Grotto of Saint Francis in Assisi (Italy), the Grotto of Lourdes in France, Cave Achbinico in Tenerife or the less known South African Motouleng cave. Certain features of the above-mentioned rituals, such as ex-votos, processions, the reappearance of saints and their miraculous effect on the patient´s body, show clearly Catholic influences, which can also be observed at sacred places in present-day Spain.

The Dominican and Cuban Cuban Spritism, Regla de Ocha and 21 Division perceive the numinous in various caverns. Although their views are sometimes stigmatized, these places are widely recognized as important sites of spiritual reflection about the mysterious invisible power of ancestral, divine and natural forces. In accordance with the respective religious frameworks, caverns are seen as dwellings or loci of manifestations of different divine beings. Curiously, the interviewed contributors did not mention an equivalent *lwa* in 21 Division for the involved patronal Saints, Saint John and Saint Francis. Maybe these two Saints do indeed not have any associated *lwa*, as occurs more often with other Catholic Saints. It is to be noticed that in Haitian Vudu Saint Francis is associated with Loco, the guardian of vegetation, who gives healing property to plants and transmits botanical knowledge to healers. The hagiography of Saint Francis – as an important healer who for a while was living in a cavern – might be sufficient for devotees to identify the values this Saint represents. The supervision of this celebration by the local church authorities may have led to greater secrecy about

397 In the 1520s some of Spaniards were consulting the piaches in Venezuela in order to know when the boat would come, and their predictions seemed to be fulfilled. One of these piaches would also go to invoke a "demon" in one of the caverns (Herrera y Tordesillas 1601, p. 111). López de Gómara (1979, p. 126 in Urbani and Urbani 2011) writes: "Invocan al diablo de esta manera: Entra el piache en una cueva o cámara secreta una noche muy oscura; lleva consigo ciertos mancebos animosos, ...

associations with non-Christian meanings, and also may have influenced the attributed meanings themselves. There were not Catholic officials were present at the Saint John feast and devotees did not refer to the celebrated saint in other terms. While it is now nearly impossible to assess whether Saint John was for Viviana de La Rosa the representation of another divine force, it is clear that at least in Baní where she came from, this Saint is now seen as associated with Indigenous Division through the water element (Lundahl & Lundius 2012).

The presence of a multiplicity of *lwas* in a context where not all healers are initiated creates a fluid and changing the atmosphere, which may lead to forgetting one or more specific characteristics or attributes.

The interpretation of caverns as dwelling places of spiritual or divine entities associated with rain may well have pre-colonial indigenous roots. We find this also in the short accounts of recent ritual cavern use in Cuban Spiritism. The cave in Antilla and the Cave of the Dead in Guara (Western Cuba) have been interpreted as places dedicated to the invocation of rain (see Rodríguez Cullel & Peña Obregón 2000; Fernández Garcell 2015).[398] Indigenous icons that were discovered after a revelation by one local spiritual medium in the cave in Antilla were used to invoke rain in times of drought (Rodríguez Cullel & Peña Obregón 2000). In Mesoamerican worldview, specific caverns are called House of Rain (*i.e.* dwelling place of the Rain God), where religious specialists communicate with the divine power to pray for and help with the production of the rain (Jansen & Perez 2017; Jiménez Osorio & Posselt Santoyo 2018). The date of the Holy Cross – 3 and 4 May -associated with the main ritual in the Cave of the Dead (Guara), coincides with the celebration of the Holy Cross as the central rain ritual of indigenous peoples throughout Mexico (Jiménez Osorio & Posselt Santoyo 2018) – in the Mexican case the ritual is clearly of pre-colonial origin: the timing coincides with the first zenith passage of the sun, which marks the beginning of the rainy season in this region. Calculations by my colleague Manuel May Castillo (using StarcCalc) show that the sun passes the zenith in the Dominican Republic on the 15th of May and the 27th of July, and in Cuba on the 24th / 25th May and the 16th/18th of July. The zenith passage on the 15th of May coincides with the very popular feast of San Isidro, the patron Saint of the agriculturalists, who is also invoked to remove the rain and make the sun shine in accordance with Spanish habit.

In the above-mentioned caverns the water aspect is often emphasized: there are man-made waterpools inside and offerings for the indigenous ancestors are deposited

---

...que hagan las preguntas sin temor. Siéntase él en un banquillo, y ellos están en pie. Llama, vocea, reza versos, tañe sonajas o caracol, y en tono lloroso dice muchas veces: `Prororure, prororure`, que son palabras de ruego". Portuondo (2016) gives us an account from the second half of 18th century by Diego Terral de Bayamo. This narrates about one of the inhabitants from Bayamo who went to explore a cave called Guysa that is located close by to this town. The motive of this visit was to explore whether it contained "enchanted treasure" because it was said that "barbarous indias" live there. During their exploration they encounter human remains from which an invisible guanajo, spirit would emerge. At that moment they could hear an "areíto". After this encounter they had to fight a large snake and got lost. After a long time without finding the way out one of them made a promise to the Virgen of Charity to visit her in her holy house. The Virgen miraculously rescued them.

398 When making a documentary about the archaeological heritage in local caverns Jorge Fernández Garcell and his team interviewed adherents of Spiritism about this celebration (presentation by Fernández Garcell at an International seminar in Santiago de Cuba 2015).

below the stalagmites or on a place where water had naturally accumulated. In one interview with an inhabitant of Bánica the cave of Saint Francis was explicitly associated with the rain, when he suggested that when one hears the drums from the caves it means that it will rain. Also in Boyá the Virgin of Boyá was suggested to be the regulator of the storms and rain. The association of indigenous people with the water element can also be directly related to the narratives about the subaquatic kingdoms where indigenous ancestors dwell.

Concluding remarks

The association of caverns with indigenous people seems to derive from a pool of knowledge in which information from different sources is mixed. Oral tradition about ancestral agencies in these places, the general association of caverns with remote past and "primitive peoples", and the extraordinary characteristics of these liminal places – eliciting the sense of entering into contact with the mysterious and dark spirit world – in combination with material remains from ancient times are likely to construct and maintain this link across the generations.

This chapter discussed how relations between the indigenous forefathers and caverns have been constructed and kept alive in the cultural memory. The local contributors to this research connected to their indigenous ancestors through various means, including oral "stories about spirits" or religiously charged histories. The oral traditions describe these places as the dwelling of the indigenous spirits, which are generally considered to be ghost stories whose objective is to excite fear (and a wish to avoid such places), but they also highlight the marvelous agency of the beings living in those places. The sacred histories, including the biographies of famous healers like Viviana or the hagiography of Saint Francis, focus also on the marvelous agency of the forces that manifested themselves at these sacred places. Adherents of 21 Division, and Cuban Spiritism but also Catholics engaged with indigenous spirits in the caverns during patronal celebrations or individual ceremonies.

The interpretation of caverns as domains of *indigenous misterios* is also encoded in the physical characteristics of the caverns. As natural shrines of rather fixed material features they are stable mnemonic tools across the generations. The "betwixt and between" characteristics of the caverns – as entrances into a earth and into a world of darkness – allow the visitors to feel a drastic break with the normality of quotidian life and to experience "time out of time" (Rappaport 1999). Their extraordinary features affects the senses, eliciting physical emotional reactions and contributing to the experience of liminality. This experience made caverns across cultures places where the visitors naturally reflect upon the threshold between the visible and invisible realms, upon the distinction and the links between past and present, upon the connections with those who have passed away but still belong to our memory. The material evidence (*e.g.* remains of ancient artefacts or rock art) recalls the ancestral presence of people dwelling in the same landscape centuries ago.

The knowledge about caverns as domains of indigenous ancestors is transmitted through collective and individual rituals as well as oral traditions, which together rely on a broad participation structure that is not restricted to a few specialists. The feast of Saint John includes not only performers who pay tribute to the indigenous *lwa*, but also a wider public audience, which supports the structure of the celebration for economic reasons. The religious traditions in these places continue also because of the influence of charismatic leaders and last but not least, as Assmann (2011) proposes, because they are meaningful to the participants and the carriers of these traditions.

The rise and continuity of these traditions are intimately connected with a specific socio-economic context, which has been influencing the religious life and the healing practices. Its role should not be seen in fully deterministic terms, but without doubt the large-scale poverty and lack of medical attention (including mental care) in Dominican society, as well as the anxieties and hope of a better future in Cuban society, have a strong influence on the choices and reactions of the people. As does the general human need for spirituality and moral guidance.

The last three chapters provided numerous examples of how the memory of the indigenous past is part of the present-day healing landscapes. The following chapter will further assess the main question of how healing landscapes encapsulate cultural memories of the indigenous past in the light of the historical and selected fieldwork data we have discussed so far.

10

Synthesis and Conclusions. At the Crossroads of Healing Landscapes

Remembrance and Oblivion

This final chapter assesses the present-day healing landscapes of the Dominican in Republic and Cuba in relation to their historical background as known from the written records and to the cultural memory of the contemporary inhabitants. Coinciding with the major objectives of the Nexus 1492 project, which focus on the histories and legacies of the indigenous peoples in the Caribbean across the historical divide, one of the objectives of this thesis was to examine present-day healing landscapes and their link to the indigenous peoples of the Caribbean. This aim led us to review some of the fragmented references to the medicinal histories of the region. Moreover, for assessing long-term historical transformation it is necessary to address contemporary perception and engagement with the past, which are an integral part of the context and mechanism of the circulation of medicinal cultures. After explaining in general terms how indigenous people (ancestors) are invoked in cultural memory, this chapter will review the associated landscape features. This will lead to a reflection upon how the image of the indigenous past is perceived and how the past practices are reinterpreted within the present. Through this discussion we will gain insights into the value of the cultural memory concept for historiography and into the value of the healing landscapes concept for landscape theories. This chapter will be rounded off by drawing some final conclusions, suggesting several follow-up avenues with future research potential.

Historical formation of Cuban and Dominican Medicinal Cultures

One of the objectives of this research was to provide more information on how the Dominican and Cuban medicinal cultures have been constructed. A review of some of the aspects of medicinal history in the region suggests that the contemporary medicinal cultures are likely to have originated from a complex multidirectional exchange of botanical, medicinal knowledge and underpinning worldviews among different populations of these islands. One crucial historical event that shaped the history of the healing landscapes was the European conquest in 1492. The subsequent colonization of the

Caribbean spurred a series of movements and multidirectional exchanges of peoples, worldviews, illnesses, and remedies. Despite the overwhelming devastation, diseases, and a large number of deaths, the present-day healing landscapes are also testimonies of survival, resilience, and creativity in finding new remedies.

Within the historical formation of contemporary medicinal cultures this study has highlighted the need of considering the particular historical developments of small locations, the role of the colonial relations, religious institutions, and individual healers.

Contrary to Fernando Ortiz's idea about a failed indigenous transculturation, indigenous descendants had various opportunities to contribute genetically and culturally to the foundation of different Cuban and Dominican settlements. Some indigenous individuals and communities survived the hostile period of the conquest and colonization in the regions of the study. As the historical overview of early colonial towns in Eastern Cuba showed, indigenous residents were present at their foundation. The spatial proximity of indigenous people and newcomers of different backgrounds enabled (but did not guarantee) the exchange of botanical knowledge and broader dispersal of medicinal cultures. In fact, indigenous descendants lived in various Cuban and Dominican locations long later after their supposed disappearance. Small pockets of indigenous inhabitants lived in both urban and rural areas throughout the colonial period. In some locations, such as Boyá and Holguín indigenous descendants were recorded even in the 19th century. This increases the probability of transmission and continuity of their medicinal knowledge. Any continuity should, however, be understood as taking place within an ongoing process of transculturation.

The analysis of changes, adaptations, and continuities in that medical history is complicated by colonial bias, which is frequently present in accounts of indigenous culture and conceals some of the meanings and uses of the landscape. Although many plants rapidly became export commodities, the registers about medicinal properties of specific plants are limited, especially when compared to the uses that are known among the contemporary population. This emphasis of one specific use of a plant could later be interpreted as a loss of information. To illustrate this, the present-day use of tobacco by Dominican and Cuban healing practitioners as a means of communication with the invisible world opposes Ortiz's suggestion that the status of tobacco shifted in the colonial period from that of a sacred plant to that of a secular leisure commodity. In fact, some of its contemporary ritual uses resemble those employed by Kalinago *boyé* (shamans) recorded in the first half of the seventeenth century (Breton 1665). Likewise, it cannot be ruled out that tobacco was already used in exchanges during the pre-colonial time (Honychurch 1997; Allaire 2013). To conclude, in a context in which a sharp distinction between sacred and profane is unlikely to have existed, a shift in the meaning of tobacco from sacred to secular seems to be far from absolute.[400]

The case of tobacco illustrates how multiple uses and meanings of plants may obscure the reconstruction of their transformation over time even when they are still relatively well documented. In other cases, the only historical information that we have about the indigenous knowledge of the ancient flora is their names. Although later

---

400 This conclusion is in fact not so far from Ortiz´ view as one might think. Ortiz spoke about changes in what he considered *the most widespread meaning or use* of tobacco. He was well aware of the fact that tobacco continues to be used in local religious practices and has also medicinal uses.

authors such as Sloane (1707) or Chateusalins (1854) included more detailed and better illustrations of medicinal use of plants, these works were created after centuries of transculturation and as such are problematic for the reconstruction of what might be considered indigenous legacy.

The critical comparison of fragmentary colonial sources with present-day traditions enables us to further assess the process of transculturation. Various aspects of medicinal history and contemporary healing practices can complement each other. Demographic history may partially explain the present-day ratios of native and exotic flora used in medicinal practices. In Boyá and Jiguaní, both locations with the long presence of indigenous descendants, we find widespread use of native medicinal plants. Given the demographic history of these locations we may interpret this use as a (partial) continuity of native plant knowledge; although we lack detailed historical sources about the concrete extension of that knowledge and about the exact modalities of its transmission. The fragmented indications that we do have, suggest that the general mobility and intercultural contacts of the population allowed for multiple possibilities of exchanging botanical and medical knowledge as well as associated ideas.

The example of tobacco demonstrates how power relations (between religions) may also have influenced the transfer of meanings. The early colonial medicinal cultures were shaped by a complex mechanism of colonial relations. The botanical knowledge was also a means of indigenous social resistance and self-protection. Indigenous peoples were aware of the colonizer´s weakness in this aspect. On the other hand, this may have hampered the colonial appropriation of their knowledge and so may have contributed to its loss. In certain locations indigenous people were recognized as botanical experts throughout the 16th century. This recognition may have facilitated the appropriation of some of their wisdom by patients who had another worldview.

The later phases of colonial medicinal history are also marked by this general power struggle, which took the form of a "spiritual conquest" by the dominating group and of an expropriation of lands and knowledge. Not surprisingly, the Spanish acquisition of indigenous botanical knowledge was highly selective, and did not necessarily include the original etiologies or beliefs about human/nature relations. Given in the general poor medical care throughout the colonial period, the common people had to rely for their health on non-institutional medicinal specialists (including those of indigenous background) and their botanical knowledge. Combined with the lack of ecclesiastical control, the medicinal practices of the past were likely to be incorporated in the non-institutional beliefs of healers and patients.

The conquest of Cuba and Hispaniola lead to a profound reinterpretation of existing landscapes according to new religious, economic, and political practices, which left material and conceptual imprints. New sacred places were consecrated and became important historical sites while others were desacralized and even demonized. In accordance with the social inequality of the colonial world, the religious views of the colonized were mentioned only incidentally. The consideration of ethnographic and historical data suggests that both the European and the African newcomers coincided with the indigenous peoples in perceiving divine powers in the Caribbean landscapes. Sometimes, as the case of Antonio Congo or, in general, the present-day notion of indigenous commissions and divisions suggest, new meanings were constructed in awareness of the historical presence of prior inhabitants. The richness of different cultural practices and meanings associated with different Caribbean landscape features today bears witness to the resilience of the colonized people and the ability of the newcomers to adapt to the new surroundings. It also indicates a complex historical process of intercultural communication, which has largely remained invisible.

The colonizers and the enslaved people alike reinterpreted radically the newly encountered landscapes in accordance with their own worldviews. Thus Cuban and Dominican flora was integrated into worldviews with underpinnings of non-local origins. As a results, African orishas are attributed power over specific local plants, places and landscape features. European Saints have manifested themselves in various natural shrines. Thus the symbolism of flora and its categorization into distinct realms of spiritual entities varies across the local population.

Some differences in the interpretation of the landscape may be explained by distinct demographic and religious developments. While Dominican plants have an 'owner' or misterio that would not be specified, in Regla de Ocha nearly every plant is attributed to an orisha. In the spiritual tradition of Jiguaní plants do not have any owners but in Managuaco all medicinal plants are seen as the domain of the indigenous commission. In European Spiritism plants generally are not considered to have a spiritual owner. The attribution of plants to indigenous commission, therefore, seems part of local epistemologies (e.g. about the indigenous predecessors being carriers of this knowledge). The widespread popularity of Spiritism in Jiguaní, Holguín and Bayamo province reflects demographic grow of European decedents in the second half of the 19th century with a great part of the population being identified in racial categories as "white". The Spiritism imported from Europe to Cuba in that same period was likely to build upon (or was at least influenced by) local religious practices, which reflected a population with a relatively small size of enslaved people of African origin (Holguín 9,5%, Bayamo 10% and Jiguaní 4%) and "free peoples of color". Espiritismo del Cordón shows that the European form of spiritism was adapted to a new context.

The volume and different moments wherein the African ancestors were brought to both islands have shaped the particular characteristic of local religions and distinct flora symbolism Regla de Ocha and Dominican 21 Division. The fact that more than 90% of the captives of the whole Transatlantic Slave Trade were brought to Cuba in the nineteenth century explains also the preservation of ritual languages, sacred narratives (patakis) and African features in religious beliefs.

Although the different African peoples (Ewe-Fon, Yoruba, Kongo) may have had distinct interpretations of specific flora, they shared the concept of the animated landscape, and often similar ideas about certain sacred trees and plants, some of which they considered as dwellings of deities and ancestors. Also the custom to ask for permission before collecting the medicinal plants in the sacred forests was widespread (*e.g.* Quiroz 2015; Herskovits 1938).

A different religious background in the area of origin, but also cultural loss or change due to enslavement may be the reason why 21 Division does not attribute *lwas* to specific plants. Keeping in mind Bastide´s argument about the importance of brotherhoods in urban areas as institutions that passed on the ancestral knowledge, we may attribute this characteristic also to cultural loss that was particular to the rural areas where the Dominican healers were interviewed.

Although, the demographic history is a good reference point for understanding the local development of spirituality and the characteristic of the medicinal cultures, the local aspects should not be seen as isolated from the situation in other locations. The individual creativity of a healer and religious groups like brotherhoods should not be underestimated. Healing specialists of non-local origin had to find ways of curing with unknown flora. The newcomers were looking for plants that were similar to known taxonomic families, but they also experimented and observed other people and animals to discover the medicinal properties of so far unknown plants. In addition, the trade, the presence of diverse religious institutions, such as the Catholic church and the brotherhoods, together with the mobility of healing practitioners and the local population at large, were likely to reinforce each other as factors that introduced and amalgamated African and European influences.

Brotherhoods (cofradías) promoted cohesion and collective action also in matters of health. Traditionally brotherhoods are discussed as important elements in the transfer of medicinal cultures of African origin, because within these institutions people could reorganize according to ethnic lines and/or regional origins. The members of Cuban and Dominican brotherhoods might consist of the same colonial categories (zapes, mandingas, biafaras, aradás) but also have quite distinct backgrounds (*e.g.* the Saint John brotherhood in Santo Domingo). The interaction of present-day brotherhoods and their members during the patronal celebrations like the one in Boyá once again show how knowledge could cross the colonial boundaries. The mobility of brotherhoods also problematizes Bastide´s (2011) observation that these institutions were less influential in rural areas. Likely, the mobility of members of *cabildos* and *cofradías* was already present during the colonial period – especially among free and freed strata of the population, and especially after the emancipation – with all its consequences for long-term intercultural communication.[401]

Based on the historical references about brotherhoods in Cuba and Hispaniola, we may expect influences from different West African peoples (principally proceeding from what is now Senegambia, Gold Coast, Bight of Benin, Bight of Biafra, Nigeria, Cameroon, Congo, and Angola) in the contemporary healing tradition. Accordingly, influences of the Lucumí brotherhood, composed by Yoruba (from what is now Nigeria and Benin) are still discernable in the present-today Regla de Ocha, as well as influences from the Bantú (Congo and Angola) in Palo Monte and Regla Conga, and from Ewe-Fon people in Regla de Arará and Fon influences in 21 Division.[402]

Brotherhoods were important for the continuation of medicinal traditions but they offer us also points of departure for tracing the changes. If we assume that certain contemporary healing practices have a long tradition, then it may be argued that the brotherhood composed of members from Allada (present-day Benin), which was dedicated to Saint Cosme and Saint Damian in 1650s in Santo Domingo, might in the same way as today be dedicated to the twin deities. Its likelyhood increases if we consider that twin deities are popular still among Fon-Egbe, Ewe, and Yoruba. However, tracing such direct parallels is complicated because of the many different symbolic

401 For more on the historical information about the historical demographic formation of communities in rural areas see (González 2011).

402 For the similarities see e.g. Bascom (1984).

elements (colors, parts of the hagiography, qualities they represent, places associated with them) that could be used to communicate the meaning of the divine personages to the devotees. Accordingly, Saint Michael, who was considered to have the power to cure smallpox in late seventeenth century Santo Domingo among Ewe and Fon speakers (the second largest group of captives at the time), might be used as a symbol of Sapata, their smallpox god.

However, many more groups of captives followed, which constantly adapted and reinterpreted the elements and meanings of their ancestral religion. These again could integrate different religious influences from West Africa but also Roman Catholic teachings. The fact that today Saint Michael is the patron of Belie Belcán in the Dominican 21 Division seems to be based on the character of Saint Michael as the archangel who fought the devil, so that he is now consulted by persons who seek protection against evil and enemies.

Thus, it is difficult to reconstruct the development of the present-day healing landscapes because it is obscured by the fragmentary characteristic of the information regarding medicinal, religious, and demographic histories. This exercise is even more complicated if we lack information about the today's healing practices and local epistemologies. Being part of a larger project that generated new data about the immediate transformations after the European invasion of the Caribbean, this study focused on some of the contemporary facets of healing landscapes. It provides an overview of the rich symbolism, paying attention to sacred and miraculous healing places, plants and other landscape features. Some of these landscape features function as mnemonic tools of the indigenous past, which might provide some contrast to the descriptions given by historical sources, but also indicate possible continuities. The concept of cultural memory was a vector for understanding people's perception of and engagement with the past as an integral part of the context and mechanism of transmitting medicinal knowledge and related cultural traditions.

Constituents of healing landscapes

Healing landscapes were defined as all agents that are said to promote physical, mental, and spiritual health. Following this definition this study has collected data that illustrate several key aspects of the rich Cuban and Dominican healing landscapes. These landscapes include healing and ritual specialists, plant remedies and in general the divine and ancestral beings residing or manifested in places, vegetation, and natural features.

Approaching healing landscapes from a holistic perspective, this study situates the general importance of the landscapes for individual health and wellbeing as well as for the quality of life of the community within the broader ecological knowledge and associated traditions of the people concerned. The intimate link between the wellbeing of rural communities, environments, and worldviews is evident in the important role that ecological and botanical knowledge plays in daily life, foodways, crafts, and agriculture.

The quality of life of these communities is linked to their surrounding landscapes. The physical health of people living in agricultural settings depends on their ecological knowledge, which they use in daily practices as well as in the time of illness. Similarly, the more psychological aspect of wellbeing is sustained through the support of divine agencies and spiritual entities. This mutual support can become materialized in, for example, offerings brought to the dwelling of these spiritual entities. Needless to stress that both aspects – the physical and the psychological, the material and the immaterial – are intimately connected, in accordance with religious worldviews, cultural memory and social ethos. The wide-spread popularity of San Isidro, the processions including collective prayers for harvest and rain, and other customs assuring the protection of the harvest, as well as ritual treatment of the flora, are just a few examples that illustrate how the vital role of the environment is reflected in cultural practices.

From the data overview emerge three particular actors that promote physical, mental, and spiritual health. Apart from the official medical care, the most important agent in promoting health and wellbeing in the Caribbean are healers, or ritual specialists, who act as mediators between the patients, the community and the divine. Spiritual mediums, religious initiates in Regla de Ocha and 21 Division literally embody the normally invisible *orishas*, *lwas*, ancestors, and spirits in order to establish diagnoses and suggest remedies.

Among the established causes of illness there are both observable and not directly observable causes. In this regard, the adjective 'healing' in 'healing landscape' might sound misleading to some readers, as we have also mentioned agents that cause illness. It is important to acknowledge, however, that many *orishas*, *lwas*, other divine beings may be both beneficial and detrimental to human health. This has been also observed in other cultural contexts (*e.g.* Reyes Gomez 2017; Artist 2016).

The remedies may include a careful application of medicinal plants, or interaction with deities, Saints, and spirits whose agencies are engaged through healing rituals at home-altars and natural shrines. From Dominican healers' biographies it is evident that the reception of the *lwas* is involuntarily and may take place anywhere. This is especially the case before the healers are initiated and before they accept the gift to heal. This should be understood in the context of a worldview wherein the Great God can be manifested in different natural elements through the *lwas*.

Directly after hospitals and doctor's surgeries, the house-temples and home altars in 21 Division, Regla de Ocha or Spiritism are the most prominent healing places in both the Dominican Republic and Cuba. The altars and house-temples are symbolically linked to outside landscapes through offerings, symbolic representations of specific places or other relevant elements. Also, in Regla de Ocha, different ritual paraphernalia, symbols, and attributes of divinities or ancestors, represent or refer to meanings of outside landscapes. Similarly, at the homes of Cuban Espiritistas we would find protective plants, stones from ancestral places and flower offerings for deceased loved ones.

In agreement with previous Adrian Gomes' explanation (chapter 8), most of the healing would take place at the healer's house-temple. Although visiting them on irregularly basis, and less frequently then the house-temples, Dominican and Cuban patients seek their recovery also in Catholic churches and chapels, or at pilgrimage sites (*e.g.* Sacred Hill, the sanctuary of the Virgen of Charity in Cobre), as well as historical sites, such as places reminiscent of the slave trade, the life of enslaved peoples, or monuments of ancestral resistance. While in many cases the integration of these sites into the religious realm could be justified by visible material human imprints, other loci were only known as dwellings of divine entities or ancestors from sacred narratives and other oral traditions.

Both in Dominican 21 Division and Regla de Ocha the *orishas* and *lwas* may manifest themselves in the four natural elements, as well as in specific places, where they may give counsel and advice about which remedies to use, including plants and ritual baths. The air together with several caves, mountains, rivers, water pools, waterfalls, sea, mountains, and hills, are identified as dwellings of *lwas*, Saints, ancestors and spirits, which might be both detrimental and beneficial. Also, in Cuba adherents of Regla de Ocha considered that certain divinities may become manifest in the landscape or may be encountered at specific places, for example: Elegua at crossroads, Chango in palm trees or in thunder, Obatala in mountains, Ogun in hills and *manigua*, Babalu Aye as guardian of the hospitals, Yemaya along the sea coast, Oshun at river banks, Oya in cemeteries. Certain divinities such as Olofi may be encountered everywhere, while nearly every tree has a specific *orisha* as its owner. Catholics pay visits to Saints at natural shrines – including caves, sacred hills, and trees – to promote health and wellbeing. Occasionally adherents of Cuban Spiritism consider specific places more apt for establishing a connection with spiritual entities.

An important component of healing landscapes are the hundreds of medicinal plants, including trees and herbs of both native and exotic origins, that are used across different religious denominations for medicinal and ritual purposes. Plants are particularly important in the countryside, where they are regularly used for curing physical, mental, and spiritual ailments. A division of the plants into broad categories of (1) ritual plants, which cure the mental and spiritual ailments, and (2) medicinal plants, which have biomedical effects on the body, would be too simple. In cases such as the described baths both ritual and medicinal plants are complementing each other and working together. Studies on Surinamese plants used in baths, potions, and rituals show that these plants also have physical healing properties, which might be one of the reasons why sacred plants are (considered) sacred (Van Andel et al. 2013). Ethnopharmacological research on ritual plant use in Benin and Gabon confirmed that the local plants used in baths also had biological effects because of their medicinal properties (Quiroz et al. 2016).

The spiritual significance of certain trees display Catholic, West African and also Caribbean indigenous notions of sacred landscapes, which have been fused in the Caribbean context. The meaning of ceiba display Catholic and African reinterpretations of indigenous symbolism. The traditional prohibition of felling certain trees such as *jobo*, *ceiba*, and *higo* because that might cause physical harm to the person should also be seen in the light of local histories, where indigenous and/or African roots may be prominent.

In contrast to the portrayal of Caribbean people as being too fragmented and uprooted to have any spiritual relationship with the local landscape, the present-day healing landscapes are rich with symbolism and expose how some elements of indigenous culture continued and how newcomers were able to adapt to the new environment, replicating some of their old worldviews and oral literary traditions in a creative manner. The newcomers reinterpreted the newly encountered landscapes according to their memory of previously known landscapes and according to the ecological insights from their homeland but also in relation to the new locale, and to the people dwelling in these landscapes before their arrival. Even though there may not have been direct contact, the ceramics from the precolonial period recovered from altars of different healers or homes of patients are an explicit indication that the precolonial past has been integrated into contemporary people's memory.

After examining how the image of indigenous peoples is invoked in the present in general terms, a review of which landscape features are associated with the indigenous peoples will help to summarize how the indigenous past is perceived and represented within the healing practices. This discussion will lead us to reflect upon the value of the concept of cultural memory for historical and ethnographic studies of the Caribbean and upon the use of the concept of healing landscapes within modern landscape theories.

Memory of indigenous ancestors

One group of agents presents in the surrounding landscapes and influential in the wellbeing of both individuals and communities is that of indigenous ancestors. In accordance with Halbwachs' observation that individual memory is shaped by interactions of individuals with others in the context of social groups, the individual memories concerning the indigenous past in both islands are shaped by the institutional and public domains of knowledge production. Consequently, the most intimate experiences such as dreaming, the perceptions of the indigenous forefathers in the landscape, or their embodiment during a trance are contextualized in that broader social framework. These domains are inseparable in oral tradition, in which information may be compared to other testimonies or traditions but often is entangled with individual memory. The individual memory is then collectively shaped by state-sponsored institutions like schools, museums, and mass-media, literature (scientific, fiction, poetry, prose), popular culture (movies, documentaries, songs), cultural artefacts (art, souvenirs, monuments, archeological artefacts, commercial products, money, city emblems, flags etc.) and places, paths, and other physical landscape features. The historical consciousness is equally codified in collective traditions, but also formed through individual interactions with the past by dwelling in (historically and/or religiously charged) landscapes.

Within the healing landscapes the indigenous past is reenacted in multiple manners. One of the most conscious ways of connecting to indigenous predecessors is the acknowledgment of their presence now (coevalness), and particularly the recognition of their agency in the context of health and wellbeing. The indigenous ancestors are believed to be present in different places and on different occasions. Indigenous ancestral forces are consulted (*e.g.* in matters of healing), commemorated, and asked for guidance, favors, or protection to benefit individuals in different situations. Indigenous ancestors may manifest themselves in dreams, through their embodiment in the healers, and by means of different signs (drumming, braided hair). Their power may also reside in certain objects, and their presence may be sensed or seen in specific places, most frequently in caverns, water pools and less frequently on mountains.

In Dominican 21 Division, the indigenous ancestors are both beneficial and potentially dangerous to one's wellbeing. The danger of the indigenous ancestral agency is exemplified by the case of children or individuals that are reported to have "*corriente del indio*". As we have seen, such individuals were warned to be cautious when around certain places such as bodies of water and caverns as these were potentially dangerous and could provoke illness, soul loss, or even death. The "*corriente*" is a spiritual link that sometimes is based on remote kinship, or phenotypical resemblances. The latter aspect is likely to have been retrieved from the official identity politics wherein the denomination "Indian" is used for a specific European determined phenotype, in close connection with the existing racism in Dominican society.

In Regla de Ocha the agency of the indigenous ancestors was acknowledged by different contributors. Within this spiritual realm, the indigenous predecessors are helping to protect against enemies and malevolent influences; they may manifest themselves at altars and some archaeological sites. Specific plants, like *acullá*, *jíba*, and *sunflower*, are attributed to them. Also, Cuban Espiritistas invoke indigenous commissions with specific prayers in general matters of wellbeing in house-temples, occasionally in caverns, or everywhere where indigenous ancestors felt well, where there was a good *fluidity*.

The memory of the indigenous forefathers is retrieved within the surrounding landscape, which is impregnated with the human past, as visible in the remains of human settlements, in living heritage or other activities, as well in ideas associated with the flora. Toponyms like Pool of Indian or Cave of Indian frequently encountered in local landscapes are an indication of how certain places remain associated with indigenous ancestors. The following paragraphs will discuss whether and how this link can be conceived as a memory of the indigenous past.

Water sources and caves as ancestral places

Despite profound material modifications and environmental changes, landscapes are constants that have had a unifying effect on people who came to the Caribbean over the last millennia. The rich cultural and religious history of their habitation has left marks on the way these landscapes are "read" and engaged with today. Some of these landmarks are directly associated with the agency of indigenous ancestors. The interpretation of this phenomenon has to take into account the cultural diversity of the social groups that dwell in the landscape and that have created their own specific cultural memory framework.

Among the prominent places that are associated with indigenous predecessors in the Dominican Republic are freshwater sources. Specific water pools in rivers, waterfalls, and rapids, are dwelling places of the indigenous spirits throughout all the Dominican regions.

Currently, waterbodies have multiple meanings: they are loci where the potentially dangerous ancestors, as well as the deceased in general, may be perceived, but they can also be the path to find the virtue to heal. The leitmotif of healing power found in the subaquatic realm is also expressed in narratives about midwives or healers travelling to the subaquatic kingdom where they received a reward (their virtue to heal). The motif of subaquatic travels following the path to the world of the deceased and to renewal, but also the figure of the Master Boa giving people the wisdom to protect and heal themselves have parallels in Kalinago narratives (1941, 1952).[403]

403 Taylor (1952): "They reached the shores of the Orinoco and plunged into its stream ... They emerged upon the opposite bank ... (as) two young lads; and upon the water ... there floated two empty turtle shells. They never came back to Dominica; and at least one of them died, but the other, was thought to be still living". The river seems to function as a liminal place. Another narrative tells about a little girl who was carried by Mama d' l'Eau (the protector of fishes) across a river to a place where she received from the Godmother the means how to mislead Fou-Fou, the kolibri bird, which was chasing her.

In general, narratives about these deep pools are like warnings to behave with caution, as these places may be dangerous for human individuals: their soul might be taken away and brought to the subaquatic domain of the spirits. The narratives about children, or persons with *corriente,* which were taken away, also resemble, at least to some degree, those from the indigenous communities on the mainland. The Ashaninka and Araweté, for example, also tell about invisible beings inhabiting the water sources which have been tricking, seducing, and abducting children, women, and travelers (their souls) to their underwater houses (Santos-Granero 1998; Viveiros Castro 1992). The same being can also potentially be beneficial by controlling the population of fish. Similarly, the Makuna Water Anaconda is the Spirit Owner of an underwater *maloca,* which is the place where the reincarnation and rebirth of people as fishes begins.

More frequently, people would engage with these freshwater sources on special occasions like a ritual bath, patron feast or healer's initiation. These celebrations are moments when gratitude is being expressed and relations with the spiritual world are renewed. The indigenous ancestors receive offerings during the feasts of Saint Francis, Carmen, or Christmas in Bánica, Saint Michael in La Jaiba, and Saint John's feast in La Mancha. In these cases, the commemoration of indigenous ancestors is part of collective celebrations of patronal *lwas* of communities or healers. The ancestral veneration within the context of collective celebrations must be understood as part of a general acknowledgment of other forces, but also as the expression of a special link with the celebrated *lwa*/Saint.

The centuries of ontological encounters and long-term transculturation, have made the waterbodies on these islands places with multiple meanings, which proceed from different origins. The indigenous sacred narratives about Great Flood, Divine Twins and possibly also the Great Serpent or the Master of the Water have not been preserved in their totality. The narrative about the Great Serpent, though, shows that there is some continuity of the indigenous worldview in the contemporary population. Therefore, also present-day narratives about indigenous ancestors or Divine Twins may echo indigenous ideas, fused with views that were imported after 1492. African-derived spiritual beings like Oshún, King of the Water, and Simbi, illustrate how diasporic communities appropriated the new spaces according to their own worldview, but also may have connected to fragmentary information stemming from the pre-colonial population. Similarly, the cult of the Virgin of Holy Waters in Boyá and the Virgin of El Cobre is to be understood as the result of long term transculturation, in which continuities and changes took place and new cultural forms emerged.

Other prominent places associated with the indigenous ancestors are caverns. Caribbean caverns have inscribed themselves into the cultural memory in multiple ways. Caverns are loci of (sacred) history, and have been calling the attention of adherents of different worldviews, of amateur and professional archaeologists, but also of looters searching for imagined treasures in these "enchanted" places. A significant number of indigenous cultural representations (in rock art or on artefacts, see Fig. 80, for more information on these pieces see Breukel 2013), objects (ritual, sacred objects), and human remains have been found in Caribbean caverns, and rock shelters (Hayward et al. 2009; Berman et al. 2013; Schaffer et al. 2012; CITMA 2007).

The examples discussed in chapter 9 highlight the caverns as places of indigenous ancestral presence with specific value for healing. Currently in Cuba and the

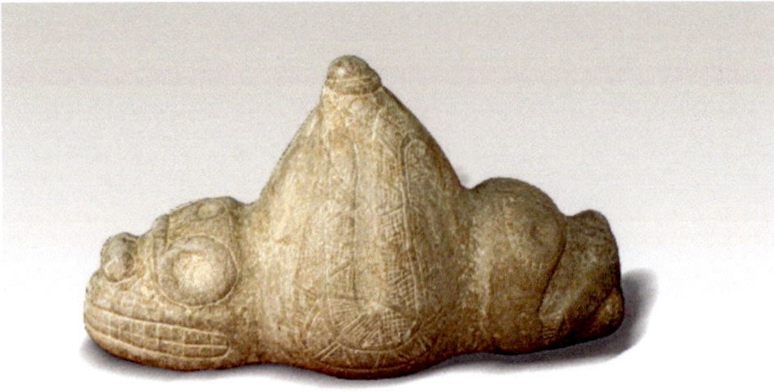

Figure 79 A threepointer with serpent-like motives found in one of Dominican caverns, the Museum of Alto de Chavón.

Dominican Republic, adherents of different religious currents (Spiritism, Dominican Vudu, *Regla de Ocha*, and Roman Catholicism) consider caves as places of manifestation or agency of divine beings, Saints, and remote predecessors, which may intervene in matters of human wellbeing.

For adherents of 21 Division and Cuban Spiritism, but also for Catholics, some caverns are empowered by indigenous ancestors. In Bánica and Mancha, cavern celebrations are devoted to Catholic Saints, but indigenous spirits (*lwa*) are expected to join in the celebration, and offerings are left for them on the ground, at specific points, at petroglyphs, or at water associated places. Being a part of a patronal celebration, these commemorations of indigenous forefathers should help establishing or maintaining a positive relationship between devotees and the Saints, spirits or *lwas*. Opinions might differ, however, about the beneficial character of the indigenous agency. The celebrations are occasions to ask for advice and remedies, but also to let the *lwa* participate in the communal feast. The interaction with ancestral forces within this context includes expressions of gratitude for ancestral guidance, warnings, and protection in times of illness or crisis. The whole is an experience and reaffirmation of a *communitas* that extends into the spirit world.

The liminal character of caves as places that permit the passage from one world to another lends itself to veneration of ancestors in general. In this respect a dead person of local origin was consulted in the Gibara cavern, and in the Mana cavern offerings were brought to Barón del Cementerio/San Elías, the head of the *guedés*, who embodies the powers of death and fertility.

The ways in which indigenous predecessors are remembered should be situated within the different modes of ancestral commemoration across 21 Division, Regla de Ocha, Roman Catholicism and Cord Spiritism. The remembrance of the indigenous past fits the ancient American and West (Central) African ancestor worship as well as European customs to commemorate deceased relatives on All Souls' Day.

The present-day beliefs in afterlife are expressed on All Souls' Day. Like in Europe, also on both islands the deceased are commemorated on November 2nd by visitation of cemeteries, where the graves are cleaned, decorated, and given offerings. Cubans and Dominicans personalize their offerings for the deceased according to what the individuals liked during the life (mostly tobacco, rum, or coffee). Within 21 Division, at this day devotees bring offerings to the earth division, the *lwas* that are in charge of the dead, to Barón del Cementerio, his daughter Saint Martha and his children, the Guedes, in the graveyards (Tejeda Ortiz 2013).[404]

Beliefs about the role of the deceased in present-day life may also be expressed during funerals. In the Dominican context we find them in customs such as placing offerings under the altar and covering mirrors to avoid that they absorb the souls of the deceased (Andújar Persinal 2013).[405]

Like indigenous ancestors, the deceased can manifest themselves in dreams, asking for the help of the living, or offering to help those alive, especially their loved ones. On special occasions the deceased can also incarnate in the body of the healer or spiritual medium. The deceased arrives with the same voice that he/she had when alive, asks about his/her family members, and answers their questions, asks for certain things, gives recommendations to resolve family problems or removes obstacles that might inhibit harmonious coexistence (Andújar Persinal 2013; Tejeda Ortiz 2013).

Beliefs in ancestral indigenous agency are also visible in Catholic liturgy, 21 Division and popular religious expressions. The devotees believe that the souls of the deceased persons may roam around in the landscape until they have done penance for their sins. According to Christian teachings, the souls of indigenous peoples like of those other non-Christians are bound to go to hell. The placement of indigenous ancestors in caverns and water bodies also fits an idea of popular Catholicism wherein some souls do not reach their final destination and remain at intermediate places in penance. Different archaeological sites scattered throughout the landscapes are material reminders of settlements and sites of past activities. These sites are often situated at riverbanks (Ulloa Hung 2014).

The indigenous antedecents are also associated with other memory places in local landscapes (*e.g.* Palenque Gibara, La Negreta, SepiSepi, El Cobre, *manigua, el monte*, hills), some of which are known only from archaeological remains, others only from oral history. As the cave of Gibara shows, a cave can also be a memory place of an African ancestor. According to historical and archaeological evidence (*e.g.* Pereira Pereira 2008) and oral testimonies of fugitives (Montejo's biography in Barnet 1966), caverns were hiding places of Maroons during the slavery period. Caverns and other memory places are of importance not only as heritage sites but may also be an interesting point of departure for archaeological surveys and historical analysis.

The identification of ancestral origins should be understood in the light of the politics of identity and personal preferences of the practitioners. Given the relatively recent kidnapping and enslavement of ancestors of African background, some of the Cuban contributors were aware of direct genetic links with specific African ancestors. Among adherents of Regla de Ocha or Cuban Espiritismo the awareness of genealogical links with Africa was not an obstacle for admitting the agency of indigenous predecessors. As we have seen, such a recognition of indigenous predecessors was also common in Dominican 21 Division, Haitian Voodoo, Brazilian Candomblé, and Surinamese Winti.

---

404 The King of the Graveyard symbolizes the first deceased who were buried in the graveyard. He is the guardian of all the deceased, a protector against negative energies, and helps in lottery. Like the whole division he works with the earth element.

405 Kalunga in Kongo means Atlantic Ocean (Brown 2012).

People's self-identification with particular ancestors is certainly influenced by both formal and informal knowledge production, which includes past colonial discourse. The association of indigenous ancestors with caves may echo, for example, the early chronicles about uncivilized people (Guanahatabeyes and Siboneyes) living in the caverns (Las Casas 1951). On the other hand, Pané registers narratives about such places being associated with ancestral emergence among the indigenous inhabitants. Similarly, among the Wayuu, the cavern Jorottuy Manna is the site of origin of the Sun (Kaí), the moon (Kashi) and the people (Perrin 1987). Together with a small well at Cabo de la Vela, this cavern is the passage through which the dead go to the sky world. The rich archaeological evidence of primary and secondary burials in caves suggests a connection with beliefs about the hereafter (La Rosa Corzo & Robaína Jaramillo 1995; CITMA 2007). In view of this complex of ideas, we suspect that the ancient mortuary depositional practices may have been directed towards ancestors. Drawing a parallel with the Kalinago cavern that was used to consult Bákamo, the Divine Serpent who gave people plants to protect them, ancient offerings in Cuban and Dominican caverns may also have been directed to such divine beings. Future studies may clarify the possible link between the testimony from Bánica that stated that the Great Serpent descended from Saint Francis hill. Saint Francis cavern illustrates how the meaning of places like this has been profoundly transformed by the last five hundred years, yet retains great importance in sacred history until today.

There is still insufficient research on the symbolism of caverns among peoples that speak an Arawakan language. According to Von Humboldt the Venezuelan Guacharo cavern, which he called the "Acheron" of the Chaimas and other indigenous peoples from the Orinoco region, was famous as a place of passage to the underworld and the hereafter. This belief even gave rise to the expression "to descend to Guacharo", which was an equivalent of "to pass away". Today the same cavern figures as an ancestral cavern in the oral tradition regarding the indigenous heroine Urimare, who until now is commemorated in Venezuelan Spiritism. Similar traditions, ideas and practices may be behind the archaeological marking of such places: nearly five hundred sites with rock art have been recorded in the Dominican Republic (López Belando 2006) and nearly two hundred in Cuba (Fernández Ortega 2006), many of which are situated in caverns. Experiences in other parts of the Americas indicate that future cooperation between researchers and indigenous experts from the mainland (native speakers) holds an important key for understanding the meanings and values encoded by the pre-colonial cultures of the Caribbean.

Healing landscapes as expressions of cultural memories of indigenous past

One of the principal questions of this investigation was: how do healing landscapes encapsulate cultural memories of the indigenous past? Needless to say, the past of all peoples and cultures is a social (re)construction by people living in the present. In many countries, such as Cuba and the Dominican Republic, as well as Mexico, Peru or Bolivia, the indigenous past is part of a foundational narrative that provides the basis for collective identity. This identity is rooted in the cultural memory that is shaped by formal institutions. In order to construct a national history, several Caribbean and

Latin American education systems tend to present an image of the indigenous past of the country as a prehistoric cultural phase, which is essentially a closed chapter of history without any continuity into the present. Throughout the Americas the pre-colonial peoples were generally interpreted in colonial terms as "uncivilized", "*not yet* Christian", etc. Their cultural heritage was seen as "primitive" and should be abandoned under the "civilizing" influence of the colonizers, who were going to instruct the natives in "true culture and religion". Similarly, the enslaved peoples were seen and treated as lower than human. This Eurocentric ideology was the justification of conquest, colonialism and slavery. Modern perspectives still suffer from this discriminatory and paternalistic mindset. Descendant populations, surviving in rural areas, are associated with poverty and underdevelopment, and may still become victims of different variants of racism and exploitation.

There are several reasons why this biased image is so persistent in present-day societies. Firstly there is the degree in which the vocabulary and concepts from primary historical resources have been incorporated in present-day texts and so keep exercising a strong influence. The perpetuation of certain vocabularies and concepts without their historical contextualization leads to a continuous transfer of ideologies and values that are biased and do not have place in the contemporary democratic societies. Secondly, it is important to acknowledge that the colonization has caused a severe fragmentation of the knowledge about the people that has suffered all this exploitation. The accidental references in many primary historical sources generated during the colonial period make the search for more information about the past of historically marginalized groups often difficult, though not an impossible or unfruitful journey. Thirdly, the old disciplinary division between the archaeologist focusing on material remains, the historian focusing on written documentary sources, and the anthropologist and sociologist focusing on present-day communities and their knowledge has reinforced the disconnection between the present and the past. The study of the cultural memory and heritage of those historically marginalized will benefit from an interdisciplinary approach.

Written history is just one way of registering and remembering the past. Following Ortiz' metaphor of counterpoint cultural memory was proposed as a counterbalance and complement to the image that emerged from the biased colonial archives and material records. Besides explicit ways of remembering the indigenous ancestors, there are at certain places more subtle connections with the indigenous past in terms of cultural continuities. While certain traditions might be recently initiated or invented, others may be continuities that have persisted during several generations, decennia or even centuries.

The past of the indigenous ancestors has been approached through archaeological studies, the primary focus of which is often disconnected from the social realities of communities living in present. Unlike in other contexts (e.g as in Mesoamerica or the Andean region), the ongoing cultural traditions in the Caribbean are generally not carried by direct descendants who have also strong linguistic continuities (indigenous people, speakers of Native American languages). The occurrence of an enormous genocide and great cultural loss, resulting in the fragmentation and even colonization of cultural memory, is undeniable in regions of this study. Although this memory cannot be separated from the colonial discourse, it may offer a new new perspectives to complete and contrast the big narratives of the shared past.

Disentangling continuities

Various elements of present-day Caribbean healing practices and ecological knowledge resemble what is reported by historical and ethnographic accounts from the Caribbean (including the Lesser Antilles) and the South American mainland. This concerns some of the concept of illness, the healers' invocation of spiritual beings, the knowledge and use of plant remedies, the selection of healing places, plants and other ingredients, as well as the ideas regarding animated landscapes and the custom of making collective pilgrimages to and performing ritual cleansing at sacred places. Yet these elements have also counterparts in Europe and Africa.[406] Particularly the African heritage is very visible (*e.g.* in the names of lwas and orishas), while the syncretism with Catholic Saints and their cult is obvious. The following section will examine this process in more detail. It will highlight the cultural traits that might be (but not necessarily are) continuities of ideas and practices deemed to be existent among indigenous peoples at the time of the conquest, and contextualize these in the demographic history of selected locations.

Boyá

Two Dominican locations, Boyá and Bánica, represent exceptions in Dominican history because of the long-term presence of indigenous descendants throughout the colonial period. In Boyá this presence has been documented from the second half of the 16th century through the 18th, and perhaps until the end of the 19th century. The local church and its patron, the Virgin of the Holy Waters, have an explicit connection with the indigenous population since the second half of 16th century when the church was founded and in the middle of the 17th century when the Virgin of the Holy Waters was highly esteemed.

According to oral history, the Virgin of the Holy Waters appeared in an orange tree in Boyá, which is said to have stood at the place where later the church was established. This manifestation has a clear parallel in the narrative about the miraculous appearance of the Virgin from nearby Higüey who also manifested itself in an orange tree. Yet the appearance of divine beings in trees or flora is a rather universal motif and has been registered also among the indigenous people of Hispaniola.

The roots of the cult of the Virgin of the Holy Waters are in Spain: she has been focus of cult in the town of Villaverde del Río (in the province of Sevilla) since the late 13th century, when Catholicism returned to that region as a consequence of the Reconquista. She is a patron of springs and flowing water and invoked as a protector against drought. Legend has it that she appeared to a shepherd. It is claimed that her cult and sanctuary go even further back in time and were founded by Saint Isidore of Seville (560-636). [407] In the 16th century the image became increasingly famous, the Virgin being brought out in processions to ask for rain. Later she came in the custody of the Franciscan order (Hernández Rodríguez and Rodríguez Becerra 2015). Obviously,

---

406 For more on the European roots of some of Cuban religious celebrations see Brea López (1998).
407 Saint Isidore of Seville (560-536) should not be confused with Saint Isidore Laborer (1070 -1130).

the connections with the area of Seville and with the Franciscans may have played an important role in the dissemination of this Virgin's veneration to the Americas.

If the Virgin travelled with the same name and hagiography from Spain to Boyá in the second half of 16th century, the small-size local indigenous population may have interpreted her character according to their own traditions, which in that period would still have preserved some traces of the pre-colonial worldview. The reference to this Virgin as an indigenous lady in the collective prayers during the patronal celebrations links her explicitly to the indigenous past. However, which elements might be identified as continuities of indigenous worldview?

As the Mother figure and the element Water are universal symbols, valued across different cultures, the Virgin of the Holy Water of Boyá may have fused with an indigenous image symbolizing the same or similar values.

De Goeje (1943) refers to comparable Virgin Mothers among the indigenous peoples of the Guyanas. One of these is said to be without beginning, without navel because she is unborn, and immortal. Among the Kaliña, Amana is the foundation of the universe: she sheds her skin continually as a serpent, she is the representation of continual change, the essence of time, mother of all things, and she can take all shapes. She is one of the water spirits, which are called Oriyo in Arawakan and Okoyumu in Kaliña (De Goeje 1943).

Friar Pané recorded the pre-colonial indigenous concept of a Divine Mother who was invisible, without beginning, and immortal in heaven. She was called by the names Atabei, Iermaoguacar, Apito and Zuimaco.[408] Arrom (1989) suggested that the name Atabeira derives from *itabo*, lagoon, and *era*, water, while De Goeje had Attabeira come from an Arawakan word for mother, *ata*, and/or beginning, *atenwa*.[409] The deciphering of the names would benefit from an emic perspective, in-depth knowledge of the languages and worldview of indigenous peoples of the Guyanas and Suriname. This, in turn, would provide a firmer base for reconstructing the way in which by the indigenous inhabitants of Boyá may have received and interpreted this Catholic image.

As Penard (2006) suggests, the concept of the Virgin Mother exists also among other indigenous peoples of America. The miraculous nature of a Virgin who is at the same time mother is, therefore, likely to be understood as a symbol across different cultures. Similarly, a female deity with the power to regulate bodies of water occurs in different cultures. The presence of such archetypical characteristics would have facilitated the integration of this image into the local belief system by the inhabitants of Boyá in the 16th century.

A plausible reconstruction would be that the syncretism or rather symbolic synergy that would have occurred in the 16th century was handed down from one generation to the next and so became gradually more and more influenced by and integrated into religious expressions from abroad. By the midst of the 17th century, when the Virgin was held in greet esteem, probably there were among her devotees indigenous people

---

408 These names are given in Whitehead´s transcription. They were earlier transcribed by Arrom in the same way; only he separated Yermao and Guacar, a division motivated by the friar's note that she had five names. D´Anghiera registered these names as Attabeira, Mamona, Guacarapita, Iiella, Guimazoa. Las Casas transcribed the name of the mother of the gods as Atabex.

409 In their analysis of Caribbean toponyms, Granberry and Vescelius 2004 have argued that water is *na* or *ne*. Pernard registered *toena* for water.

of local and non-local origins (*e.g.* from La Tortuga). The circulation of indigenous beliefs took place in a context in which the indigenous population fluctuated strongly through successive periods. In addition, local religions were likely to be exposed to external religious influences, including those of nearby Monte Plata, where enslaved peoples were living in the 18th century or those of the brotherhoods from Bayaguana.

The present-day reference to the Virgin as an indigenous lady is likely derived from the widespread traditions about indigenous people living under water. This association can be based on her name and hagiography, which belong to the water domain. The connection with the indigenous past is obviously rooted in the general awareness that Boyá's first inhabitants were indigenous people, who are also said to have built the church. The material reminders, such as Enrique's grave, statues of indigenous faces at the church, ceramics displayed among the church's holy relics, or San Isidro holding a *coa* (digging stick), together with publications about the local history (Zambrano 2009) and the local collection of some indigenous artefacts, all reinforce this historical consciousness. The memory of the indigenous past is reenacted in explicit ways through patronal celebrations, oral traditions and oral history referring to the foundation of the settlement.

The cultural memory of the indigenous past is also more subtly embedded in daily practices and traditions. Ancestral indigenous knowledge could in part be passed down through living material heritage like kitchen utensils (calabash plates, *bateas*), alimentation, and pottery making. Some inhabitants make pottery from local clay sources, a tradition which should be further examined for identifying possible indigenous continuities in its manufacturing process. And last but not least, one of the important continuities in the oral tradition is the story that seems to contain elements of the Great Serpent narrative.

In Boyá, the continuity of ancient medicinal culture is difficult to evaluate because the only active healer discontinued her practices a few years ago as her son destroyed her altar after converting to the Pentecostal faith. From the information gathered, it is clear that the majority of the recorded plants used for medicinal practices were native to the New World. Some of the native plants were also used to treat smallpox. The exotic species from Africa, and from Europe are applied to matters of spiritual protection, cleansing and improving one's fortune or love life. Besides the orange tree in which the Virgin manifested herself, also the guano, piñon and ceiba are considered to be mysterious and sacred, but only the latter has also a negative association. When collecting the plants prayers are directed to the Virgin of Remedies and Jesus, but also to the plant itself with the *misterio* that empowers it and gives it strength for healing. As previously mentioned, indigenous communities in the Guyanas also acknowledge the animating force of trees and plants (De Goeje 1943). Similar use of apazote, ceiba, or Jatropha spp. in Boyá has been earlier recorded also in Dominica.

Within this context, Mrs. González Moreno's self-identification as one of the indigenous descendants may be justified by her having the same last name as one of the indigenous families in the beginning of the 17th century (suggesting that knowledge may have passed through her family line from one generation to another), but can also be seen as a more general metaphor for her personal spiritual connection with the ancestral powers and knowledge of green remedies (which is not limited to Boyá).

Bánica

The rock-art in the Saint Francis cave suggests that the first human settlements in the Bánica region likely date from before the arrival of the Europeans. The circumstances and date of the foundation of Bánica are unclear. Although it is widely accepted that the town was founded by Canarian families, the hypothesis that it was one of the first villas founded by Velazquez cannot be ruled out. It is interesting in this respect that Moreau de Saint-Méry at the end of 18th century mentioned that Baniqueros continued to identify with their indigenous ancestry and that this historical link could be proven. Saint-Méry's account should be viewed in the context of several inhabitants having Canarian and West African roots. These diverse origins are also reflected in present-day religious life and medicinal cultures.

The celebration of Saint Francis follows the Roman Catholic tradition of patronal feasts. The selection of both Saint Francis and Virgen del Carmen, whose hagiographies are both related to mountains and caves, could be interpreted as a careful choice in conjunction with the characteristics of the local landscape. The selection of a cavern as a holy place might follow a tradition of the Islas Canarias, where one of the caverns was a dwelling place of the Virgen de la Candelaria, continuing the spiritual meaning it had among the Guanche prior to the religious conquest. The different elements of the feast of Saint Francis – such as processions, circumventing the calvario, ex-votos, vows expressed in humble attire identifying them with Saint Francis, and the general idea of pilgrimages to sacred places in order to recover health – are also known from Spain and other European countries.

Saint Francis' teachings about the human relation with nature, and about the sun, moon and animals being our relatives, would have been appealing to indigenous and African peoples. Similarly, the part of his hagiography, where this Saint resided in a cave on his journey to achieve divine power (or his divine power to heal), would have been recognizable for indigenous people. One of the miracles attributed to Saint Francis was that he cured a man by washing off his affliction with skin disease (leprosis). This miracle could remind indigenous people of similar acts of their own Divine healer, one of the Divine Twin brothers (Caracaracoli), Bákamo or other divine beings/zemí. The selection of the patronal Saint may also have been the consequence of an identification with the *lwa* Loko, who is the guardian of vegetation, who gives healing properties to plants and transmits botanical knowledge to healers – his representation in neighboring Haiti is precisely the image of Saint Francis.

Some Baniqueros and pilgrims perceived the ancestral agency at the cavern and certain parts of the river Aitibonito and some surrounding springs. The association of indigenous forefathers with earth and water can be explained as a consequence of the fusion of indigenous traditions with Kongo beliefs about Simbi and Dahomeyan beliefs about Toxosu. Names such as *Dorsú, marasás,* Simbi an dlo, Simbi Macaya, King of Earth, King of Water, together with the importance of Divine Twins, suggest connections to Ancient Dahomey and Kongo. These are also prominent regions of the first two hundred years of the Transatlantic Slave Trade to this part of the world. Other components of the celebration can be considered as African influences: the collection of white calcic powder from the wall of caverns, the manifestation of indigenous ancestors through the head of the devotees, or the importance of drumming (type of *palos*) to make the *lwa*s descend.

The present-day importance of the holy cavern and the river Aitibonito, and their link to indigenous predecessors may also derive from the narrative about the Great Serpent, which was known by at least three Baniqueros. This narrative has clear links with the sacred narrative of the Kalinago about the origin of plants for protection. As this narrative identifies a cavern and a river, these might have a symbolical value within the indigenous worldview. Inhabitants of the Bánica region may have been in contact with indigenous people of the Lesser Antilles in the 16th century because enslaving voyages to the Kalinago territories were organized during that period (Deive 1995). Yet, the local presence of indigenous people in that period remains to be confirmed. The Great Serpent narrative might also have arrived in the Greater Antilles through pre-colonial exchanges of ideas and peoples (see chapter 7).

The role of the indigenous ancestors in the Saint Francis celebration may reflect indigenous beliefs about the role of ancestors in health, and their association with the subaquatic and subterranean realm as the eternal world of invisible beings (De Goeje 1943). The present-day symbolism of subaquatic kingdoms as ancestral places, sources of regeneration and cures, has parallels among indigenous peoples on the South American mainland (see chapter 2). A further parallel is the conceptualization of rivers as loci where the art of healing comes from, or as symbolizing the road or journey to another sacred place (cave).

If the commemoration of the indigenous ancestors has any pre-colonial roots, it seems to survive until the present day because of its incorporation into the Catholic tradition of patronal celebrations. Regardless of the many unanswered questions that remain, it is clear that certain places have inspired peoples across cultural differences and through the centuries to reflect upon the mysterious workings of the universe.

Other locally mentioned components of medicinal cultures, like etiologies, have also parallels elsewere. For example the concept of bad air (mal aire) is well documented for medieval Spain, but may also involve indigenous ideas about negative influences of the wind deities (documented for Mexico). Soul loss because of the violation of a prohibition has parallels among indigenous peoples of South America and in Africa. In the particular context of the visit of the spring in La Descubierta, the idea of soul loss is closely related to features of African origin. The incarnation of an indigenous spirit, the experience of being devoured might be influenced by Haitian ideas about an attack by the *lwa* (compare also the predatory relations mentioned by de Castro 1998 or Århem 2001). The prohibition of cutting the jobo tree has similarities with cases documented in the Guyanas and Suriname, and teaches us about respecting the life (spirit) of the vegetation and securing the natural balance.

Other medicinal customs like the use of tobacco and maracas to invoke *lwas* are most likely derived from native Caribbean heritage (De Goeje 1943). Among the selection of sacred trees are Catholic and West African influences, but also possible American influences. The crops for offerings were native (corn, peanuts, beans), but also exotic (coffee), and strongly integrated in the local economy. The animals brought to Saint Francis were delivered like a live offering. Local plants are awakened and asked permission before their collection. The prayers aren't directed to a specific owner of the plant like in Regla de Ocha.

In contrast to the situation in Boyá, there are no individuals in Bánica who would identify as indigenous descendants. Some inhabitants, however, feel a strong spiritual link with the indigenous forefathers. The historical consciousness about the indigenous past is expressed in the belief that the church of the Patron Saint was built by indigenous people and in the recognition of their agency in the cavern, where together with Saint Francis, they occasionally manifest themselves. Like in Boyá, material reminders of ancestral presence are scattered throughout many households in Bánica, where we encounter hammocks, kitchen utensils (like calabash plates and spoons), culinary traditions like cassava making, and the use of *bixa*. Last but not least, indigenous words survive in some names of flora and fauna, toponyms, or technical vocabulary (*e.g.* related to cassava making) – a study of the local lexicon may yield more insights in the future.

Boca de Mana

Compared to Bánica and Boyá, we know even less details about the colonial history of the indigenous descendants in Boca de Mana. While indigenous descendants were living in Baní and Buenaventura in the early decades of the 16th century, their presence afterwards is unclear. If there were any in the later period, the provincial histories suggest that they were integrated into the population, where people of African and European ancestry and Creoles predominated. Yet, the possible contact between indigenous descendants and newcomers at the beginning of the 16th century invites us to reflect upon whether any elements of the indigenous worldview may have played a role in the motivations to select the cavern as a place for the celebration of Saint John's feast, as it contains an aspect of ancestral commemoration.

Again, any possible indigenous influences may have been integrated into or fused with the beliefs of African and European origins. The commemoration of the indigenous predecessors as part of Saint John's feast may have its origin in pre-colonial Caribbean ancestor cult as well as in West African respect for the deceased. According to Catholic models, caverns were miraculous and sacred places, and sometimes they were conceived as entrances to the purgatory.[410]

A first, most obvious factors in the selection of the cavern for ceremonial activities in the past and present may be the impact of such liminal places on the human body and psyche, as it is apt to create a sense of transcendence. The precise motives for the selection of Saint John as patron Saint for this location remain unclear, but most likely they stem from the spirituality of Mrs. Viviana de La Rosa, who came from Baní where Saint John is the patronal Saint. Whether the figure of Saint John was previously associated with any other spiritual entity, which in the meantime has been lost or changed, remains unclear. Like in the case of Saint Francis, the biography of Saint John the Baptist may have appealed to people of different religious backgrounds as a symbol of the healing and cleansing power of water, of both the destructive and the regenerative power of water, or simply of water as life force, of crucial importance for humans and other beings in this world.

The selection of the cavern as a place for the celebration of Saint John's feast might be rooted in pre-colonial worldview. There have been more components of the celebration in Mana that have parallels among different indigenous peoples of the Americas. Among these were: seeking health through pilgrimages to the sacred places such as

410 See for the European conception of caverns as entrances to the purgatory Walsh Pashulka (2015).

caverns, asking permission before entering sacred places, physical presence of divine beings at the celebration, the ritual use of tobacco, drums and chanting, food offerings, together with the general beliefs about caves as sacred liminal places where contact with divine powers and ancestors can be established.

The belief in the healing power of the water from the cavern, the accommodation of offerings for indigenous ancestors at places where water accumulates could all refer to pre-colonial beliefs about water as a dwelling place of deities and ancestors, as a symbol of the flow of time and for regeneration, or as a connecting element between the visible and invisible worlds. In Jamaica many caverns that in the past have been used in indigenous rituals are situated close to water sources or contain a water source. In some cases (*e.g.* in Mona) caverns were the only source of freshwater (Samson et al. 2017).

Another factor in the selection of this Saint may have been his feast day (24 June), which, as a counterpart to Christmas (24 December), is associated with the summer solstice, a phenomenon that, of course, is observed worldwide as a key element for distinguishing the seasons. A study by Jansen & Perez (2015) shows that such coincidences in time organization facilitated the process of fusion and synergy between Mesoamerican and European time perceptions and related symbolism in the Mexican context. Accordingly, the summer solstice may have been a point of mutual recognition and facilitated the process of transculturation of indigenous, European and African beliefs in Mana.

In Boca de Mana, like in other locations on the island, present-day agricultural activities are guided by the lunar calendar, integrated into the European liturgical calendar, which serves to organize Caribbean patronal celebrations and other ritual activities. The lunar calendar seems to have been in use in West Africa, Europe, and the Caribbean at the time of European colonization of the Caribbean. The celebration of Our Lady of Mercy falls two days after the September equinox. In Boca de Mana, however, this Virgen is celebrated on the same day as the Virgen of Charity in Cuba: on the 9th of September. Such anomalies merit further attention to identify their possible seasonal, astronomical or symbolic reasons.

Simultaneously, some of these features may have African roots. More details are necessary to establish this link. To illustrate this point: the idea about the physical presence of divine or spiritual entities (*lwas*) may come from different cultures. Its form, however, indicates African roots. Within the 21 division *lwas* incarnate in the head of the *caballos*. In addition, the spatial proximity of small points of other *lwas* (Barón del Cementerio, Santa Marta) to the place where the indigenous forefathers reside in the cavern indicate an African incorporation of indigenous ancestors into their own pantheon of deified deceased persons. The plentiful images of *lwas*, including their names like Tindjo (probably from Haitian Creole Simbi dlo), traditionally respected among the 21 Division, only further confirm that these places have been sacralized according to West African beliefs. This is only to be expected, given the history of Haina and Nigua, which were for a long period sugar plantation regions.

Spanish (Canarian) influences are obvious in the very figure of Saint John, a very popular Catholic Saint until the present. Other components of the feast such as messianic figures, the circumventing crosses, stones representing penance, the importance of the holy images, the use of water from sacred places as a blessing and for healing, all can be found also in European pilgrimages to sacred places.

Traditional foodways (including the preparation of cassava bread, the culinary use of guayiga, corn or bixa), with the use of basketry (from guano), and kitchen utensils (bateas, plates of calabash) indicate continuity of indigenous legacy in this sphere. Such material culture was common in rural areas in the 18th century and has been observed until today in different locations.

La Jaiba

In the location La Jaiba archaeological surveys (Ulloa Hung & Herrera Malatesta 2015) have established a long-term pre-colonial occupation. Elements of the indigenous culture in this region may have been transferred to the newcomers at the time of first colonial encounters and the subsequent *encomienda* period, and possibly even much later in the 17th century and the first half of the 18th century when some indigenous descendants (*mestizos*) were still living in Satiago region.

The name of the pool Tamare strongly reminds us of Tamare, one of the main personages from the Venezuelan narrative about the origin of Maracaibo (which emerged from a great flood caused by the great lord Zapara) (Peréz Escalarin 1996). While none of the inhabitants of La Jaiba mentioned this narrative, many suggested that Tamare was an indigenous name. This pool may have been named by the healer who was known to have used it three generations ago. As there is very little known about the biography of this healer we must take into account the possibility that was inspired by the Venezuelan narrative. It is difficult, however, to assess to what extent this narrative was known at the time or available as a published text in the Dominican Republic. It should be noted that indigenous people from the surroundings of the lake Maracaibo were also victims of the slave trading voyages that captured people and brought them to Hispaniola during the first half of 16th century.

The ingredients of the bath reveal also Old world origins (Europe, Asia), New World (especially those aromatic aromatic herbs resembling European ones), or those symbolic such as sunflower that imported to Europe from (North) America during the early 16th century.

The cavern La Iglesia and Poza Encantada at El Burén were places where Saints and *lwas* could manifest themselves and where they were invoked in cleansing ceremonies. During such ceremonies both Catholic saints (Virgen Altagracia, *San Gregorio/Santo Medico*), and *lwas* such as Ogún, Anaisa Pie, and Metreselí, but also the *indigenous misterios* were invoked. The selection of *lwas* that is invoked in here was dependent on the healers training, and problem that is in need of being solved. The mentioned lwas and saint invoked at El Burén are popular among the Catholic devotees and those of 21 Division.

Like in Bánica, indigenous ancestors were commemorated on occasions near pools and in caverns. The justification for consulting deified indigenous heroes is rooted in the historical consciousness of the religious specialist, who might not have this spiritual link but would recognize the ancestral agency at certain places, especially where tangible signs (archaeological findings) of ancestral dwellings have been encountered. Archaeological findings at the site El Burén suggest that these places had spiritual importance for the pre-colonial inhabitants. Further analysis of the objects via carbon dating may yield more historical depth and inform us about the successive phases of their functioning.

The present-day association of indigenous ancestors with the subaquatic domain as the place where they have originated from, and departed to after passing away has parallels in the origin narratives of various linguistically related peoples on the South-American mainland. These beliefs may also be reinforced by the observation that many of the archaeological sites are situated at riverbanks.

The idea of mutual caring between man and the invisible world often materializes in food; flower offerings are rather universal and found not only among different indigenous peoples of the Americas, but also in Africa. The long term importance of cavern in religious realm of indigenous ancestors in Caribbean is supported by residues of possible offerings which were found in Caribbean caverns and sinkholes.[411] These offerings often miss dating and were in general associated with indigenous ancestors and their cemís. However, dating of some of these sites is likely to disclose its long term use also throughout the colonial period including the power dynamics and how this could be reflected in these spaces. Some of these findings could evidence of religious change which was described already by Martyr d' Anghiera who suggested that the indigenous ancestors were bringing offerings (necklaces and ceramic vessels with food and water) to one of the first icons of the Virgin brought by Hojeda to Cuba. Perhaps future interdisciplinary studies will bring more insights into Martyr d' Anghiera's reflection upon that these acts were reminiscent of the ancestral cult to the cemís in Cuba.

Jiguaní

Like in the above-mentioned cases, indigenous people lived in the Jiguaní region long before the first Cuban colonial encounters. One of the first historical references to an indigenous community here comes from the 1530s and there is a later one from the 1680s, thirty years before the town was officially established by a founder of indigenous ancestry. Based on the subsequent demographic development, it is again likely that indigenous cultural elements have fused with European and West African heritage.

The foundation of Jiguaní implied also the selection of the patronal Saint for its church. Jiguaní is the only known Cuban town where reportedly an indigenous descendant engaged himself in that selection. Can we discern in the choice of Saint Paul a nexus between the religions of the Old and the New World? Did his fame as the Apostle of the Gentiles, as the person who first persecuted the Christians and later converted himself to Christianity play any role? Again, what Manuel de Rojas´, the founder of Jiguaní of indigenous origin, real motives were to choose Saint Paul is purely a matter of speculation.

The strong tradition of Cord Spiritism suggests that local spirituality has developed in its own unique way, in which the spiritual entities of the deceased are very much respected. Cord Spiritism is based on the European model of Kardec´ Spiritism but includes a local expression of collective prayers through the cord. Some popular knowledge sources such as Ecured indicated that the cord formed by the attendees of the spiritists´mass resembles the *areíto* (circular dance) described by the early chronicles.[412] In my view, the Cord Spiritism mass displays some features that are present in

411 For example guácima seed in La Aleta (Beeker et al. 2002).

412 See in Ecured part on Espiritismo de Cordón en Guisa retrieved from https://www.ecured.cu/Espiritismo_de_Cordón_en_Guisa [accessed on 31 April.2018].

Kaliña ceremonial dances.[413] However, such features can also be found in ceremonial dances that do not have any historical relationship with the Caribbean.

The surrounding landscapes – including elements such as San Pedruscón, sacred trees like the ceiba, anacagüita, symbolism of pumpkin, and medicinal flora – are other ways in which local spirituality is expressed. Different native and exotic plants serve for spiritual protection of houses and their inhabitants, as remedies against different diseases and are of great value in daily activities. Some uses of these medicinal plants (apazote, bixa, cotton, guyaba, jaboncillo, verveine, tabacco) in Jiguaní overlap with indigenous practices found on Dominica (See Table 9).

There are more traditions that display similarities with indigenous worldviews. Among these are the appearances of deceased persons in dreams, the act of transforming oneself in a dream into an animal, the narratives about *cagüeyros*. Like different female contributors from the Dominican Republic, Jiguaní women were prohibited in the past to enter the field when being in their period. Other possible continuities we find in the application of the lunar calendar to different activities such as: collecting cocoa clay for making a burén, painting house walls, or cleaning the floor, as well as selecting the wood for building a house, collecting plants, planting crops, and cutting hair.

Continuities are evident in foodways (cassava, great variety of corn dishes including ayaca, atol, chicha), material culture (basketry, pottery, *piraguas, jibe, batea, canoa, burén*), fishing with poisonous plants, using fishing traps like *nasas*, the use of *fotuto* (conch shell) for announcing messages, the use of *maracas* in healing and the use of loan-words (technical and biological terms) from indigenous languages.[414] All these examples, including those traditionally recognized as indigenous heritage (such as the basketry, pottery, and fishing) need more research in order verify the details and developments of these continuities, as all these may have been modified according to the skills and knowledge of other populations arriving in later colonial periods.

The memory of indigenous ancestors is supported by the active role of the local historian, family histories, the local museum, or publications about the foundation of the town. Rich oral traditions, including the use of songs to recall and transmit historical events, narratives about great *majás, jigües* and owls announcing death, and dogs bringing bad luck … all these may communicate some of the indigenous messages in modified versions today. Especially, the story about the boas seems to be a secularized version of the religiously charged narrative about the Great Serpent.

Barajagua and Managuaco

Indigenous people lived in small settlements like Barajagua before the Spanish conquest and their descendants continued to do so much later, through the 16th, the 17th, the

413 The circular cord that is formed by the attendees of the spiritual mass has reminded some investigators of the historical description of the pre-colonial ritual dance (*areíto*). Indeed, the collective experience of dancers, rhythmically leaning and bending, beating with their feet, stepping forward and backward, swinging their arms, connecting with other dancers while singing in chorus, among devotees of Espiritismo del Cordón may be compared to the ritual practice of, for example, Kaliña dancers.

414 Among these linguistic continuities are words like: ayaca, babiney, cativía, caguayo, cuchubey, naiboa, ñape, jiribía, macana, quaniquiqui, guacaica.

18th, until the second half of the 19th century. Indigenous offspring lived in both urban and rural settings of the region, and co-existed with indigenous people of non-local, and mixed backgrounds. Simultaneously, different lines of evidence suggest that the Catholic faith transformed but did not completely obliterate all continuities of indigenous culture (*e.g.* in mortuary treatment at Chorro de Maíta). In Barajagua and Managuaco indigenous descendants were exposed to institutional instruction in the Catholic faith, since the foundation of the first hermitage of the miraculous Virgin of Charity in the early the 17th century or since that of the hermitage in Managuaco at the end of the 17th century. The numerous registers of events of "spiritual conquest", such as the baptisms of indigenous people, suggest that these were not the first or last encounters with the Catholic Church. The fragmented picture of the past of these locations offer us points for reflection about the continuities within rural areas marked by a history of small-scale agriculture, animal husbandry and illicit trade.

Various authors have discussed the Virgen of Charity as an example of a Catholic image with echoes of indigenous beliefs (Trincado 1997; Oliver 2009; Ortiz 2012; Peña et al. 2014). These authors have suggested several points of coincidence as indications of syncretism. In my view, the co-existence of features from worldviews that resemble each other in their meaning or form is likely to facilitate a process of transculturation, which may be the reason why the image has been incorporated. We must keep in mind, however, that such co-existence does not automatically or necessarily lead to symbolic synergy and that what now may appear to us as coincidences was not necessarily perceived as such by the indigenous people in those days.

Different attributes may be used to find symbolic or religious parallels between the Virgen of Charity and pre-colonial deities: *e.g.* being protector (from a storm), being mother, being the Mother of a Divine Being, being associated with the moon (in her image), or having a link to water. Some parallels are part of her hagiography. The Virgin was found by three children, two of which had an indigenous background and one an African background. This suggests the on-going presence of indigenous people (probably acculturated into colonial society) in Barajagua at the time (like in some other places in this region in the same period). The selection of the waterfall with a small pool as the first place for building the small hermitage for the Virgen might indeed be rooted in (remains of) indigenous worldview.

As the plurality of meanings of the Saltadero for present inhabitants of Barajagua indicates, this place is sacred: multiple divine and spiritual beings dwell here. The present-day symbolic associations (the river being Ochún, or the bay being sacred because it is the place where Yemayá and Ochún meet) would suggest that the selection of the first hermitage might also have been inspirited by beliefs of African and Creole origin. Under the supervision of the indigenous boy the Virgin disappeared on various occasions and returned repeatedly with wet clothes to her altar at the Saltadero. The returning water symbolism could be a reference to a fusion of the values associated with water and with the Virgin.

The significance of the waterfall for the indigenous people in the 16th century remains an enigma. The contemporary meaning is closely related to the oral history of the settlement as being the first hermitage of the Virgen of Charity. As such it holds a great spiritual value until today, even though the official Mass is celebrated in the church. According to oral tradition, this place is also linked to Great Boa. Although the narratives of the Virgin and the Great Majá (who is here considered beneficial) are connected to the same place, these are by no means considered as related or fused: one (that of the serpent) is considered a legend while the other (that of the Virgin) is a truthful story about a divine being. According to one of the contributors, the Virgin may be a representation of Simbi, the Lady of Waters, whose description displays similarities with the Great Serpent narrative. Contemporary oral tradition about the Mother of Water, the Great Majá living in this place, also recognized as Simbi, supports the hypothesis about a synergy of worldviews.

For the inhabitants of Barajagua the Virgin is a caring mother during droughts, sickness, or other periods of crisis. This archetypical role of the Virgin/Mother seems to be appealing across different religions. Therefore, the image of the Catholic Virgin should neither be understood as a replacement of some "pagan idol", imposed by the missionaries, nor as a "mask" or "veneer" to cover the continued veneration of an indigenous deity under another name. This image, like so many similar cases, is the result of a complex interaction of religious ideas from different cultural backgrounds: syncretism in the sense that different ideas fused into a new unity, or rather symbolic synergy in the sense that one religious interpretation reinforces the other.[415] These cases allow us to contemplate universal values that humans have in common regardless of their religious background.

The present-day interpretation of the appearance of a Great Serpent as a sign of prohibition to contaminate this place, as retold by inhabitant from Managuaco, may again reflect the continuity of the indigenous teachings about the balance between people and natural forces, but at the same time may express modern ecological concerns or just a preoccupation or feeling of guilt on the part of the contributors. In a similar fashion, the connection that Mr. De Los Santos made between the narrative about the Great Serpent in Pedro Santana and the destructive power of Aitibonito during the cyclone David, reminds us of the dangerous character of the river in the Dominican Republic. Thus, the message included in the narrative about the Great Majás living in Cuban rivers, or the jigües, may have a didactic function even though its status has shifted from a sacred text, containing a symbolic narrative, to a "legend", "myth" or "folktale" because of the secularization of society and because of the marginalization of the beliefs of the colonized peoples.

The meaning of the Saltadero has to be situated in the context of beliefs of a community where also Spiritism plays an important role and where followers of Regla de Ocha are present. In this location too we find that ceiba and anacaüita have a spiritual meaning, while the ritual use of tobacco and maracas are important components of local medicinal practices.

In Managuaco, among the adherents of Cord Spritism the spiritual development, health recovery, and spiritual protection is sought through the contact with ancestors, which include groups of indigenous and African spiritual entities. On special occasions, people seek the advice of indigenous predecessors in the surrounding landscape, including a small cavern because indigenous people are thought to reside in these

415 See also the examples of the Virgin of Boyá, Saint Francis in Bánica, the Virgin icon by the cacique at Cueybá, the Virgin of Guadalupe venerated by indigenous descendants in Caney (and, of course, in Mexico).

places. Sitochi, Queen of Waters, provides guidance through dreams and in private expressions of spirituality, embedded in the local landscape. Other spiritual activities, such as ritual cleansing performed with the help of Oshun (the river flow), or asking permission before entering sacred places like Monte, have also parallels in Regla de Ocha. The Jiguaní, Barajagua and Managuaco rivers and especially their deep pools are dwellings of *jigües*, which adds yet another layer to the meaning of local landscapes with their long religious history.

We have seen the importance of the oral tradition about the Great Serpent as an emblematic identifier of indigenous cultural memory. This narrative, earlier registered only in the Lesser Antilles, Suriname and Guyanas, offers new insights into the religious and medicinal history of Cuba and the Dominican Republic. The continuity of this narrative until today in Boyá and Bánica is likely related to the long-term presence of indigenous descendants in these locations. The present-day continuity of this narrative in Managuaco, Barajagua and also Fray Benito might be the result of specific transmission by indigenous inhabitants (either local or from other locations), but may also be indicative of the wide distribution of narratives with this motif. Anyway it seems to reflect the presence of indigenous offspring in diverse locations in the East Cuba, including Holguín province, which is also suggested in the most recent studies of Valcárcel Rojas and Pérez Concepción (2014) and Válcarcel Rojas (2016). In addition, it suggests a pre-colonial or colonial exchange of ideas and peoples between Cuba and Hispaniola on the one side and other islands (specifically Dominica, where this narrative has been well documented) and the mainland on the other.

In Barajagua the aforementioned cultural practices deserve further analysis in order to assess any possible continuities in more depth. One of the practices found both in Barajagua and Managuaco is the collective healing, wherein various members of the groups enter into communication with the invisible world, so that the medium may transmit the diagnosis and the remedy to the patients. In these healing practices tobacco and maracas were important elements for making this contact with the other world. Also here we encounter more material continuities in basketry (including *jibe, catauro*), craftwork (*batea, coa, burén, jícara*, wood colorants), lunar calendar, alimentation (cassave, masamoro, tamales, pinol, corn wine, other dishes), the technique of fishing through poisoning the water with plants, and the presence of loanwords from indigenous languages in the local vocabulary (*e.g. macuyo, catibilla*). Another such element is the general notion of animated landscapes in which specific sacred trees are important, such as ciguaraya, cedro, piñon, and ceiba (in which the Virgin was hidden). Lastly, like in other locations, we can find narratives about *cagüeyros*, and the idea that owls announce death.

Continuities and heritage loss

The previous presentation of the data from islands might direct some readers to wonder whether continuities and loss of the indigenous heritage can be explained by different historical trajectories. As comparison was not the aim of this study I will briefly elaborate on a few ideas about the pool and caves.

The symbolism of pools as gateways to subaquatic kingdoms where the indigenous ancestors live is to be find in many Dominican locations where no prior historical records to the indigenous descedants are known. Its widespread character can be related to the moment when this information might be passed on by the indigenous people to other ancestors, the integration of its symbolism in 21 Division, the relevance of this information through the generations or just general preservation of oral traditions in rural regions of the Dominican Republic. The Great Serpent and boa narratives have been encountered in both regions of the study where indigenous descedants were living during the colonial period. Oral traditions evidently are not bound to one place but may travel freely across regions. When the knowledge from oral tradition has also other means of transfer (ritual offerings to the Virgen of Barajagua, offerings brought at Charco Tamare, or physical reminders of ancestral agency) its likelihood for preservation seems to increase.

The discussed celebrations in cavern setting illustrate that other factors important in this transfer are: the accessibility of the caverns (which was more restricted in different Cuban places), the organization relying on authorities which mantains influence in the place (Bibiana de la Rosa, the church in Bánica), its long-durée use and the cross-cultural liminal character of these places. Continuities and loss might be furthermore explained by the intra-and-inter-island heterogenous cultural and religious histories, including differences in industrialization, urbanization and literacy rate. These are related to general shifts in the means of transfer of cultural memory (in Assmann's term from oral to literal society to perhaps mass media oriented society). Differences have also been caused by historical contingencies.

When highlighting the continuities of the indigenous heritage one of the first striking features is the continuous perpetuation of stereotypes in the representation of indigenous and formally enslaved peoples.[416] The main sources perpetuating this negative representation are according to my observation the school textbooks. These are important formative sources shaping how individuals position themselves vis-à-vis the problematic past as well as the continuity and protection of their cultural heritage. The colonial discourse is enweaved in the oral tradition at large. An example is the narrative about naked "Indian women" combing their golden hair at the river pools and enchanting passersby with their beauty. This semi-erotic image of the deceitful beauty of indigenous women reoccurs in stories about *ciguapas*, mythical creatures, naked, with long hair, whose feet facing backward reveal their magical character. *Ciguapas*, depicted as creatures that lurk men into their dwellings in order to kill them, resemble the ancient narratives about Amazons, which according to Martyr D' Anghiera were living in Martinique (called Madanina or Matinino in the indigenous language). Whatever its origin – it could be based on indigenous beliefs and then influenced by Ashanti oral tradition, European imagination or Creole folklore – this narrative is clearly influenced by the colonial categories of race.

I would like to close this paragraph with stressing that the tendency of both colonial Christianity and western modernity to disqualify other worldviews in terms of "superstition" ("witchcraft", "magic", "primitive, pre-logic or mythical thinking" etc.) only impedes adequate understanding. In order to learn from each other, a respectful intercultural translation is necessary. Phenomena described as spiritual or religious by a

416 Some of the present-day stereotypes may also be influenced by images of the indigenous peoples from North America, because of their relatively prominent presence in Hollywood movies, popular literature etc.

traditional culture actually often are comparable with what is defined as psychological in a western vocabulary. Different cultural expressions to describe illness such as those of feeling of being consumed from inside should first be seen as comparable also how for example also European patients in time of spiritual crisis use symbols and metaphors to convey their experience and impact of the disease (see *e.g.* Harrington 2012). Often these metaphors are embedded in our terms *e.g.* cancer is derived from the Greek word for crab, cancers, like crabs, creeping along and eating away the flesh and the lives of patients (Harrington 2012). The soul loss or feeling of being possessed by the lwa could also be compared to the western idiom to emotional and psychological trauma and sometimes psychiatric illness, which would be addressed through psychotherapy, cognitive behavioral therapy etc (see *e.g.* Hanwela et al. 2012). Similarly, the references to ancestors, deities, spirits and misterios in Dominican and Cuban cultures, may for a non-local readers correspond to memories, awe with the natural beauty and fascination with hidden, extraordinary, beyond conception and understanding workings of the universe (creature feeling, mysterium in Otto's vocabulary, see Turner & MacKenzie 1977). When reading these accounts it is important to keep in mind that different cultures define etiologies and healing in their own specific vocabularies, but often seem to address the same aspects of human experience.

The interpretation of any Caribbean living heritage in terms of indigenous cultural continuity remains a highly speculative endeavor. The impact of the European invasion of the Caribbean was enormously detrimental to the indigenous communities. The illnesses, violent oppression and exploitation led to a nearly total erasure of peoples, languages and worldviews, including ancient medicinal knowledge. Fragmentation by conquest, colonization, and forced assimilation together with the profound demographic and cultural changes, have created an obstacle for deconstructing the colonial bias included in the written texts and for reconstructing the history, which often lacks detailed accounts, so that cultural continuity is difficult to pinpoint. This study has shown that the voyage seeking such continuities in the Greater Antilles is highly complex and without definitive conclusions. It does suggest, however, that one of the important vehicles of continuity is the ability of parties to identify key concepts and features that resemble (and make sense in) their own cultural universe. This co-occurrence leads to strategies to mask the preservation of own values, but also to create new symbolic synergies. Cultural memory has two aspects: it may serve to contrast the biased colonial archives, but it also carries in itself the imprints of five hundred years of cultural hegemony.

Systematic excavations of cavern settings may in the future verify the historical depth of the relation between the water element and the offerings. Certainly, many discontinuities and ruptures in the cultural memory are to be expected. Oblivion is part of the colonization of memory. But we find also a process of transculturation in which the creativity and the convictions of other populations rewrote (and contributed to) the meanings of these places – even so, these new layers of meaning are shaped in conjunction with the memory of the indigenous predecessors.

Healing landscapes within landscape theories

A final research question brings us to reflect upon how interpretations of healing landscapes can be situated within current landscape theories. The concept of healing landscape was used as an umbrella term to integrate approaches to human health from a holistic perspective. The term combined insights from previous botanical and anthropological studies (Cabrera 1954; Roig y Mesa 1974; Portorreal 2011; Germosén-Robineau 2005; Ososki 2004; Roersch 2016; Bolívar Aróstegui 1998; Quiroz-Moran 2009; Deive 1988; Tejeda Ortíz 2013; Brendbekken 1998), which addressed medicinal plants, some facets of religious views of landscape features, or present-day healing practices in the region.

When looking at all agents that at present have an active role in the health and wellbeing of the contributors, I have tried to highlight the relation between these different components of landscapes. The concept 'landscape' has been used to bridge the dichotomies between nature/culture and time/space, and to describe the relational character of the human wellbeing and health and the historical dwelling in the landscape. The health of people and their quality of life are inextricably linked to the health of their environment. Cultural practices both constitute and are constituted by the relationship between the physical aspects of the environment (physical, environmental factors, and man-made objects) and the immaterial cultural aspects (the spectator's view of landscapes, *e.g.* as a painting, involving specific perspectives, rituals, narratives, knowledge etc.).

The intimate relationship between people and the landscape they feel a part of has profound consequences for concepts of illness and health.[417] This awareness of the interdependency of humans and the environment is culturally expressed and codified. Some of these local examples were: the concept of illness (*e.g.* deriving from a violation of the prohibition of cutting trees), the doctrine of signatures in order to identify the cures, the divine manifestation in landscapes features involving Saints, *orishas*, *lwas*, and other divine beings. These cultural expressions of contiguity between the social and natural have been observed in teachings of diverse religious systems about the origin of the world, including how and why the invisible beings or forces can manifest themselves in the material surroundings. These teachings, including sacred narratives like *patakis*, or biographies of famous healers, establish links between the community and different landscape features, which are periodically reaffirmed during pilgrimages, communal celebrations or other ritual engagements with these places or landscape features.

Unlike the approach followed by several previous studies, the definition of healing landscapes used here includes also human agents. The inclusion of healers, plants, places, but also other landscape features like airs into one category serves to overcome the modern anthropocentric separations between nature and culture, between positivist notions of inanimate objects and animated subjects, divine beings and other manifestations of nature as a divine creation. These boundaries were trespassed by the very concept of illness, as well as by the ability of healers to incorporate the *lwas*, *orishas*, ancestors, and other normally invisible forces that may reside in landscape features.

---

417 In particular the concept of illness as being taken away, being devoured by the *lwa* or impacted by the evil eye, being bewitched, as a disturbance of the balance between hot and cold element, or a disturbance of community harmony caused by societal conflicts among persons or an imbalance occurring in the relationships among the divine realm, intermediaries and patients.

This study did not collect sufficient examples to also address the symbolism related to the animal world in a systematic manner. Various animals (about owls, cocuyos, dogs, snakes, and turtles) are told in narratives including the spiritual references. Given the fact that pre-colonial material culture is often decorated with zoomorphic and anthropo-zoomorphic motives the understanding of present-day animal symbolism may bring new insights into an analysis of their importance in spiritual realm.

The concept of landscape was only used to summarize and translate, not to replace local expressions. The examples used here to illustrate the mutual relation between people and environment, were selected by the author from the available information collected during her fieldwork and not by the contributors themselves. The focus on the healing landscape is one of various approaches to agency and life-giving sources in landscapes, highlighting the relevance of these for health and wellbeing.

Many of the aforementioned aspects were earlier described under the heading of sacred landscapes in for example the Mesoamerican context (Jansen & Pérez Jiménez 2008; Jansen & Pérez Jiménez 2016; Jiménez Osorio & Posselt Santoyo 2018; Aguilar Sanchez 2017). With the exception of the cavern of Saint Francis, which was consecrated by the local Church authorities, none of the previously discussed places, plants, or healers were said to be "holy" or "sacred". These terms have been used within institutionalized religion (as an aspect of colonial rule) for more than five hundred years in the region. This historical context affects their meaning and associations. For devotees these terms did not encompass all non-consecrated, intrinsic, invisible powers, which also might be potentially dangerous for health. The most common description of these aspects that devotees used in the Dominican Republic was: *"tiene un misterio"*.

The long-term process of discriminating and downgrading the religions of the historically marginalized populations has influenced the definition of their official status. As a consequence many places, reliquaries or acts performed by adherent of 21 division are still considered by many as clandestine witchcraft and perceived as incompatible with terms as "sacred" or "holy", which are generally used in the Catholic context. Consequently, some sacred narratives became secularized or downgraded to "myths" and "(folk)tales".[418]

Given the often-contested nature of practices whose religious underpinnings and values belonged to different religious groups, I opted first to focus on the therapeutic potential of the landscape in order to create more empathy and understanding among atheists, agnostics and members of other religious groups. At the end of the day, many of the aforementioned testimonies do not reflect the atheistic views, which are held by a large part of the Cuban and Dominican population. Different accounts exemplified the deep spiritual value attributed to aspects of nature and their importance to the

418 The exotic divine and normally invisible beings might have been incorporated within indigenous worldviews, which regardless of their differences shared several universal principles of human spirituality with the newcomers. The status of these divine beings might of course vary but their animating forces whether perceived as positive or negative fitted with the ideas about nature animated by *orishas*, ancestors, spirits, *jigües* living in the river pools situated in wider landscapes animated by *cagüeyros, bakás, cucuyos*, owls and other mysterious and metamorphic beings whose meaning in the meantime may have become subject to secularization. Some of these beings (again, like owls) were believed to be bad omen also in Spain, but might also relate to pre-colonial beliefs about these – possibly spiritual – beings (see Arrom 1989 on the symbolism of the owl).

health and wellbeing of individuals and communities. The faith in plant, remedy, and deity was an important element in the process of recovery.

History has taught us that faith can be beneficial for health and wellbeing, but that, when being manipulated in order to legitimize xenophobic and extremist ideas, and oppress other beliefs, it can also cause violence and death. The negative attitudes towards 21 Division in the Dominican Republic today display many similarities with the biases of colonialism, which demonized such practices in order to justify its own religious and political order.[419] Future studies from an emic perspective should however consider and address how to decolonize and enhance the emancipatory value of terms such as "sacred" and "holy". It is possible that other terms might be more apt to communicate the meanings they stand for in order to achieve more recognition for some of the historically marginalized beliefs.

The concept of healing landscapes was also based on the concept of illness, which is included in the general awareness of the interconnectivity and interdependence of humans and nature. By emphasizing the healing aspect, my attention is focused on the potential of some healing landscapes to improve physical, mental and communal wellbeing. When reading about the Caribbean healing landscapes, readers may also think of the worldwide beliefs in the salutary effects of the environment exemplified in curative waters, spas or sacred sites of religious pilgrimages in Europe itself, in Africa or elsewhere in the Americas. The concept of healing landscapes brings together various sacred places like Lourdes, Bath, sacred groves of Ghana or Benin, Ceiba in Cuba, but also extend the observation to other natural elements including winds (winti, Greek: airs), and those of other invisible beings dwelling in our landscape. The comparative aspect of this concept helps to recognize the common values and shared preoccupation with basic needs of our becoming, such as own health and a healthy environment.

The aim of this dissertation was not to prove the effectiveness of these practices. The evaluation of many holistic practices including the medicinal properties of plants, their dispensing practices, and dosage has yet to be carried out. While the value of plants has been traditionally well acknowledged – it has been the objective of centuries of colonial exploitation and bio-piracy, which continues to be a reoccurring problem across the world – the effectiveness of other healing traditions, such as ritual baths or visitation of healing places, merits attention as well and should be studied seriously rather than a priori discredited. The baths at the Sulphur spring La Zurza used at least for two hundred years indicate that ancestral knowledge can be beneficial both as a cure of physical ailments (Sulphur used for skin ailments) and as a factor promoting psychological wellbeing (a relaxing environment, the psychological sense of support because of having the divine on our site).

---

419 In the past, much criticism has been directed at traditional healing practices and its practitioners. This criticism seems to be rooted not only in religious bias, but also in the often unregulated nature of these practices, which sometimes enables individuals lacking proper knowledge of medicinal plants to lure vulnerable and ill people into paying for unwarranted therapies. The majority of healers interviewed during this study acknowledged the limits of their abilities and of the efficacy of their remedies. In the case that the client needed licensed medical attention that they were not able to offer, they suggested to the patient to seek medical aid at an appropriate institution. Many healers focused on mental care and health rather than on physical ailments.

As earlier studies about Africa, the Americas, and Europe indicate, several of these practices might indeed be valuable for improving mental and/or physical health of individuals and communities. Similarly, the consults with traditional healers should be also more appreciated for their therapeutic function in their psychological support of individuals and communities. The pilgrimages to various sites could be argued to have a positive effect by removing patients from daily stress and by creating a sustained concentration on the ethical principles of the community and the comfort of ancestral religious faith. As Post et al. (2014) suggested for the pilgrimage to the South African Motouleng cave, *"the movement from station to station under the guidance of a spiritual leader constitutes a profound spiritual experience for the pilgrim and a transformed sense of healing and reunion with culture and belief"*. In addition, other authors like Talbot (2002) have emphasized the potential of pilgrimage for recovery from physical and mental ailments.

Many rituals aiming to improve wellbeing actually created a sense of security, self-esteem, control over social difficulties for the contributors to this study, who often are living in (extreme) poverty, with lack of access to medical care, low literacy rates (among the elderly), unemployment, violence (especially high rates of domestic violence against women), epidemics (*zika, chikungunya*), continuous environmental degradation, and natural disasters. In particular, people depending economically on their agricultural work have been among the most vulnerable to the effects of climatic change. This became apparent as a series of hurricanes (Irma, María, and Mathew), extensive droughts, floods, and coastal erosion hit the visited region on numerous occasions during the time of the study. Although the perceived social differences were much less pronounced in the affected Cuban communities, the local economy, agricultural production, and health care have been hugely disadvantaged by the embargo and state of Cuban economy. The lack of certain medical drugs on the Cuban market provoked governmental attempts to integrate holistic medicine into conventional medicine.[420]

My approach to healing landscapes from a cultural memory perspective was first motivated by the observation of the role of ancestors in the health of the descendants in diasporic communities. Ancestral commemoration and the participation in communal celebrations have potential for improving mental health by providing people with a sense of belonging to a community and place. The sense of belonging is considered in social psychology as a fundamental human need, a powerful factor that influences people's health (Baumeister & Leary 1995; Walton & Cohen 2011). In connection with this view, communal celebrations are meaningful for creating social cohesion and a sense of stability, which builds upon the balance, reciprocity and harmony that is required among the visible and invisible beings.

Approaching landscapes from a cultural memory perspective allowed us also to address their role as a mnemonic tool. Being seemingly constant features, landscapes are unifying factors for the different population groups that came to these Caribbean islands. Despite profound material modifications, the Caribbean landscapes were and are a rather stable background and matrix for human activities, lifeways, and worldviews. Landscapes are an integral part of a people's becoming and cultural memory,

420 In 2017 there has been again a drug shortage. In cities like Holguin and Santiago one can find green pharmacies, which sell some remedies from plants such as anamú, romerillo, tilo, garlic, onion etc.

incorporating continuities, multi-directional changes related to historical process and events, connecting the contemporary inhabitants to the past as well as to the visible and invisible worlds. The cultural memory perspective allows us also to address the connections of the present-day dwellers in these landscapes with their ancestors and with the heritage that they have left behind.

Perhaps one of the most important aspects of healing landscapes in the Caribbean was their capacity to contrast colonization, including long-term dehumanization, displacement, disintegration, and violent oppression. Healing landscapes encoded the cultural memory, which speaks about ancestral resilience, creativity, cohesion, and ways to heal as individuals but also as a society. Healing landscapes are also testimonies of how communities preserved some of their ancestral beliefs and wisdoms, created new and rich religious ideas and practices, and cultivated healing traditions emplaced in new loci. The history of these landscapes also reveals how diasporic communities appropriated new landscapes, transformed them into places of habitus, ceremonies, and pilgrimages, thus giving them new layers of significance, often in relation to the history of their forefathers. The rich religious and literary symbolism that animates the Cuban and Dominican landscapes together with multiple meanings of certain places, such as Barajagua, show that, in spite of a constant creation of differences by the colonial authorities, creole populations shared important common values and were able to create new communities in which different meanings could coexist. Finally, healing landscapes manifestly contradict the still popular simplified notions about the Caribbean communities as being without profound roots in their landscapes, therefore lacking any spiritual relation with their surroundings. From this perspective, landscapes are not sources of alienation; on the contrary, landscapes have been connecting contemporary inhabitants with their ancestors, and thus help us to remember our common past.

The creativity, resilience, and strength that local communities have developed to overcome these hardships in both areas do not erase the suffering or underestimate ongoing social conflicts. There is much room for improvement of wellbeing and the health of communities and individuals in this region. In spite of the world-fame of Cuban medical care, Cubans suffer from large shortages of pharmaceutical medicines. The rich botanical knowledge and medicinal cultures should be cherished, and could serve as an inspiration for constructing more equal and sustainable futures with collective knowledge empowering these communities. One of the steps towards this development is to comprehend the value of present-day healing landscapes, because these have potential of to be cultural codification of insights that emerge from long, intimate interactions with the environment. Joint interdisciplinary efforts in cooperation with local institutions, while respecting local epistemologies, are a key approach for enhancing the wellbeing and health of the communities.[421]

421 Among these institutions are for example: Experimental Station of Medicinal Plants «Dr. Roig» – Cuba, Botanical Garden Dr. Rafael Moscoso, UASD, Lab. Central de Farmacología, Facultad de Ciencias Médicas de la Habana, and Caribbean collaborative efforts like TRAMIL.

Future directions of research

This study elaborated several aspects of medicinal cultures and their past. The focus on indigenous legacies should not distract the reader from the rich heritage of multiple origins in present-day medicinal cultures of both islands. As the biography of Onesimus, the enslaved individual who introduced the practice of inoculation (against smallpox) from Africa to North America, illustrates, important medical discoveries are also owed to the knowledge of those most marginalized.

As healing traditions still constitute an important part of daily life and are often combined with the modern medicine prescribed by physicians, more research should be conducted in order to establish the phytochemical and pharmacological evaluation of herbal medicine, their dispensing practices, dosage and effect in combination with other herbs or medicines. Such research should also advocate and promote the concrete recognition of the intellectual property rights of the communities involved. In a similar way, the future approaches of medicinal histories in the Caribbean will benefit from interdisciplinary approaches integrating paleopharmacological, phytochemistry, ethnographic, historic, and archeological data.

This study once more highlights the richness of the reservoir of historical information enmeshed in oral traditions. The works on oral histories of Maroon communities in other parts of the Caribbean, like Suriname (Price 1983) or Jamaica (Tanna 1993) demonstrate their potential as sources of historical data. Previous publications by Lydia Cabrera, Barnet, and Feijoó are examples of seminal works that illustrate the diverse genres of rich oral tradition in the Cuban context.[422] As Vansina (1987) proposed, not all information of oral tradition can be seen as a reliable source for history, but it has rather to be understood for what it is, a unique source of evidence upon which the historical process has left its traces. Price (1983) reflected upon the value of special forms of oral tradition among the Maroons for their ability to preserve and transmit historical knowledge. The significance of oral tradition has been recognized in the research of Caribbean history, though the losses have been enormous (Alleyne 1999). From a memory perspective, oral traditions are to be considered as continuous reflections upon the past, and they indicate what past is believed to be relevant in the present. A future study on landscape biography would benefit from research on toponyms like that of Higman (2009), or Granberry and Vescelius (2004), or the work of linguists such as Valdés Bernal (1991).

The spatial character of remembering, combined with various cognitions of time, is an important avenue to explore for future heritage studies and for policies aiming at the preservation of tangible and intangible heritage. Different examples of memory sites and healing landscapes may guide scholars, readers and the national authorities to appreciate their universal value as cultural heritage and their importance for local histories and identities. These examples, together with recognized heritage sites such as Viñales Valley, First Coffee Plantations in Southeast Cuba, Jamaican Blue and John Crow Mountains, show the richness and worldwide importance of non-monumental mixed heritage sites in the Caribbean. Before any nominations of these places on the UNESCO's World Heritage List, it should be carefully assessed what the impact of

422 For more valuable sources see http://docsouth.unc.edu/neh/manzano/manzano.html#p102.

such a registration will be on ongoing cultural practices and on their value for the wellbeing and health of the carriers of these traditions.

Future investigation of intangible cultural heritage should pay attention to divergent demands among the local people with regard to the publication of certain information. Some aspects of their worldview may be profoundly religious, therefore secret and prohibited to publish. As my colleague, Adrian Gomes (2016) explained in another context, the publication of such secret knowledge in violation of this principle amounts to a destructive attack on the indigenous culture and the indigenous community:

"Knowledge pertaining to spiritual healing which is linked to sacred sites does not belong to the individual alone, but also to the community. By respecting the sites, we protect and control them. Thus, any developmental project for the community will not function well without the full participation of the community. Researchers should take note of this. Also, if development of the land must take place, resource management is crucial so that future generations can benefit from the resources including the sacred sites... The narratives associated with the water bodies and other sacred sites are not secret...Publication of certain information about Wapishana knowledge is not allowed by the Wapishana people, though I am not sure if this has been adhered to in the past by "western" researchers. Over a decade ago, a "western" researcher gained the confidence of our villagers and was shown parts of the forest our villagers traversed. He was given information on the locations of some valued plants, including medicinal ones."

This Wapishana scholar continues to explain: *"At the request of the people, he was not allowed to published where exactly they are found...Also, the publication of spiritual prayers of the Wapishana in Guyana is prohibited. For this reason I was taken aback when I saw some Wapishana spiritual prayers alongside some Wapishana and Portuguese Christian prayers/hymns in a booklet, published in Brazil. It could be that some Wapishanas over there, for one reason or another, divulged information on Wapishana spiritual prayers and gave permission to the missionaries to publish them in the booklet. By the Wapishana standards I know, this should not have happened. Based on our belief that our spiritual prayers are passed on orally, I would go as far to say that the spiritual prayers in Wapishana may not be effective if one attempts to apply them from the written material. I am not sure if our Wapishana leaders together with our marunao healers would ever allow the publication of our spiritual prayers. On the Guyana side, such publication by Wapishana themselves and non-Wapishanas is strictly prohibited."*

We share the view that restrictions for disclosure of religious and medicinal knowledge should be respected when writing about 21 Division, Regla de Ocha, Palo de Monte and where applicable.

Therefore, future research in the Caribbean and Circum-Caribbean areas should take into account the principles and standards of the U.N. Declaration on the Rights of Indigenous Peoples (2007), which demands the full respect for the intellectual property rights of the communities and for their right to determine, co-design and co-direct research as part of giving their Free, Prior and Informed Consent. Although these guidelines were developed for the Indigenous Peoples as instruments to protect their rights, which have been violated on a large scale, it is recommendable to further assess their relevance as standards in the case of all historically marginalized populations, also those in the Greater Antilles, which might not be direct descendants of the original inhabitants with preserved languages but are (also) descendants of enslaved and diasporic populations. These standards were designed to secure the rights of those who share the experience of colonialism in the past and suffer equally its consequences in the presence.

This study set out to examine in what way the knowledge of the present-day societies can provide us better insights into the pre-colonial and colonial past and vice versa. The concept of memory offers us an interdisciplinary bridge over the barriers that separate the present from the past. Throughout the study I have considered the voices of contributors as crucial epistemological factors that underpin the relevance of the past in the present with a potential to decolonize contemporary ideas about the past. They show the room for resistance, the coping mechanism with those colonial legacies, and, most importantly, they offer an emic view of the past. This approach was by no means meant to exploit the present-day medicinal cultures, or to make contemporary societies a mere object of study with the aim of creating some grand theory about cultural developments. This reflection does, however, bring us closer to an understanding of the impact of the colonial past on the indigenous inhabitants, the present-day population, and the large cultural transformations that were triggered by the European invasion. Knowledge of the interests of present-day communities and of the context in which the past is being (re-) interpreted is a necessary premise for making studies of history and heritage socially relevant.

From a holistic perspective healing in societies with colonial history lies first and foremost in overcoming the social division created by colonialism and by its justification through pretentions of racial and religious superiority. From the same perspective our communal wellbeing is only possible if we are going to reconstruct relations with each other and our ancestors in a caring and respective way. This implies improving social justice and the participation of historically marginalized segments of the population, as well as doing away with the stereotypes and stigmas that emerge from (neo)colonial relations. It is an essential condition to recognize all human rights including those of freedom of belief.

Remedies in the Caribbean landscape can also be envisioned as rhizome in which the connection between self and other transforms into a hybrid force that challenges the colonial rule. The Cuban and Dominican rivers are pathways to the re-membering of *our common* ancestors, acknowledging them as an important source of inspiration, wisdom, and moral guidance in order to reinforce our collective wellbeing. The traumatic colonial history, which is haunting the consciousness and affecting the wellbeing of many people (Fanon 1952), does not disappear if suppressed through cultural amnesia; rather as Morales (2001) has stated, active remembering may produce remedies for the present and future generations.

Bibliography

Acevedo-Rodríguez, P. & T. Strong, M. 2012. *The Catalogue of Seed Plants of West Indies.* Washington: Smithonian Institution Scholarly Press.

Ackerknecht, E. H. 1978. Primitive Surgery. In M. H. Logan & E. E. Hunt (eds), *Health and the Human Condition: Perspectives on Medical Anthropology.* North Scituate: Duxbury.

Aguilar Sanchez, O. 2017. El Paisaje Sagrado de Santo Tomás Ocotepec. In M. May Castillo & A. Strecker (eds), *Heritage and Rights of Indigenous Peoples.* Leiden: Leiden University Press.

Albelo Ginnart, R., Valdés López, M., Gallo González, G. Molina Martínez, M. 2011. *Historia de Cuba. Quinto Grado.* La Habana: Editorial Pueblo y Educación.

Alcocer, L.J. 1942 [1650]. *Relación sumaria del estado presente de la Isla Española en las lndias Occidentales y cosas notables que hay en ella, de sus frutos y de algunos sucesos que han acontecido en ella, del Arzobispado de la ciudad de Santo Domingo de la dicha Isla y vidas de sus Arzobispos hasta el año de 1650. BAGN 5,* 20-21.

Alderete, W. E. 1999. *The Health of Indigenous Peoples: Sustainable Development and Healthy Environments.* Geneva: WHO.

Alexander VI 1493. *Demarcation Bull Granting Spain Possession of Lands Discovered of Pope Alexander VI.* Reproduced with English translation in The Gilder Lehrman Collection. Retrieved from *www.gilderlehrman.org.*

Alexiades, M. 1996. Collecting Ethnobotanical Data: An Introduction to Basic Concepts and Techniques. In M. Alexiades (ed.), *Selected Guidelines for Ethnobotanical Research: A Field Manual.* Bronx: New York Botanical Garden Press.

Allaire, L. 2013. Ethnohistory of the Caribs. In W. F. Keegan, C. L. Hofman & R. Rodríguez Ramos (eds), *The Oxford handbook of Caribbean archaeology.* Oxford: Oxford University Press.

Alleyne, M. C. 1999. Linguistics and the oral tradition. In B. W. Higman (ed.), *General History of the Caribbean. Methodology and Historiography of the Caribbean* (Vol. VI). London and Oxford: UNESCO Publishing.

Amin, S. & Moore, R. 1989. *Eurocentrism.* London: New York: Zed Books, Monthly Review Press.

Andel, van, T. & Ruysschaert, S. 2011. *Medicinale en rituele planten van Suriname.* Amsterdam: KIT.

Andel, van, T. 2013. What makes a plant magical? Symbolism and sacred herbs in Afro-Surinamese winti rituals. In R. Voeks & J. Rashford (eds), *African ethnobotany in the Americas* (pp. 247-284). New York, London: Springer.

Andel, van, T. 2015. African names for American plants: Slaves brought plant knowledge with them that remains in communities of African descent in the New World. *American Scientist, 103*(4), 268-275.

Andel, van, T., Ruysschaert, S., Boven, K. & Daly, L. 2015. The use of Amerindian charm plants in the Guianas. *Journal of Ethnobiology and Ethnomedicine, 11*(1).

Anderson-Cordova, K. F. 1990. *Hispaniola and Puerto Rico: Indian Acculturation and Heterogeneity 1492-1550*. Ph.D. dissertation, Yale University. Ann Arbor: University Microfilms.

Anderson-Córdova, K. F. 2017. *Surviving Spanish Conquest: Indian Fight, Flight, and Cultural Transformation in Hispaniola and Puerto Rico*. Tuscaloosa: University of Alabama Press.

Andújar Persinal, C. 2013. *Diálogos Cruzados con La Dominicanidad.* Santo Domingo: Editora de UASD.

Angel Bello, S. T., Delgado Ceballos, L., Álvarez de La Paz, O. & Eguiguren, T. 2002. Estudio arqueológico del sitio Birama. Trinidad Sancti Spíritus. *El Caribe Arqueológico 6*, 56-70.

Anwana, E. D., Cheke, R. A., Martin, A. M., Obireke, L., Asei, M., Otufu, P. & Otobotekere, D. 2010. The Crocodile is our Brother: Sacred Lakes of the Niger Delta, Implications for Conservation Management. In B. Verschuuren, R. Wild, J. McNeely & G. Oviedo (eds), *Sacred Natural Sites Conserving Nature and Culture.* London/Washington: Earthscan.

Arens, W. 1979. *The Man -Eating Myth. Anthropology & Anthropophagy.* New York: Oxford Unversity Press.

Århem, K. 1996. The Cosmic food web. Human-nature relatedness in the Northwest Amazon. In P. Descola & G. Pálsson (eds), *Nature and Society. Anthropological Perspectives*. London and New York: Routledge.

Århem, K. 2001. Ecocosmología y chamanismo en el Amazonas: variaciones sobre un tema. *Revista Colombiana de Antropología, 37*, 268-288.

Århem, K. 2016. Southeast Asian animism: a dialogue with Amerindian perspectivism. In K. Århem & G. Sprenger (eds), *Animism in Southeast Asia*. London: Routledge.

Arranz, L. 1991. *Repartimientos y encomiendas en la Isla Española: el repartimiento de Albuquerque de 1514.* Madrid: Editora Fundación García Arévalo.

Arrom, J. 1975. *Mitología y artes prehispánicas de las Antillas (Arqueología).* México: Siglo Veintiuno Editores.

Arrom, J. 1989. *Mitología y artes prehispánicas de las Antillas (2nd Edit.).* México: Siglo XXI.

Artist, R. 2016. *Indiaans Verhaal. In de schaduw van twee beschavingen*. Zuthpen: Walburg Press.

Assmann, J. 2011. *Cultural Memory and Early Civilization: Writing, Remembrance, and Political Imagination*. Cambridge: Cambridge University Press.

Atiles Bidó, J. G. 2011. *Panorama histórico de los estudios del arte rupestre en República Dominicana.* Retrieved from http://www.rupestreweb.info/panorama.html.

Atkinson, L. 2010. Taíno Influence of Jamaican Folk Traditions. Retrieved from http://www.jnht.com/download/influence.pdf.

Azam, A. (2016, October 17). Haitians, Battered by Hurricane, Huddle in Caves: 'This Is the Only Shelter We Have', Retrieved from http://www.nytimes.com/2016/10/18/world/americas/haiti-hurricane-matthew-caves.html?_r=0.

Bachiller y Morales, A. 1881. *Tipos y costumbre de la isla Cuba. Por los mejores autores de este genero.* Habana: Avisador Comercial.

Backer, L. 2008. From Hatuey to Che: Indigenous Cuba without Indians and the U.N. Declaration on the Rights of Indigenous Peoples. *American Indian Law Review, 33*(1), 201-238. doi:10.2307/20455380

Baďura, B. 2013. *Páginas de la historia del pueblo del Caney.* Praga: Karolinum.

Barandián, D. 2011. *Los Hijos de La Luna. Monografía Antropológica sobre los Indios Sanemá-Yanoama. Kindley Edition.*

Barcia Zequeira, M. C. 2004. *El tema negro en la historiografía cubana del siglo XX. Del Caribe (44),* 102-110.

Barnes, J., Cleveland, D., Coombe, R., Descola, P., Hiatt, L., Jackson, J. & Brown, M. 1998. Can culture be copyrighted? *Current anthropology, 39*(2), 193-222.

Barnet, M. 2012. *Biografía de un cimarrón.* La Habana: Editorial Letras Cubanas.

Barreiro, J. 2001. *Panchito. Cacique de la montaña.* Santiago de Cuba: Ediciones Catedral.

Barreiro, J. 2002. Words of a Cacique: Panchito Ramirez (Cuba). *Biodiversity, 3*(3), 6-7.

Barreiro, J. 2006. Taíno Survivals: Cacique Panchito, Caridad de los Indios, Cuba. In M. C. Forte (ed.), *Indigenous resurgence in the contemporary Caribbean: Amerindian survival and revival.* New York, NY: Peter Lang.

Barrow, L. 1992. Family land and development in St. Lucia. Cave Hill, Barbados: Institute for Social and Economic Research, University of the West Indies.

Bascom, J. W. 1984. *The Yoruba of Southwestern Nigeria.* Illinois: Waveland Press.

Bascom, W. R. 1942. Ifa Divination: Comments On The Paper By J. D. Clarke. *Journal Of The Royal Anthropological Institute Of Great Britain And Ireland, Man* (69) 235-56, 41-43. Retrieved from http://ehrafworldcultures.yale.edu/document?id=ff62-024.

Bastide, R. 2011. From The African Religions of Brazil: Toward a Sociology of the Interpenetration of Civilizations. In J.K. Olick & L.D. Vinitzky-Seroussi (eds), *The Collective Memory Reader.* Oxford: Oxford University Press.

Baumeister, R. F. & Leary, M. R. 1995. The Need to Belong: Desire for Interpersonal Attachments as a Fundamental Human Motivation. *Psychological Bulletin, 117*(3), 497-529.

Beauvoir-Dominique, R. 2009. *The rock images of Haiti: A living heritage.* In M. Hayward, L. G. Atkinson & M. A. Cinquino (eds), *Rock Art of the Caribbean.* Tuscaloosa: The University of Alabama Press.

Beauvoir-Dominique, R 2008. Tradities in de vormgeving van vodou-Makaya in het Haïtiaans erfgood. In J. Hainard, P. Mathez & O. Schinz (eds), *Vodou kunst en mystiek uit Haïti.* Amsterdam: KIT.

Beeker, C. D., Conrad, G. W. & Foster, J. W. 2002. Taíno use of flooded caverns in the East National Park region, *Dominican Republic Journal of Caribbean Archaeology, 3,* 1-26.

Bender, B. 2002. Time and landscape. *Current Anthropology, 43*, 103-S112.
Benzo de Ferrer, V. 2005. *La Real Villa de Bánica.* Santo Domingo: Alcázar de Colón.
Berman, M., Gnivecki, P. & Pateman, M. 2013. The Bahama Archipelago. In W. F. Keegan, C.L. Hofman, R. Rodríguez Ramos (eds), *The Oxford handbook of Caribbean archaeology*. Oxford: Oxford University Press.
Bhabba, H. K. 1994. *The Location of Culture.* London: Routledge.
Bianchi, C. C. 1988. *Gubida Illness And Religious Ritual Among The Garifuna Of Santa Fe, Honduras: An Ethnopsychiatric Analysis*. Ann Arbor, Michigan: University Microfilms International.
Bisnauth, D. 1996. *A history of religions in the Caribbean.* Kingston: Kingston Publishers.
Blanco Díaz, A. (ed.) 2009. *Escritos Históricos* Santo Domingo: Búho.
Bolívar Aróstegui, N. 1994. *Los Orishas en Cuba.* La Habana: PM Ediciones.
Bolívar Aróstegui, N., González Díaz de Villegas, C., Del Río Bolívar, N. 1998. *Ta Makuende Yaya y Las Reglas de Palo Monte. Mayonbe, Brillumba, Kimbisa y Shamalongo*. Habana: Instituto Cubano Del Libro Editorial José Martí.
Bollig, M. & Bubenzer, O. (eds) 2009. *African Landscapes: Interdisciplinary Approaches.* New York: Springer.
Boomert, A. 2000. *Trinidad, Tobago and the Lower Orinoco Interaction Sphere: an / ethnohistorical study*. Leiden: University Leiden.
Bourdieu, P. 1990. *The Logic of Practice.* Cambridge: Polity Press.
Bouton, J., McKusick, M. B. & Verin, P. 1640. Concerning The Savages Called Caribs. *Account Of The Establishment Of The French In The Year 1635 On The Island Of Martinique*. A Paris: Chez S. Cramoisy. Retrieved from http://ehrafworldcultures.yale.edu/document?id=st13-003.
Boven, K. 1996. Sukutumulu: initiatieproeven bij de Wayana. *Oso, 15*(1), 18-29.
Boven, K. 2006. *Overleven in een grensgebied: veranderingsprocessen bij de Wayana in Suriname en Frans Guyana. PhD thesis*. Utrecht University: Netherlands.
Brathwaite, E. 1971. The Development of Creole Society in Jamaica 1770- 1820. Oxford: Clarendon Press.
Brea López, R. 1998. Huella hispánica en fiestas de Cuba. *Del Caribe, 28*, 65-71.
Brendbekken, M. 1998. *Hablando con la Mata.* Santo Domingo: Instituto de Medicina Dominicana.
Breton, R. 2015 [1665]. *Dictionnaire caraïbe-francais.* (D. Troiani transl). El caribe insular del siglo XVII. Tratado sobre la lengua y la cultura de los Callínago. Muenchen: LINCOM.
Breton, R., la Paix, A. de & Turner, T. 1929. Account Of The Island Of Guadaloupe. *Historie Coloniale*. Paris: Librairie GTnTrale et Internationale. Retrieved://ehrafworldcultures.yale.edu/document?id=st13-001.
Breukel, T. 2013. *Threepointers on Trial: A biographical study of Amerindian ritual artefacts from the pre-Columbian Caribbean*. Research Master Thesis.
Bry, de, Th. 1979 [16th century]. *De Ontdekking Van De Nieuwe Wereld. Grand Voyages.* Amsterdam: Van Hoeve.
Bry, Theodor de, 1528-1598, engraver (1594). *The religious ceremony of the Indians.* Theodor de Bry's America. Special Collections, University of Houston Libraries. Retrieved from https://digital.lib.uh.edu/collection/p15195coll39/item/74.

Cabrera, L. 1993 [1953]. *El Monte.* Havana: Letras Cubanas.
Cabrera, L. 2004 [1940]. *Afro-Cuban Tales.* Lincoln and London: University of Nebraska Press.
Cain, A. 2015. Slavery and Memory in the Netherlands: Who Needs Commemoration? *Journal of African Diaspora Archaeology and Heritage, 4*(3), 227-242.
Callejas Opisso, S. 2010. Capítulo 1. In J. A. Rodríguez Ben et al. (eds), *Historia de Cuba. Nivel Medio Superior.* La Habana: Editorial Pueblo y Educación.
Campbell, A. T. 1982. *Themes for translating: An account of the Wayapi Indians of Amapa, Northern Brazil.* UK: University of Oxford.
Carney, J. A. 2003. African Traditional Plant Knowledge In the Circum-Caribbean Region. *Journal of Ethnobiology 23*(2): 167-185.
Caro Baroja, J. 2003. *The witches and their world.* Madrid: Alianza Editorial.
Cassá, R. 1999. Historiography of the Dominican Republic. In B. W. Higman (ed.), *General History of the Caribbean. Methodology and Historiography of the Caribbean* (Vol. VI). London and Oxford: UNESCO Publishing.
Castañega, De, M. 1997 [1529]. *Tratado de las supersticiones y hechicerías.* Argentina: Universidad de Buenos Aires.
Castro, E. & Howard, C. 1992. *From the enemy's point of view: Humanity and divinity in an Amazonian society.* Chicago: University of Chicago Press.
Césaire, A. 1972 [1955]. *Discourse on Colonialism.* New York and London: Monthly Review Press.
Chanca, D. 1494 [2011]. The Report of Diego Chanca on Columbu´s Second Voyage to America. In N. L. Whitehead (ed.), *Of Cannibals and Kings. Primal Anthropology in Americas.* Pennsylvania State University: University Press.
Charmaz, K. 2001. Grounded Theory: Methodology and Theory Construction. In *International Encyclopedia of Social & Behavioral Sciences*, 6396-6399.
Chateusalins, de, B. 1854. *El Vademecum de los Hacendados Cubanos ó Guia Práctica Para Curar La Parte de las Enfermedades.* Habana: Imprenta de Manuel Soler.
Chatterjee, H., Vreeland, S. & Noble, G. 2009. Museopathy: Exploring the Healing Potential of Handling Museum Objects. *Museum and Society, 7*(3), 164-177.
Chevalier, J. M. & Sánchez Bain, A. 2003. *The Hot and the Cold: Ills of Humans and Maize in Native Mexico.* Toronto: Univ. Toronto Press.
Chiarelli, B. & Luna Calderón, F. 1987. The excavations of La Isabela, the first European city of the New World. *Int. J. Anthropol. 2* (3), 199-210.
Chouin, G. 2002. Sacred Groves in History: Pathways to the Social Shaping of Forest Landscapes in Coastal Ghana. *IDS Bulletin 33*(1).
Christian, W. A. 1989. *Local Religion in sixteenth-century Spain.* USA: Princeton University Press.
CITMA, 2007. Catálogo de las Cavernas Arqueológicas de la Provincia de Granma. Not Published.
Coelho, R. G. D. A. 1955. *Black Carib Of Honduras: A Study In Acculturation.* Ann Arbor, Mich.: Microfilms.
Colón, C. 1961. *Diario de Navegación.* La Habana: Comisión Nacional Cubana de la Unesco.
Columbus, C. & Varela, C. (ed.), 1982. *Textos y documentos completes: Relaciones de Viajes, Cartas y Memoriales.*, Madrid: Alianza.

Con Aguilar, E. Forthcoming. A dissertation within Nexus 1943. Leiden University.
Con Aguilar, E., Álvarez, A., Frederick, C., Hofman & C.L. 2017. Teaching Indigenous History and Heritage. Reviving the Past in the Present: Caribbean Experiences from the Dominican Republic and Dominica. *Creative Education* 83(3): 333-346.
Corbea Calzado J. 1996. La Virgen de la Caridad del Cobre: construcción simbólica y cultura popular. *Del Caribe 24,* 4-11.
Córdova Martínez, C. & Barzaga Sablón, O. 2000. *El Espiritismo de Cordón.* Habana: Fundación Fernando Ortiz.
Coster, W. & Spicer, A. 2011. *Sacred Space in Early Modern Europe.* Cambridge: Cambridge University Press.
Courlander, H. 1960. *Drum and the Hoe: Life and Lore of the Haitian People.* Berkeley and Los Angeles: University of California Press.
Crespo Vargas, P. L. 2011. *La Inquisición Española y Las Supersticiones En El Caribe Hispano a Principios Del Siglo XVII: Un Recuento de Creencias Según Las Relaciones De Fe Del Tribunal De Cartagena De Indias.* Kindle Edition: Palibrio.
Croll, E. & Parkin, D. 2002. *Bush Base, Forest Farm: Culture, Environment, and Development.* London: Routledge.
Crosby, A. 1972. *The Columbian exchange: Biological and cultural consequences of 1492.* Westport, Conn.: Greenwood Press.
Curet, A. 2015. Indigenous Revival, Indigeneity and the Jíbaro in Borinquen. *Centro Journal, 1,* 206-246.
D'Aghiera, P. M. 1912. *De Orbe Novo. The Eight Decadas of Peter Martyr D'Aghiera.* (F.A. MacNutt transl.). New York and London: G.P. Putnams Sons.
Daly, L. 2015. *What kind of people are plants? The challenges of researching human-plant relations in Amazonian Guyana.* Retrieved https://aesengagement. wordpress. com/2015/12/08/what-kind-of-people-areplants-the-challenges-of-researchinghu-man-plant-relations-in-amazonianguyana/.
David, B., Isaacs, P., Angelbert J., Johnson, L., Pugsley, M., Ramacindo, C., Winter, G. & Winter, Y. 2006. *Wa Wiizi – Wa Kaduzu Our territory – Our Custom. Customary Use of Biological Resources and Related Traditional Practices within Wapichan Territory in Guyana. An indigenous case study.* Retrieved from https://www.forestpeoples.org/.
De Castro, E. 1998. Cosmological deixis and Amerindian perspectivism. *J. R. Anthropol. Inst., 4*(3), 469-488.
De Goeje, C. H. 1942. 'De inwijding tot medicijnman bij de Arawakken (Guyana) in tekst en mythe', in: *Bijdragen tot de Taal-, Land- en Volkenkunde van Nederlandsch-Indië,* 101, 211-276.
De Goeje, C. H. 1943. *Philosophy, Initiation and Myths of The Indians of Guiana and Adjacent Countries.* Leiden: Brill.
De Jesús de Galván, M. 1882. *Enriquillo, Leyenda Histórica Dominicana (1502-1533).* Santo Domingo: De Garcia Hermanos.
De La Fuente, A. 2007. Población libre y estratificación social, 1510-1770. In Naranjo Orovio, C. (ed.), *Historia de Cuba* (Vol. 1), España: Editorial Doce Calles.
De La Sagra, R. 1861. *Historia física, política y natural de la isla de Cuba* (Vol. 2). Paris: A. Bertrand.
Deagan, K. 1995. *Puerto Real: the archaeology of a sixteenth-century Spanish town in Hispaniola.* Gainesville etc.: University Press of Florida.

Deagan, K. 1996. Colonial Transformation: Euro-American Cultural Genesis in the Early Spanish-American Colonies. *Journal of Anthropological Research, 52*(2), 135-160.

Deagan, K. 2014. Reconsidering Taino Social Dynamic after Spanish conquest: gender and Clas in Cultures Contac Studies. *American Antiquity, 69* (4), 597-626.

Deagan, K. 1988. The Archeology of the Spanish Contact Period in the Caribbean. *Journal of World Prehistory, 2* (2), 34.

Deagan, K. & Cruxent, J. 2002. *Columbus's Outpost among the Taínos.* Yale: Yale University Press.

Deive, C. E. 1985. *Los Cimarrones Del Maniel De Neiba. Historia y Etnografía.* Santo Domingo: Banco Central de la República Dominicana.

Deive, C. E. 1988. *Vodú y magia en Santo Domingo.* Santo Domingo: Fundación Cultural Dominicana.

Deive, C. E. 1989. *Los guerrilleros negros: esclavos fugitivos y cimarrones en Santo Domingo*, Santo Domingo, Ediciones Cultural Dominicana.

Deive, C. E. 1995. *La Española y la esclavitud del indio.* Santo Domingo: Fundación García Arévalo.

Deive, C. E. 2002. *Antología de la flora y fauna de Santo Domingo en cronista y viajeros (Siglo XV-XX).* Santo Domingo: Amigo del Hogar.

Deive, C. E. 2009. *Los dominicanos vistos por extranjeros (1730-1929).* Santo Domingo: Publicaciones del Banco Central de la República Dominicana.

Deive, C.E. 1976. *Vodú y Magia en Santo Domingo.* Santo Domingo: Museo del hombre dominicano.

Deive, C.E. 1981. *La esclavitud del negro en Santo Domingo.* Santo Domingo: Museo del Hombre Dominicano.

Deive, E. 1982. *Heterodoxia e inquisición en Santo Domingo 1492 – 1822.* Taller Isabel la Católica 309, Santo Domingo: República Dominicana.

Deive, E. 1991. *Las emigraciones Canarias a Santo Domingo, siglo XVII and XVII.* Santo Domingo: Fundación Cultura Dominicana.

Del Río Moreno, J. L. 2012. *Los inicios de la agricultura europea en el Nuevo Mundo, 1492-154.* Santo Domingo: Academia Dominicana de la Historia.

Descola, P. & Pálsson, G. 1996. *Nature and Society. Anthropological perspectives.* London: Routledge.

Díaz de Castillo, B. 1844 [1568]. *Memoirs, of the Conquistador Bernal Diaz del Castillo written by himself containing a true and full account of the discovery and conquest of Mexico and New Spain.* (J. I. Lockhart transl.). London: J. Hatchard and Son.

Dodson, J. & Millet Batista, J. 2008. *Sacred spaces and religious traditions in Oriente Cuba* (Religions of the Americas Series). Albuquerque: University of New Mexico Press.

Domínguez, L. 1980. Cerámica transcultural en el sitio colonia Casa de la Obrapía. In *Cuba Arqueológica I,* 15-19.

Echagoian, J. 1942 [1568]. Relación de La Isla Española. In E. Rodríguez Demorizi (ed.), *Relaciones Históricas de Santo Domingo.* Ciudad Trujillo: Montalvo.

Edmonds, E. B. & Gonzalez, M. A. 2010. *Caribbean Religious History. An Introduction.* New York: New York University Press.

Eng Menendéz, Y. G. 2003. Los culíes chinos en Cuba: esclavos contratados. *Del Caribe 42.*

Engerman, S. L. & Higman, B.W. 1997. The demographic structure of the Caribbean slave societies in the eighteenth and nineteenth centuries. In F. W. Knight, *General History of the Caribbean – III* (ed.), Hong Kong: Unesco Publishing.

Erll, A. 2008. Cultural Memory Studies: An Introduction. In Erll, A., Nünning, A. & S. B. Young (eds), *A Companion to Cultural Memory Studies*. De Gruyter: Medien Und Kulturelle Erinnerung.

Estevez, J. 2013. Taíno Spirituality Today. A Practionair's perspective. In S. Meighoo, Case, F. I. & P. Taylor (eds), *The Encyclopedia of Caribbean Religions* (Vol.1). Champaign, IL: University of Illinois Press.

Exquemelin, A. O. 1971 [1678]. *De Americaensche zee-rovers beschreven door A. O. Exquemelin die self alle dese roveryen, door noodt, bygewoont heeft.* Laren, The Netherlands: A. J. Luitingh.

Fabian, J. 1983. *Time and the Other. How anthropology make its object.* New York: Columbia University Press.

Fairclough, N. 2003. *Analysing Discourse. Textual analysis for social research.* Oxford: Routledge.

Fanon, F. 1952 [2012]. Černá kůže, bílé masky. Praha: Tranzit.cz.

Fanon, F. 1961 [2015]. *Psanci této země*. Praha: Tranzit.cz.

Fariñas Gutiérrez, D. 1995. *Religión en las Antillas: Paralelismos y transculturación*. La Habana: Editorial Academia.

Feijóo, S. 1986. *Mitología Cubana.* La Habana: Editorial Letras Cubanas.

Ferdinand, M. 2017. 'Living in contaminated land: Struggle for a decolonial environmental justice in contemporary Martinique and Guadeloupe'. In M. May Castillo & A. Strecker (eds), *Heritage and Rights of Indigenous Peoples.* Leiden: Leiden University Press.

Fernández de Oviedo, G. 2002 [1535-1557]. Historia General y Natural De Las Indias. In C. E. Deive (ed.), *Antología de la flora y fauna de Santo Domingo en cronista y viajeros (Siglo XV-XX)*. Santo Domingo: Amigo del Hogar.

Fernández Olmos, P. G. & Paravisini-Gebert, L. 1997. *Sacred possessions: Vodou, Santería, Obeah and the Caribbean*. New Brunswick, N.J.: Rutgers University Press.

Fernández Ortega, R., González Tendero, J. B., Gutierrez Calvache, D. A. 2006. History, Survey, Conservation, and Interpretation of Cuban Rock Art. In M. Hayward, L. G. Atkinson & M. A. Cinquino (eds), *Rock Art of the Caribbean.* Tuscaloosa: The University of Alabama Press.

Finol, J. E. 2007. *Mito y Cultura Guajira. Contribución a la semiótica del mito guajiro.* Venezuela: Ediciones del Vice Rectorado Académico.

Fischer, E. J. 1999. Cultural Logic and Maya Identity: Rethinking constructivism and essentialism. *Current Anthropology 40* (4), 473-499.

Fitzpatrick, S. M. & Keegan, W. F. 2007. Human impact and adaptation in the Caribbean Islands: an historical ecology approach. *Earth and Environmental Science Transaction of the Royal Society of Edingburgh 87(1):* 29-45.

Font, M. A. & Quiroz, A. W. 2005. *Cuban counterpoints: The legacy of Fernando Ortiz* (Western hemisphere studies 273382535). Lanham, MA [etc.]: Lexington Books.

Fornaris, J. 1862. *Cantos del Siboney*. Havana: La Antilla.

Forte, M. C. 2006. Extinction: Ideologies against Indigeneity in the Caribbean. *Southern Quarterly, 43*(4), 46-69.
Forte, M. Ch. 2006. *Indigenous resurgence in the contemporary Caribbean: Amerindian survival and revival.* New York, NY [etc.]: Peter Lang.
Foster, B. 1986. *Heart Drum: Spirit Possession In The Communities Of Belize.* Belize: Cubola Productions.
Foster, G. M. 1953. Relationships between Spanish and Spanish-American folk medicine. *Journal of American Folklore, 66* (261), 201-217.
Foster, G. M. 1960. *Conquest and Culture: America's Spanish Heritage.* Chicago: Quadrangle Books Chicago.
Foucault, M. 1970. The Order of the Things: An Archeology of the Human Sciences. New York: Pantheon Books.
Fouchard, J. 1979. The slave trade and the peopling of Santo Domingo. In UNESCO, *The African Slave Trade from the Fifteenth to the Nineteenth Century.* Paris: UNESCO.
Françozo, M. & Strecker, A. 2017. Caribbean Collections in European Museums and the Question of Returns. *24*(4), 451-477.
Freire, G. V. ed. 2011. *Perspectivas en salud indígena. Cosmovisión, enfermedad y políticas públicas.* Ecuador: Abya-Yala.
Freyre, G. 1933. Casa-grande e senzala: formaçao de familia brasileira so o régimen de economía patriarcal, Rio de Janeiro: Maia and Schmidt. Published in English as The Masters and the Slaves: A Study in the Development of Brazilian Civilization, New York: A.A. Knopf. Berkeley: University of California Press.
Frómeta Suárez, S. 2003. *Imagen en el tiempo Jiguani.* Bayamo: Ediciones Bayamo.
García Arevalo, M. 1988. *El Indigenismo, arqueología, identidad nacional.* Santo Domingo: Museo del Hombre Dominicano: Fundación García Arévalo.
García Arevalo, M. 2008. El Indigenismo dominicano. Mar Oceana. Revista del Humanismo Español e Iberoamericano, no. 24.
García Castañeda, J. A. 1949. La transculturación indo-española en Holguín. *Revista de Arqueología y Etnología 8 y 9 año IV época II,* pp.195-205.
García Molina, J.A., Garrido Mazorra, M. & Fariñas Gutierrez, D. 2007. *Huellas vivas del indocubano.* La Habana: Editorial de Ciencias Sociales.
Gemi-Iordanou, E. 2014. *Medicine, Healing and Performance.* Oxford: Oxbow Books.
Germeten, von, N. 2007. Alonso de Sandoval. Treatise on Slavery: Selections rom De Instauranda Aethiopum Salute. Hackett Publishing.
Germosén-Robineau, G. 2005. *Farmacopea Vegatal Caribeña.* Nicaragua: Editorial Universitaria, Unana.
Gesler, W. 1993. Therapeutic Landscapes – Theory and a case-study of Epidauros, Greece. *Environ. Plan. D-Soc. Space, 11*(2), 171-189.
Gesler, W. 1996. Lourdes: Healing in a place of pilgrimage. *Health and Place, 2*(2), 95-105.
Gesler, W. M. 2003. *Healing Places*: Rowman & Littlefield.
Gil-Bermejo García, J. 1983. *La Española Anotaciones Históricas (1600-1650).* Sevilla: Escuela de Estudios Hispano-Americanos de Sevilla.

Gillin, J. 1936. The Barama River Caribs of British Guiana. Papers of the Peabody Museum 14. 1948 Tribes of the Guianas and the Left Amazon Tributaries. In Handbook of South American Indians. J. H. Steward, ed. Smithsonian Institution, Bureau of American Ethnology Bulletin 143, 3:799-860.
Glissant, E. & Dash, J. 1996. *Caribbean discourse: Selected essays*. Charlottesville: University Press of Virginia.
Glissant, E. & Wing, B. 1997. *Poetics of relation*. Ann Arbor: University of Michigan Press.
Godo, P. P. 2016. El problema del indio en Cuba. In Jorge Ulloa Hung & Roberto Valcárcel Rojas (eds), *Indígenas e indios en el Caribe. Presencia, legado y estudio*. Santo Domingo: Instituto tecnológico de Santo Domingo.
Godwin, J. 2002. *The Pagan Dream of the Renaissance*. Boston: Red. Wheel and Weiser.
Gómez, P. 2017. *The experiential Caribbean: Creating knowledge and healing in the early modern Atlantic*. Chapel Hill: The University of North Carolina Press.
González Peréz, J. 1997. Ellos están muertos y me eligieron a mí. *Del Caribe 26*, 56-63.
González, N. L. & Castillo, G. 2004. Garifuna. In C. R. Ember & M. Ember (eds), *Encyclopedia of Medical Anthropology: Health and Illness in the World's Cultures Volume I: Topics Volume II: Cultures* (pp. 672-681). Boston, MA: Springer US.
Górdon y Acosta, A. 1894. Medicina indígena de Cuba y su valor histórico: trabajo leído en la sesión celebrada el día 28 de octubre de 1894 por Antonio de Górdon y de Acosta. Habana: Sarachaga y H. Miyares.
Gosden, C. 1999. *Anthropology and Archaeology: A Changing Relationship*: Florence, KY, USA: Routledge.
Grafton, A. Shelford, A., Siraisi, N. 1992. *New Worlds, Ancient Texts: The Power of Tradition and the Shock of Discovery.* Cambridge, Mass.: Belknap Press of Harvard University Press.
Granberry, J. & Vescelius, G. 2004. *Languages of the pre-Columbian Antilles*. Tuscaloosa, AL: University of Alabama Press.
Greene, S. 2002. Sacred Sites and the Colonial Encounter. A History of Meaning and Memory in Ghana. Bloomington: Indiana University Press.
Guanche, J. 2011. Componentes étnicos de la nación cubana. Habana: Editorial Sciencias Sociales.
Guitar, L. 2013. Taíno Classic Taíno Spiritual Beliefs and Practices. In Meighoo, S., Case, F. I. & Taylor, P. (2013). *The Encyclopedia of Caribbean Religions: Volume 1: A-L; Volume 2: M-Z*. Champaign, IL: University of Illinois Press.
Gullick, C. J. M. R. 1976. *Exiled From St. Vincent: The Development Of Black Carib Culture In Central America Up To 1945*. Malta: Progress Press.
Gutierrez Calvache, D.; Fernández Ortega, R. & González Tendero, J. 2009. *Arte Rupestre Cubano*. La Habana: Ediciones Geo and Fundación Fernando Ortíz.
Halbmayer, E. 2012. Debating animism, perspectivism and the construction of ontologies. *Indiana 29*, 9-23.
Halbwachs, E. & Coser, L. A. 1992 [1941]. *On collective memory*. Chicago, IL [etc.]: University of Chicago Press.
Hall, S. 1992. The West and the Rest: discourse and power. In S. Hall, B. Gieben & U. Open (eds), *Formations of modernity* (Vol. Understanding modern societies, pp. 276-280, 291-320, 328-329). Oxford: Polity in association with Open University.

Hall, S. 1997. *Cultural Representations and Signifying Practices.* London: Sage Publication.
Hanwella, R., De Silva, V., Yoosuf, A., Karunaratne, S. & De Silva, P. 2012. Religious Beliefs, Possession States, and Spirits: Three Case Studies from Sri Lanka. *Case Reports in Psychiatry, 2012*, 3.
Harner, M. J. 1973. "Jívaro: People Of The Sacred Waterfalls." Garden City, N.Y.: Anchor Press / Doubleday. http://ehrafworldcultures.yale.edu/document?id=sd09-034
Harrington, K. J. 2012. The Use of Metaphor in Discourse About Cancer: A Review of the Literature. *Clinical Journal of Oncology Nursing, 16*(4), 408-12.
Haslam, N. 2006. Dehumanization: An integrative review. Personality and Social Psychology Review. 10. 252-264.
Hayward, M., Calvache, D. A. G., Ortega, R. F., Layos, P. A. A., Belando, A. L., Allsworth-Jones, P. 2009. *Rock Art of the Caribbean.* Tuscaloosa: The University of Alabama Press.
Heller Anderson, S. 1969. Three Relations of the West Indies, 1659-1660. Transactions of the American Philosophical Society, *New Series, 59* (6): 1-49.
Henfrey, T. 2002. *Ethnoecology, Resource Use, Conservation and Development in a Wapishana Community in the South Rupununi, Guyana* (Dissertation). UK: University of Kent at Canterbury.
Hermans, R., Kolen, J. & Renes, H. 2013. *Landscape Biographies: Geographical, Historical and Archaeological Perspectives on the Production and Transmission of Landscapes: Geographical, Historical and Archaeological Perspectives on the Production and Transmission of Landscapes.* Amsterdam: Amsterdam University Press.
Hernández González, M.V. 2006. La Colonización de la Frontera Dominicana. Santo Domingo: Búho.
Hernández González, M.V. 2007. Expansión fundacional y desarrollo del norte dominicano (1680-1795). El Cibao y la Bahía de SaMana. Santo Domingo: Búho.
Hernández Rodríguez, S. & Rodríguez Becerra, S. 2015. La Virgen de Aguas Santas de Villaverde y la ciudad de Sevilla. Análisis de una devoción mariana en la periferia hispalense. *Archivo hispalense: Revista histórica, literaria y artística, 98,* 297-299, 47-76.
Herrera Malatesta, E. N. 2018. Una isla, dos mundos: estudio arqueológico sobre el paisaje indígena de Haytí y su transformación al paisaje colonial de La Española (1200-1550). Leiden: Sidestone Press.
Herrera Martinez, E. 2017. Reflexiones sobre el Territorio y la construcción del "bien estar" entre los ñuu savi (mixtecos) de la Montaña de Guerrero, México. In M. May Castillo & A. Strecker (Eds), *Heritage and Rights of Indigenous Peoples.* Leiden: Leiden University Press.
Herskovits, M. 1937. African Gods and Catholic Saints in New World Negro Belief. *American, 39*(4), 635-643.
Herskovits, M. J. 1933. *An outline of Dahomean religious belief.* Menasha, WI: American Anthropological Association.
Herskovits, M. J. & Herskovits, F. S. 1933. Outline Of Dahomean Religious Belief. *Memoirs Of The American Anthropological Association.* Menasha, Wis.: The American Anthropological Association. Retrieved from http://ehrafworldcultures.yale.edu/document?id=fa18-003.

Herskovits, M. J. 1941. Some Comments on the Study of Cultural Contact. *American Anthropologist (43) 1*, 1-10.
Herskovits, M. J. 1937. *Life In A Haitian Valley*. NewYork: http://ehrafworldcultures.yale.edu/document?id=sv03-001.
Heywood, L.M. 2001. Introduction. In L. M. Heywood (ed.), *Central Africans and Cultural Transformations in the American Diaspora:* Cambridge: Cambridge University Press.
Higuera-Gundy, A., Brenner, M., Hodell, D. A., Curtis, J. H., Leyden, B. W., Binford, M. W. 1999. A 10,300 14C yr Record of Climate and Vegetation Change from Haiti. *Quaternary Research, 52*(2), 159-170.
Hill, J. (ed.) 1988. *Rethinking History and Myth. Indigenous South American Perspectives on the Past*. Urbana and Chicago: University of Illinois Press.
Hippocrates. ca. 400 B.C.E. *Airs Water Places*. Transl. Francis Adamss. Retrieved from: http://classics.mit.edu/Hippocrates/airwatpl.html.
Hirsch, E. & O'Hanlon, M. 1995. *The anthropology of landscape: perspectives on place and space*: Oxford etc.: Clarendon Press.
Hirsch, M. & Smith, V. 2002. Feminism and Cultural Memory: An Introduction. *Signs: Journal of Women in Culture and Society, 28*(1), 1-19.
Hodge, W. H. & Taylor, D. M. 1957. Ethnobotany Of The Island Caribs Of Dominica. *Webbia, 12*, 513-644. Retrieved from http://ehrafworldcultures.yale.edu/document?id=st13-013.
Hoffman, B. 2013. Exploring Biocultural Contexts: Comparative Woody Plant Knowledge of an Indigenous and Afro-American Maroon Community in Suriname, South America. In R.Voeks & J. Rashford, *African ethnobotany in the Americas*. New York; London: Springer.
Hofman C.L. & Duijvenbode A. van 2011. *Communities in Contact: Essays in Archaeology, Ethnohistory and Ethnography of the Amerindian circum-Caribbean.* Leiden: Sidestone Press.
Hofman C.L. 18 March 2008, *'Indianenverhalen' : het kwetsbare verleden van de Antillen* (Inaugural address). Leiden: Universiteit Leiden.
Hofman, C. L., Ulloa Hung, J. & Hoogland, M.L.P. 2016. El paisaje social indígena al momento del encuentro colonial: nuevas investigaciones en el norte de la República Dominicana. *Boletín del Museo del Hombre Dominicano, 47*, 300-310.
Hofman, C., Hung, J., Malatesta, E., Jean, J., Sonnemann, T. & Hoogland, M. 2018. Indigenous Caribbean perspectives: Archaeologies and legacies of the first colonised region in the New World. *Antiquity, 92*(361), 200-216.
Hofman, C. L, Davies, G. R., Brandes, U. & Willems, W. J. H. 2012. NEXUS 1492: New World Encounters in a Globalising World. ERC Synergy Grant 2012. Research proposal. Leiden: Leiden University.
Hofman, C., Mol, A., Hoogland, M. & Valcárcel Rojas, R. 2014. Stage of encounters: Migration, mobility and interaction in the pre-colonial and early colonial Caribbean. *World Archaeology, 46*(4), 590-609.
Hofman, C.L. & Bright, A. J. 2010. Mobility and exchange from a Pan-Caribbean perspective. *Journal of Caribbean archaeology*, Special Publication 3.

Hofmann, B. 2013. Exploring Biocultural Contexts: Comparative Woody Plant Knowledge of an INdigneou snad Afro-American Maroon Community in Suriname, South America. In R. Voeks & J. Rashford, African ethnobotany in the Americas. New York; London: Springer.
Honychurch, L. 1997. Crossroads in the Caribbean: a site of encounter and exchange on Dominica, *World Archaeology*, 28 (3): 291-304.
Horta García, F. 2012. A la sombra de los árboles mágicos. Artemisa: Editorial Unicornio.
Hough, K. 2008. The expression & perception of space in Wayana. Leiden: Sidestone Press.
Houlberg, M. 1996. Sirens and Snakes: Water Spirits in the Arts of Haitian Vodou. African Arts, 29(2), 30-101.
Hoyos Sainz & de Hoyos Sancho, N. 1947. Manual de Folklore: La Vida Popular Tradicional en España. Spain: Istmo Ediciones.
Hugh – Jones, S. 1974. Barasana Initiation: Male Initiation and Cosmology among the Barasana. Ph.D. diss., Cambridge University.
Hugh-Jones, C. 1980. *From the Milk River: Spatial and temporal processes in Northwest Amazonia.* Cambridge: Cambridge University Press.
Hulme, P. 1986. *Colonial Encounters. Europe and the Native Caribbean, 1492 – 1797.* London: Methuen.
Huracán Matthew in Gibara. 10 October 2016. Retrieved from://adisgib.cubava.cu/2016/10/06/huracanes/.
Ingold, T. 1993. Companion Encyclopedia of Anthropology. London/New York: Routledge.
Ingold, T. 2000. The perception of the environment: essays on livelihood, dwelling and skill: London etc.: Routledge.
Ingold, T. 2002. Culture and the Perception of the Environment. In edit. By Croll, E. & Parkin, D. Bush Base, Forest Farm: Culture, Environment, and Development. London/New York: Routledge.
Insoll, T. 2011. The Oxford Handbook of the Archeology of Ritual Religion. Oxford: Oxford University Press.
James Figarola, J. 1999. *La muerte en Cuba.* La Habana: Ediciones Unión.
James Figarola, J. 1989. *Sobre Muerto y Dioses.* Santiago de Cuba: Caserón.
James Figarola, J. 1993a. La vida y la muerte en el espiritismo de cordón. *Del Caribe, 20,* 14-25.
James Figarola, J. 1993b. Presencia de la muerte en la cultura cubana. *Del Caribe 22,* 14 -25.
Jansen M.E.R.G.N. & Pérez G.A. 2015. Tiempo, Religión e Interculturalidad en la Colonia: los catecismos pictográficos de México. In M.E.R.G.N., Jansen & V. Raffa (eds), *Tiempo y Comunidad. Herencias e interacciones socioculturales en Mesoamérica y Occidente.* Archaeological Studies Leiden University no. 29 Leiden: Leiden University Press.
Jansen M.E.R.G.N. & Pérez Jiménez G.A. 2017. *Time and the Ancestors: Aztec and Mixtec Ritual Art.* Leiden: Brill.
Jansen, M.E.R.G.N. & Peréz Jimenez, G A. 2008. Sacred Landscapes: Codices and Archaeology of Ñuu Dzaui. *Itinerarios 8,* 83-112.

Jardines Macías, J. 2014. Peña Obregón, Á., Rojas Espinosa, Y. Fernández Batista, Y. El Rastro del aborigen en la ciudad de Holguín visto a través de las investigaciones Arqueológicas. In R. Valcárcel Rojas & H. Pérez Concepción (eds), *Indios de Holguín*. Holguín: La Mezquita.

Jiménez Osorio, L. I. & Posselt Santoyo, E. 2018. *Tiempo, Paisaje y Líneas de Vida en la Arquelogía de Ñuu Savi (La Mixteca, Mexico)*. Leiden: ASLU.

JMP 2017. *WHO/UNICEF Joint Monitoring Programme for Water Supply and Sanitation*. Retrieved from https://washdata.org/.

Juhé-Beaulaton, D. & Roussel, B. 2003. May vodun sacred spaces be considered as a natural patrimony? In T. Gardner & D. Moritz (eds), *Creating and Representing Sacred Spaces*. Göttingen: Peust & Gutschmidt Verlag.

Kambel, E.R. & de Jong, C. (eds) 2006. *Marauny Na'na Emandobo Lokono Shikwabana. "Marowijne – our territory". Traditional use and management of the Lower Marowijne area by the Kaliña and Lokono.* Retrieved from www.forestspeoples.org.

Kavari, J. U. & Bleckmann, L. E. 2009. Otjiherero Praises of Places: Collective Memory Embedded in Landscape and the Aesthetic Sense ofa Pastoral People. In M. Bollig & O. Bubenzer (eds), *African Landscapes: Interdisciplinary Approaches*. New York: Springer.

Keegan, W. F., Hofman, C. L. & Rodríguez Ramos, R. 2013. *The Oxford handbook of Caribbean archaeology*. Oxford: Oxford University Press.

Keegan, W. & Carlson, L. 2008. *Talking Taíno: Essays on Caribbean natural history from a native perspective*. Tuscaloosa: University of Alabama Press.

Keegan, W. & Hofman, C. 2017. *The Caribbean before Columbus*. Oxford & New York: Oxford University Press.

Khachatourians, A. 2006. *Therapeutic landscapes: A critical analysis*. ProQuest Dissertations Publishing.

Knight, F. 1970. *Slave society in Cuba: During the nineteenth century*. Madison; London: University of Wisconsin Press.

Koelewijn, C. 1987. *Oral literature of the trio Indians of Surinam*. Dordrecht etc.: Foris Publications.

Kuschick, I. 1995. *Medicina popular en España*. Madrid: Siglo XXI De España Editores.

La Rosa Corzo, G. 1991. La Cueva de la Cachimba: Estudio arqueológico de un refugiode cimarrones. *Estudios Arqueológicos*, Havana: Editorial Academia.

La Rosa Corzo, G. & Robaína Jaramillo, R. 1995. *Costumbres funerarias de los aborígenes de Cuba*. La Habana: Editorial Academia.

Lago Vieito, Á. 1996. El espiritismo de cordón en el Bayamo colonial. Santiago de Cuba: *Del Caribe, 25*, 16-18.

Lalung, H. d. 1948. Les Caraïbes un peuple étrange aujourd'hui disparu: Paris: Bourrelier.

Lanceley, A., Noble, G., Johnson, M., Balogun, N., Chatterjee, H. & Menon, U. 2012. Investigating the therapeutic potential of a heritage-object focused intervention: A qualitative study. *Journal Of Health Psychology, 17*(6), 809-820.

Land, K. v. t., Nijdam, H. & Baker, P. A. 2012. *Medicine and Space: Body, Surroundings and Borders in Antiquity and the Middle Ages*. Leiden: Brill.

Landers, J. 2001. The Central African Presence in Spanish Maroon Communities. In L.M. Heywood (ed.), *Central Africans and Cultural Transformations in the American Diaspora*. Cambridge: Cambridge University Press.

Langham, W. 1597. *The garden of health conteyning the sundry rare and hidden vertues and properties of all kindes of simples and plants, together with the maner how they are to be vsed and applyed in medicine for the health of mans body, against diuers diseases and infirmities most common amongst men. Gathered by the long experience and industrie of William Langham, practitioner in phisicke* (Early English books online). Imprinted at London: By the deputies of Christopher Barker.

Las Casas, B., de 1992. *Historia de las Indias.* 3 vols. Edited by A. Saint-Lu. Caracas: Fundación Biblioteca Ayacucho.

Las Casas, B., de, 1967 [1875-1876]. *Apologética historia sumaria.* 3 Vol. México City: UNAM.

Layng, A. 1983. *Carib Reserve: Identity And Security In The West Indies*. Washington, D.C.: University Press of America. Retrieved from http://ehrafworldcultures.yale.edu/document?id=st13-014.

Vidal, L. 1993. *Concepto yoruba de la muerte. Del Caribe, 22,* 29-31.

Lemaire, T. 1986. *The Indiaan in ons bewustzijn*. Baarn: Ambo.

Levin, H. 1969. The myth of the Golden Age in the Renaissance. Bloomington: Indiana University Press.

Levin, J. 2010. Religion and Mental Health: Theory and Research. *International Journal of Applied Psychoanalytic Studies 7(2)*: 102-115.

Levi-Strauss. C. 1962. *The Savage Mind.* Lechtworth, Hertfordshire: The Garden City Press.

Llavarías y Martínez, 1931. Papeles existentes en el Archivo General de Indias relativos a Cuba y muy particularmente a la Habana (donativo Néstor Carbonell). London: Johns Hopkins University Press.

Loomba, A. 1997. *Colonialism/postcolonialism*. London [etc.]: Routledge.

López Belando, A. 2006. El arte rupestre en el Parque Nacional los Haitises. Retrieved from http://www.rupestreweb.info/haitises2.html.

López de Gómara, F. 2002 [1552]. Historia General de Las Indias. In C. E. Deive (ed.), *Antología de la flora y fauna de Santo Domingo en cronista y viajeros (Siglo XV-XX)*. Santo Domingo: Amigo del Hogar.

López Sánchez J. 1970. La medicina en la Habana. 1550-1730. *Cuad Hist Sal Pub 47.*

López Sánchez, J. 1997. *Cuba. Medicina y civilización: siglos XVII y XVIII.* La Habana: Editorial Científico-Técnica.

López Velansco, J. 2002 [1571]. Geografía y Descripción Universal de Las Indias. In C. E. Deive (ed.), *Antología de la flora y fauna de Santo Domingo en cronista y viajeros (Siglo XV-XX)*. Santo Domingo: Amigo del Hogar.

Luengo López, A. A. 2009. La cosmogonía Añú. *Revista de Artes y Humanidades UNICA, 10* (1), 105-127.

Lundahl, M. & Lundius, J. 2012. *Peasants and Religion: A Socioeconomic Study of Dios Olivorio and the Palma Sola Religion in the Dominican Republic*. London: Taylor & Francis.

MacGaffey, W. 2001. Twins, Simbi Spirits, and Lwas in Kongo and Haiti. In L. M. Heywood (ed.), *Central Africans and Cultural Transformations in the American Diaspora*. Cambridge: Cambridge University Press.

MacGregor, A. 1994. *Sir Hans Sloane: Collector, scientist, antiquary, founding father of the British Museum*. London: British Museum Press.

Macuil Martínez, R. 2017. *Los Tlamatque, guardianes del patrimonio: Dinámicas interculturales en la sociedad naua (México)*. Leiden: Archaeological Studies Leiden University.

Malinowki, B. 1995 [1963]. Introducción. In Ortiz, F. *Cuban counterpoint, tobacco and sugar*. Durham etc.: Duke University Press.

Mans, J. 2012. *Amotopoan trails a recent archaeology of Trio movements*. Leiden: Sidestone Press.

Marquina-Márquez, A., Virchez, J. & Ruiz-Callado, R. 2016. Postcolonial healing landscapes and mental health in a remote Indigenous community in subarctic Ontario, Canada. Polar Geography, 39(1), 20-39.

Martí, J. 1889. Las Ruinas Indias. *La Edad de Oro, 2*.

Martin, G. J. 2005. All possible worlds: a history of geographical ideas (4th ed.): New York etc.: Oxford University Press.

Martínez Fortún, J. A. 1958. *Historia de la medicina en Cuba*. La Habana: Edición mimeografiada.

Mason, P. 1990. *Deconstructing America: representations of the other*. Oxford: Routledge.

Mather, C. 2003. Shrines and the Domestication of Landscape. *Journal of Anthropological Research, 59*(1), 23-45.

May Castillo M., Strecker A. (eds) 2017. *Heritage and Rights of Indigenous Peoples*. Leiden: Leiden University Press.

McCallum, J. 1985. *Folk medicine in the Caribbean: An annotated bibliography*. Mona, Jamaica: Medical Library, University of the West Indies.

McCann, J. 2001. Maize and Grace: History, Corn, and Africa's New Landscapes, 1500-1999. *Comparative Studies in Society and History, 43*(2), 246-272.

McLeod, J. 2007. *The Routledge Companion To Postcolonial Studies*. London: Taylor & Francis.

McNiven, I. M. & Russel, L. 2005. *Appropriated Pasts: Indigenous Peoples and the Colonial Culture of Archaeology*. Oxford: AltaMira Press.

Meighoo, S., Case, F. I. & Taylor, P. 2013. *The Encyclopedia of Caribbean Religions: Volume 1: A-L; Volume 2: M-Z*. Champaign, IL: University of Illinois Press.

Memén Pérez, F. 2000. *La Utopía Colombina*. In J. G. Guerrero & H. Olsen Bogaert (eds), *Cristóbal Colón. Antropología e Historia del Encuentro de Dos Mundos*. Santo Domingo: Museo del Hombre Domincano.

Memmi, A. 1957. *Portrait du colonisé précédé de Portrait du colonisateur*. Paris: Buchet/Chastel.

Méndez Nieto, J. 1989. *Discursos medicinales*. Salamanca, España: Universidad de Salamanca.

Mendieta, J. 2006 [1870]. *Historia eclesiástica Indiana*. Retrieved from: //www.cervantesvirtual.com/obra/historia-eclesiastica-indiana--0/.

Mintz, S. 1989. *Caribbean transformations*. New York: Columbia University Press.

Mintz, S.W. & Price, R. 1992. *The Birth Of Afro-American Culture. An Anthropological Perspective.* Boston: Beacon Press. Kindle Edition.
Mira Caballos, E. 1997a. *El indio antillano: repartimiento, encomienda y esclavitud: (1492-1542).* Sevilla: Muñoz Moya y Montraveta.
Mira Caballos, E. 1997b. La medicina indígena en la Española y su comercialización (1492-1550). *Asclepio: Revista de historia de la medicina y de la ciencia, 2,* 185-198
Mira Caballos, E. 2000. *Indios y mestizos americanos en la España del siglo XVI.* Madrid: Iberoamericana.
Mira Caballos, E. 2009. *Conquista y Destrucción de Las Indias (1492-1573).* Monz Moya: Editores Extremos.
Mitchell, L. & Scheiber, M. D. 2010. *Across a Great Divide. Continuity and Change in Native North America.* Tucson: The University of the Arizona Press.
Mitchell, M. 2006. *Crucial issues in Caribbean religions.* New York, NY: Peter Lang.
Monardes, N. 1580. *Primera, y segunda y tercera partes de la Historia medicinal de las cosas que se traen de nuestras Indias Occidentales,* Sevilla. Retrieved from://archive.org/details/bub_gb_eAtm3cE1smAC.
Monte y Tejada, del, A. 1890. *Historia de Santo Domingo.* Santo Domingo: Imp. García.
Morales Patiño, O. &. Pérez Acevedo, A. 1945. El Período de Transculturación Indo-hispánica. In Contribuciones del Grupo Guama. *La Habana Antropología, 4,* 5 – 6.
Morales, A. L. 2001. *Remedios: Stories of Earth and Iron from the History of Puertorriqueñas.* Cambridge, Massachussets: South End Press.
Moreau de Saint-Méry, L. E. 1796. *Description topographique et politique de la partie espagnole de l'isle Saint-Domingue.* Philadelphie: L'auteur.
Moreno Rodríguez, E., Bermúdez, A. & Herrera Oliver, P. P. 1995. Las plantas y el Espiritismo Cruzado en Cuba. *Fontqueria 42,* 289-308.
Moreno, D. 1998. Forma y tradición en la Artesanía popular Cubana. La Habana: José Martí.
Moreno, J. S. 2007. *Cuba: un pueblo nuevo: herencias etnoculturales indígenas en la región oriental.* Mexico City: UNAM.
Moret, E. S. 2013. Trans-Atlantic Diaspora Ethnobotany: Legacies of West African and Iberian Mediterranean Migration in Central Cuba. In Voeks, R. & J. Rashford (eds), *African ethnobotany in the Americas.* New York; London: Springer.
Morillo Peréz, A. 2014. *El Mapa de la Pobreza de la Republica Dominicana.* Santo Domingo: UAAES.
Morphy, H. 1995. Landscape and the reproduction of the ancestral past. In E. Hirsch & M. O'Hanlon (eds), *The anthropology of landscape: Perspectives on place and space.* Clarendon Press, Oxford.
Moya Pons, F. & Flores Paz, R. 2013. *Los Taínos en 1492, el debate demográfico.* Santo Domingo: Academia Dominicana de la Historia.
Moya Pons, F. 2009. *Historia de la República Dominicana.* Madrid]: [S.l.]: Consejo Superior de Investigaciones Científicas.
Moya Pons, F. 2010. *The Dominican Republic: A national history* (3rd edit.). Princeton, NJ: Wiener.

Nacher 8 September 2017. Holguineros evacuados en una cueva de las FAR ante proximidad de huracán Irma. Retrieved from https://www.cibercuba.com/noticias/2017-09-08-u157374-e157374-holguineros-evacuados-cueva-far.

Naranjo Orovio, C. 2009. *Historia de Cuba.* Madrid: Consejo Superior de Investigaciones Científicas.

NCMMA, National Commision for Museums and Monuments Abuja. 2004. Nomination to the World Heritage List Osun- Osogbo Sacred Grove, Osun State, Nigeria. Retrieved from*://whc.unesco.org/uploads/nominations/1118.pdf.*

Newcomb, S. 1992. Five Hundred Years of Injustice: The Legacy of Fifteenth Century Religious Prejudice. *Shaman's Drum.* 18-20. Retrieved from http://ili.nativeweb.org/sdrm_art.html on 6 June 2017.

Newsom, L. A. 2008. Caribbean Paleoethnobotany: Present Status and New Horizons (Understanding the Evolution of an Indigenous Ethnobotany). In C.L. Hofman, M. Hoogland & A.L. Gijn van (eds), *Crossing the Borders: New Methods and Techniques in the Study of Archaeological Materials from the Caribbean.* Tuscaloosa: The University of Alabama Press.

Newson, L. 1993. *Native West Indian Plant Use.* Dissertation published at The University of Florida.

Nora, P. 1997. *Les lieux de mémoire.* Paris: Gallimard.

Nünning, A., Erll, A. & Young, S. 2008. *Cultural memory studies an international and interdisciplinary handbook.* Berlin; New York: Walter de Gruyter.

O'Brien, S. C. 2013. *Coming Full Circle: Spirituality and Wellness among Native Communities in the Pacific Northwest.* Lincoln, Nebraska: UNP Nebraska.

Oliver, J., McEwan C. & Casas Giberga, A. 2009. *El Caribe precolombino. Fray Ramón Pané y el universo taino.* Barcelona: Ministerio de Cultura, Museu Barbier-Mueller Art Precolombí y Fundación Caixagalicia.

Oliver, J.R. 2009. *Caciques and Cemi Idols. The Web Spun by Taino Rulers Between Hispaniola and Puerto Rico.* Tuscaloosa: University of Alabama Press.

Oostindie, G. 2013. Intellectual Wastelands? Scholarship in and for the Dutch West Indies up ca. 1800. In P. Boomgaard (ed.), *Empire and Science in the Making. Dutch colonial scholarship in Comparative Global Perspective.* New York: Palgrave Macmilan.

Ortega, E. 2005. *Compendio General Arqueológico de Santo Domingo.* Volumen I. Santo Domingo: Academia de Ciencias de la República Dominicana.

Ortiz Monasterio, F. 1975. *Historia de una pelea cubana contra los demonios (2nd Edition).* Habana: Editorial de Ciencias Sociales.

Ortiz, F. 1995 [1947]. *Cuban counterpoint, tobacco and sugar.* Durham etc.: Duke University Press.

Ortus Sanitatis. 1491. Germany: Jacob Meydenbach. Available on: http://cudl.lib.cam.ac.uk/view/PR-INC-00003-A-00001-00008-00037/1#.

Ososki, A. L. 2004. *Ethnobotany of rural and urban Dominican Republic: medicinal plants, women, and health.* S.l.: s.n.

Ostapkowicz, J., C.B. Ramsey, F., Brock, T., Higham, A. C., Wiedenhoeft, E., Ribechini, J. J. & Lucejko, S. 2012. Chronologies in wood and resin: AMS ^{14}C dating of pre-Hispanic Caribbean wood sculpture, *Journal of Archaeological Science 39*, 2238-2251.

Overing, J. 2004. The Grotesque Landscape of Mythic "Before Time": the Folly of Sociality in "today time". An egalitarian aesthetics of human existence. In Kultur, Raum, Landschaft. Zur Bedeutung des Raumes in Zeiten der Globalität *Atención! Jahrbuch des Österreichischen Lateinamerika-Instituts, 6,* 71-92.

Oviedo y Valdéz, G. F. 1851 [1525-1585]. *Historia general y natural de las Indias. Islas y tierra-firme del mar océano.* Madrid: Imprenta de Real Academia de la Historia.

Pagán Jiménez, J. R. & Oliver, J. R. 2008. Starch Residues on Lithic Artifacts from Two Contrasting Contexts in North Central Puerto Rico: Los Muertos Cave and Vega Nelo Vargas Farmstead. In C.L. Hofman, M. Hoogland & A.L. Gijn van (eds), *Crossing the Borders: New Methods and Techniques in the Study of Archaeological Materials from the Caribbean.* Tuscaloosa: The University of Alabama Press.

Pagán Jiménez, J. R. 2002. Agricultura precolombina de las Antillas: retrospección y análisis, *Anales de Antropología 36,* 43-91.

Pagán Jiménez, J. R. 2007. *De antiguos pueblos y culturas botánicas en el Puerto Rico indígena. El archipiélago borincano y la llegada de los primeros pobladores agroceramistas.* Oxford: Archaeopress.

Pagán Jiménez, J. R. 2009. Nuevas perspectivas sobre las culturas botánicas precolombinas de Puerto Rico: Implicaciones del estudio de almidones en herramientas líticas, cerámicas y de concha Cuba *Arqueol. II* (2), 7-23.

Pagán-Jiménez, J. R. 2013. Human-Plant Dynamics in the Precolonial Antilles: A Synthetic Update. In W.F Keegan, C.L. Hofman & R. Rodríguez Ramos (eds), *The Oxford Handbook of Caribbean Archaeology.* New York: Oxford University Press.

Pagán-Jimenéz, J. R. & Carlson, L. A. 2014. Recent archaeobotanical findings of the hallucinogenic snuff cojoba (Anadenanthera peregrina (L.) Spec.) in precolonial Puerto Rico. *Latin American Antiquity, 25*(1), 101-116.

Pagán-Jiménez, J. R. & Oliver, J. 2008. Starch Residues and Lithic Artifacts from Two Contrasting Contexts in Central Puerto Rico: Cueva de los Muertos and Vega Nelo Vargas. In C.L. Hofman, M. Hoogland& A.L. Gijn van (eds), Crossing the borders, new methods and techniques in the study of archaeological materials from the Caribbean. Tuscaloosa: The University of Alabama Press.

Pagden, A. 1987. *The Fall of Natural Man: The American Indian and the Origins of Comparative Ethnology.* Cambridge: Cambridge University Press.

Palacio, J. O. 1982. *Food And Social Relations In A Garifuna Village.* Ann Arbor, Mich.: University Microfilms International.

Palka, E. 1999. Accessible Wilderness as a Therapeutic Landscape: Experiencing the Nature of Denali National Park, Alaska. *Therapeutic Landscapes: The Dynamic Between Place and Wellness.* MD: University Press of America.

Pané, R. 1498. Writings of Friar Roman on the Antiquities of the Indians, Which He Collected on Request of the Admiral with Diligence, as a Man Who Knows Their Language (ca. 1498). Transl. Whitehead, N. L. 2011. Of Cannibals and Kings. Primal Anthropology in Americas. Pennsylvania State University: University Press.

Pané, R. & Arrom, J. 1498 [1974]. *«Relación acerca de las antigüedades de los indios»: El primer tratado escrito en América* (Nueva versión, con notas, mapas y apéndices / José Juan Arrom. (ed.), México]: Siglo XXI.

Pardo Tomás, J., López Terrada, M. A. L. & Slater, J. 2014. *Medical Cultures of the Early Modern Spanish Empire.* Farnham, Surrey: Routledge.

Paulino Ramos, A. 2008. *Censos municipales del siglo XIX y otras estadísticas de la población.* Santo Domingo: Archivo General de la Nación.
Penard, F. P. & Penard, A. P. 2006 [1907]. *De menschetende aanbidders der zonneslang.* Paramaribo: H.B. Heyde. Accesible on:http://www.dbnl.org/tekst/pena002mens01_01/colofon.htm.
Peña Herrera, A. R. 2006. *Santa Cruz de Yaguate. Prov. San Cristóbal: Sus cosas y Casos.* Santo Domingo: Velos Impresos y Vallas.
Peña Obregón, A., Varcárcel Rojas, R., Urbina Herrán, M.A. 2012. *La Virgen cubana en Nipe y Barajagua.* Holguín: Editorial La Mezquita.
Perara, M. A. 1991. Cuevas y cerros en la tradición oral y ceremonial de los amerindios de Venezuela. *Revista de Indias, 51* (193). ProQuest Copyright.
Pereira Pereira, O. 2007. Las rebeldías esclavas del siglo XVI y el contacto interétnico entre aborígenes y esclavos africanos en Cuba. *Boletín Museo del Hombre Dominicano, 41.*
Pereira Pereira, O. 2008. La confluencia del arte rupestre aborigen y de esclavos cimarrones en las cuevas de Cuba. Santiago de Cuba: *El Caribe Arquelogico, 11.*
Peréz Cruz, F. J. 2014. *Los Indioamericanos en Cuba Estudios abiertos al presente.* Habana: Editorial de Ciencias Sociales.
Peréz Escalarin, A. 1996. *Leyendas y tradiciones Venezolanas.* Caracas: Distribuidora Estudios.
Peréz Jimenéz, A. 2015. Descolonizar memoria, mentalidad e investigación. In M.E.R.G.N. Jansen & V. Raffa (eds), *Tiempo y Comunidad. Herencias e interacciones socioculturales en Mesoamérica y Occidente.* Leiden: Leiden University Press.
Perrin, M. 1987. Shamanistic Symptoms Or Symbols? A Case Of Indetermination (The Body Of The Guajiro Shaman). *Anthropos, 82*, 567-580.
Perrin, M. 2011. Cura chamánica, sueños y eficacia terapéutica: el ejemplo de los wayuu. In G. V. Freire (ed.), *Perspectivas en salud indígena. Cosmovisión, enfermedad y políticas públicas.* Ecuador: Abya-Yala.
Petitjean Roget, H. 1995. Les calebasses peintes, la poterie et l'arc-en-ciel chez les Caraïbes insulaires. Actes du XVIe Congrès international d'archéologie de la Caraïbe, Basse-Terre, 1, 159-175.
Phulgence, W. 2015. African Warriors, Insurgent Fighters, and the Memory of Slavery in the Anglophone Caribbean. *Journal of African Diaspora Archaeology and Heritage, 4*(3), 214-226.
Pichardo Moya, F. 1945. *Los Indios de Cuba en Sus Tiempos Históricos.* La Habana: Academia de Historia de Cuba.
Pineda Giraldo, R. & Muirden, J. S. 1950. Aspects Of Magic In La Guajira. *Revista Del Instituto Etnologico Nacional.* Bogota: [s.n.]. Retrieved from http://ehrafworldcultures.yale.edu/document?id=sc13-002.
Portorreal, F. 2011. *Plantas medicinales en el Este dominicano. Estudio etnobotánico en las provincias de Monte Plata, Hato Mayor y El Seibo de la República Dominicana.* Santo Domingo: Instituto de Investigaciones Científicas Universidad Central del Este.
Portuondo Zúñiga, O. 2008. *La Virgen de la Caridad del Cobre. Símbolo de cubanía.* Santiago de Cuba: Editorial Oriente.
Portuondo Zúñiga, O. 2012a. *El Departamento Oriental en Documentos, Tomo I (1510-1799).* Santiago de Cuba: Editorial Oriente.

Portuondo Zúñiga, O. 2012b. *El Departamento Oriental en Documentos, Tomo II (1800-1868).* Santiago de Cuba: Editorial Oriente.

Portuondo Zúñiga, O. 2012c. *El Departamento Oriental. 1510-1868: dos temas de historia económica.* Santiago de Cuba: Ediciones Santiago.

Portuondo Zúñiga, O. 2016. No solo novedades en la ciencia arqueológica. In J. Ulloa Hung & R. Valcárel Rojas (ed.), *Los Indígenas más allá de Colón. Indígenas e indios en el Caribe Presencia, legado y estudio.* Santo Domingo: Búho.

Posselt Santoyo, E. & Jiménez Osorio, L. I. 2015. El ritual como restablecimiento del paisaje sagrado. In M.E.R.G.N. Jansen & V. Raffa (eds), *Tiempo y Comunidad. Herencias e interacciones socioculturales en Mesoamérica y Occidente.* Leiden: Leiden University Press.

Post, P., Nel, P. & Beek, W.E.A. van. 2014. *Sacred spaces and contested identities: Space and ritual dynamics in Europe and Africa.* Trenton, NJ: Africa World Press.

Preiswerk, R. & Perrot, D. 1978. *Ethnocentrism and history, Africa, Asia and Indian America in Western textbooks.* New York etc.: Nok International.

Pressley-Sanon, T. 2013. One Plus One Equals Three: *Marasa* Consciousness, the *Lwa*, and Three Stories. *Research in African Literatures 44*(3), 119-137.

Price, R. 1976. *An Anthropological Approach To The Afro-american Past: A Caribbean Perspective.* Boston: Beacon Press.

Price, R. 1983. *First-time: The historical vision of an Afro-American people.* Baltimore, London: Johns Hopkins University Press.

Prins, F. E. & Hall, S. 1994. Expressions of fertility, in the rock art of Bantu-speaking agriculturists. *The African Archaeological Review 12*: 171-203.

Puello Nina, R. & Tavarez, M. C. 2013. Un estudio Preliminar de la fiesta de San Francisco. *Boletín del Museo del Hombre Dominicano, 45.*

Puello Nina, R. & Tavarez M. C. 2016. Creencias, curaciones, promesas y milagros en la festividad de San Francisco en Bánica, Provincia Elías Piña. *Boletín del Museo del Hombre Dominicano, 47.*

Quiros-Moran, D. 2009. *Guide to Afro-Cuban Herbalism.* Bloomington, Indiana: Author House.

Quiroz, D. 2015. *Do not fear the supernatural! The relevance of ritual plant use for traditional culture, nature conservation, and human health in western Africa.* PhD thesis, Wageningen: Wageningen University.

RAH, Real Academia de la Historia. 1885. Coleccion de Documentos Inéditos Relativos al Descubrimiento, Conquista y la Organización de las Antiguas Posiciones Españolas. Tomo I. Madrid: Impresores de la Real Casa.

Ramsey, K. 2012. *The spirits and the law: vodou and power in Haiti.* Chicago and London: The University of Chicaco Press.

Rappaport, R. 1999. *Ritual and Religion in the Making of Humanity.* Cambridge: Cambridge University Press.

Rawley, J. A. & Behrendt, S. D. 2005. *The Transatlantic Slave Trade: A History.* Nebraska: University of Nebraska Press.

Real Cédula de Felipe II, 1841 [1570]. In *Recopilación de leyes de los reinos de las Indias: mandadas imprimir y publicar por la magestad católica del rey don Carlos II.* Madrid: Boix.

Regino y Espinal, F. B. 2006. Conucos, hatos y habitaciones en Santo Domingo, 1764-1827. *Boletín Archivo General de la Nación 31* (116), 487-555.
Restall, M. (ed.) 2005. *Beyond Black and Red. African – Native relations in colonial Latin America.* USA: UNM Press.
Ricourt, M. 2016. *The Dominican Racial Imaginary: Surveying the Landscape of Race and Nation in Hispaniola.* New Brunswick, New Jersey: Rutgers University Press.
Rival, L. 2012. Animism and the meanings of life: reflections from Amazonia. In M. Brightman, V. E. Grotti, O. Ulturgasheva (eds), *Animism in rainforest and tundra: personhood, animals, plants and things in contemporary Amazonia and Siberia* (pp. 69-81). New York/Oxford: Berghahn Books.
Rochas Vivas, M. 2010. *Antes del amanecer. Antología de los Andes y la sierra nevada de Santa Marta.* Bogotá: Biblioteca Básica de Los Indígenas de Colombia.
Rodríguez Bruzón, Y. 2015. *Estudio histórico de las haciendas holguineras de Guayacán, Managuaco y Yareniquén hasta el siglo XVIII, como parte de la dinámica del poblamiento de las Tierras Altas de Maniabón.* Tesis de Master en Historia y Cultura en Cuba. Universidad de Holguín Oscar Lucero Moya.
Rodriguez Cullel, C. & Peña Obregon, A. 2000. Taguabo y Maicabó: Un Testimonio e torno al elemento aborigen en el sincretismo religioso Cubano. *El Caribe Arqueológico, 4.*
Rodríguez Demorizi, E. 1944. *Documentos para la Histoira de la República Dominicana.* Vol. I. Ciudad Trujillo: Montalvo.
Rodríguez Demorizi, E. 1945. *Relaciones Históricas de Santo Domingo.* Vol. II. Ciudad Trujillo: Montalvo.
Rodríguez Demorizi, E. 1945. *Samaná, pasado y porvenir.* Ciudad Trujillo: Montalvo.
Rodríguez Demorizi, E. 1947. *Documentos para la Histoira de la República Dominicana.* Vol. II. Ciudad Trujillo: Montalvo.
Rodríguez Demorizi, E. 1957. *Relaciones Históricas de Santo Domingo.* Vol. III. Ciudad Trujillo: Montalvo.
Rodríguez Demorizi, E. 1978. *Fray Cipriano de Utrera. Noticias Historicas de Santo Domingo.* Santo Domingo: Editora Taller.
Rodríguez Morel, G. 2007. *Cartas de Cabildo de Santo Domingo en el siglo XVII.* Archivo General de la Nacion Vol. XXXIV. Santo Domingo: Búho.
Rodríguez Morel, G. 2007. *Cartas de la Real Audiencia de Santo Domingo (1530-1546).* Santo Domingo: Archivo General de la Nación.
Rodriguez Morel, G. 2011. *Cartas de la Real Audiencia de Santo Domingo (1547-1575).* Santo Domingo: Archivo General de la Nación.
Rodriguez Morel, G. 2015. *Cartas de la Real Audiencia de Santo Domingo (1575-1578).* Santo Domingo: Archivo General de la Nación.
Rodriguéz Ramos, R. & Pagán Jiménez, J. R. 2016. Sobre nuestras indigenidades boricuas. In J. Ulloa Hung & R. Valcárcel Rojas (eds), *Los Indígenas más allá de Colón. Indígenas e indios en el Caribe Presencia, legado y estudio.*
Rodríguez Ramos, R., Pagán-Jiménez, J. R., Narganes Storde, Y. & Lace, M. J. (Forthcoming). Guácaras in early precolonial Puerto Rico: the case of Cueva Ventana. In C.L. Hofman and A. Antczak (eds), *Middle to Late Holocene settlers of the Circum-Caribbean.* The University of Alabama Press, Tuscaloos.
Rodriguez Reyes, A. 1993. La Muerte, los muertos y los santeros. *Del Caribe 22*, 19-25.

Rodriguez Reyes, A. 1998. El Entorno y la Santería Cubana. *Del Caribe 27*, 24-30.

Rodríguez Suárez, R. & Pagán Jiménez J. R. 2006. Primeras evidencias directas del uso de plantas en la dieta de los grupos agroalfareros del Oriente de Cuba. *Catauro, Revista Cubana de Antropología 8*(14): 100-120.

Rodríguez Suárez, R. & Pagán Jiménez, J. R. 2008. The Burén in Cuban Precolumbian Archaeology: New Insights about Plant and Clay Griddle Use During the Late Ceramic Age of Western Caribbean through Starch Analysis. In C.L. Hofman, M. Hoogland & A.L. van Gijn (eds), *Crossing the Borders: New Methods and Techniques in the Study of Archaeological Materials from the Caribbean.* Tuscaloosa: The University of Alabama Press.

Rodriguez Suarez, R. & Pagán Jimenéz, J. R. 2009. The Burén in Precolonial Cuban Archeology. New Information Regarding The use of Plants during the Late Ceramic Age of Eastern Cuba Gathered through Starch Analysis. In C.L. Hofman, M. Hoogland & A.L. van Gijn (eds), *Crossing the Borders: New Methods and Techniques in the Study of Archaeological Materials from the Caribbean.* Tuscaloosa: The University of Alabama Press.

Roe, P. 1982. *Indians of the Vaupés Area of Colombia. The Cosmic Zygote. Cosmology in the Amazon Basin.* New Brunswick, New Jersey: Rutgers University Press.

Roersch, C., Tavares de Andrade, J. M. & Menédez, E. 1993. *Medicina Tradicional 500 años después. Historia y Consecuencias Actuales.* Santo Domingo: Búho.

Roersch, C. 2016. Medicinal plants in the Dominican Republic and their possible role in public health care. *Acta Hortic. 1125*, 249-254.

Roig y Mesa, T. 1974. *Plantas medicinales, aromáticas o venenosas de Cuba.* La Habana: Instituto del libro.

Romero Rodríguez, D. N. 24 October 2016. Historias tras Matthew: Refugiados en las cuevas. Retrieved from http://www.cubadebate.cu/noticias/2016/10/24/historias-tras-matthew-refugiados-en-las-cuevas/.

Roque, R. & Wagner, K. A. 2012. *Engaging Colonial Knowledge. Reading European Archives in World History.* Great Britain: Palgrave MacMillan.

Rosengarten, D. 2013. By the Rivers of Babylon: The Lowcountry Basket in Slavery and Freedom. In R. Voeks & J. Rashford (eds), *African Ethnobotany in the Americas.* New York: Springer.

Roth, W. E. 2011 [1915]. The Animism and the Folklore of The Guayana Indians. Guyana: The Caribbean Press.

Roura Álvarez, L. 2011. Supervivencia aborigen en la Habana Cuba Arqueológica. *Revista de Espeleología y Arqueología, 1(4)*, 29-37.

Rouse, I. 1992. The Taínos: Rise & decline of the people who greeted Columbus. New Haven [etc.]: Yale University Press.

Rousseau, J. J. 1761. *Upon the Origin and foundation of the Inequality among Mankind.* London: R. J. Dodsley. Retrieved from https://archive.org/details/discourseuponori00rous.

Russo, K. 2008. *Healing landscapes: An historical perspective.* ProQuest Dissertations Publishing.

Sáez, J. L. 1996. Los hospitales de la ciudad colonial de Santo Domingo: tres siglos de medicina dominicana (1503-1883). Santo Domingo: Organización Panamericana de la Salud.

Sáez, J. L. 2008. *Libro de bautismos de esclavos (1637-1670).* Santo Domingo: Archivo General de la Nación.

Said, E.W. 1978. *Orientalism.* New York: Vintage Books.

Samson, A. V. M., Wrapson, L. J., Cartwright, C. R., Sahy, D., Stacey, R. J. & Cooper. J. 2017. Artists before Columbus: A multi-method characterization of the materials and practices of Caribbean cave art. *Journal of Archaeological Science, 88*, 24-36.

Samson, A., Cooper, J. & Caamano-Dones, J. 2016. European visitors in native spaces: Using paleography to investigate early religious dynamics in the New World. *Latin American Antiquity, 27*(4), 443-461.

Samson, A.V. M. 2010. *Renewing the House: Trajectories of Social Life in the Yucayeque (community) of El Cabo, Higüey, Dominican Republic, AD 800 to 1504.* Leiden: Sidestone Press.

Santos-Granero, F. 1998. Writing History into the Landscape: Space, Myth, and Ritual in Contemporary Amazonia. American Ethnologist, 25(2), 128-148.

Santos-Granero, F. 2002. The Arawakan Matrix: Ethos, Language, and History in Native South America. In J. D. Hill & F. Santos-Granero (eds), *Comparative Arawakan Histories. Rethinking Language Family and Culture Area in Amazonia.* Urbana and Chicago: University of Illinoius.

Santos-Granero, F. 2009. *The Occult Life of Things.* Arizona: University of Arizona Press.

Sauer, C. O. 1925. The Morphology of Landscape. In J. Agnew, D. N. Livingstone & A. Rogers, *Human geography: an essential anthology* (ed.), Great Britain: T. J. International Limited.

Schaffer, W., Carr, R., Day, J. & Pateman, M. 2012. Lucayan-Taíno burials from Preacher's cave, Eleuthera, Bahamas. *International Journal of Osteoarchaeology, 22*(1), 45-69.

Schiebinger, L. 2017. *Secret cures of slaves: People, plants, and medicine in the eighteen-th-century Atlantic world.* Stanford, California: Stanford University Press.

SEE, Secretaría de Estado de Educación, 2007. *Ciencias Sociales 3. Educación básica.* Santo Domingo: Centario.

SEH, Sociedad Economica Habana, 1847. Real Junta de Fomento de Agricultura y Comercio y Sociedad Economica Habana. Estadistica. Referente á la Tenecia de Gobierno de Giguaní en el Departamento Oriental de la isla de Cuba. In Anales de las Reales Junta de Fomento Real Junta de Fomento de Agricultura y Comercio y Sociedad Economica Habana, Habana: Imprenta del Gobierno y Capitania general por S.M.

Siegel, P. 2005. *Ancient Bonriquen. Archeology and Ethnohistory of Native Puerto Rico.* Tuscaloosa, Alabama: The University of Alabama Press.

Siegel, P. E. (ed.) 2018. *Island Historical Ecology: Socionatural Landscapes of the Eastern and Southern Caribbean.* Oxford and New York: Berghahn.

Siegel, P. E., Jones, J. G., Pearsall, D. M., Dunning N. P., Farrell, P., Duncan, N.A., Curtis, J. H. & Singh S. K. 2018. Humanizing the Landscapes of the Lesser Antilles during the Archaic. In B. A. Reid, *The Archaeology of Caribbean and Circum-Caribbean Farmers (5000 BC – AD 1500)* (pp. 55-70). London: Routledge.

Silliman, S. W. 2009. Change and Continuity, Practice and Memory: Native American Persistence in Colonial New England. *American Antiquity, 74*(2), 211-230.

Slater, J. 2014. *Medical Cultures of the Early Modern Spanish Empire*. Farnham: Ashgate Publishing Ltd.

Sloane, H. 1707. *A voyage to the islands Madera, Barbados, Nieves, S. Christophers and Jamaica with the natural history … of the last of those islands; to which is prefix'd an introduction, wherein is an account of the inhabitants, air, waters, diseases, trade.* London: Printed by B. M. for the author.

Sluyter, A. 2001. Colonialism and Landscape in the Americas: Material/Conceptual Transformations and Continuing Consequences. Annals of Association of American Geographers 91 (2): 410 – 428.

Snelders, S. 2012. *Vrijbuiters van de heelkunde: Op zoek naar medische kennis in de tropen, 1600-1800.* Amsterdam [etc.]: Atlas.

Sonnemann, T. F., Ulloa Hung, J. & Hofman, C. L. 2016. Mapping Indigenous Settlement Topography in the Caribbean Using Drones. *Remote Sensing, 8* (10), 791.

Stephen, H. 2002. *Winti: Levenshouding en religie.* Kampen: Kok.

Sued Badillo, J. 1978. *Los caribes: realidad o fábula.* Río Piedras: Editorial Antillana.

Sued Badillo, J. 2003. The Indigenous societies in the time of conquest. In B. W. Higman (ed.), *General History of the Caribbean. Methodology and Historiography of the Caribbean (Vol. VI).* London and Oxford: UNESCO Publishing.

SVD, Slave Voyage Database. Retrieved from slavevoyages.org, accessed on 1 August 2017.

Taçon, P. S. C. 2010. Identifying ancient sacred landscapes in Australia. From physical to social. In R. W. P. & S. A. Mrozowski (ed.), *Contemporary archaeology in theory: the new pragmatism* (pp. 77-91). United Kingdom: Wiley-Blackwell.

Taíno Legacies Project. Retrieved from http://www.tainolegacies.com/ (Accessed on 10 October 2014).

Talbot, A. 2002. Pilgrimage to Healing Shrines: The Evidence of Miracle Accounts. *Dumbarton Oaks Papers, 56*, 153-173.

Tanna, L. 1993. *Jamaican folk tales and oral histories (2nd Edit.).* Kingston: Institute of Jamaica Publ.

Tausiet, M. 2014. *Urban Magic in Early Modern Spain. Abracadabra Omnipotens*, Hampshire and New York: Palgrave Macmillan.

Taylor, D. 1952. Tales and Legends of the Dominican Caribs. *The Journal of American Folklore, 65*, 267-279.

Taylor, D. 1945. Carib Folk-Beliefs and Customs from Dominica. *Southwestern Journal of Anthropology. 1* (4), 507 -530.

Taylor, D. M. 1938. Caribs Of Dominica. *Bulletin; Anthropological Papers*, 103-159.
Retrieved from: http://ehrafworldcultures.yale.edu/document?id=st13-006.

Taylor, D. M. & Moore, H. C. 1948. "Note On Dominican Basketry And Its Analogues." *Southwestern Journal Of Anthropology, 4* 328-43. http://ehrafworld-cultures.yale.edu/document?id=st13-007.

Taylor, P. & Case, F. I. 2013. The Encyclopedia of Caribbean Religions: Volume 1: A – L; Volume 2: M – Z: University of Illinois Press.

Tedlock, B. 1987. An interpretive solution to the problem of humoral medicine in Latin America. *Social Science & Medicine, 24*(12), 1069-1083.

Tejeda Ortiz, D. 1978. *Mana, monografía de un movimiento mesiánico abortado.* República Dominicana: Alfa y Omega.

Tejeda Ortiz, D. 2013. *El Vudú en Dominicana y en Haití.* Republica Dominicana: Indefolk.

Tertre, J. B. Du, McKusick, M. B. & Verin, P. 1667. Concerning The Natives Of The Antilles. *General History Of The Antilles Occupied By The French ....* Paris: T. Iolly. Retrieved from: http://ehrafworldcultures.yale.edu/document?id=st13-004 (Accessed on 3 March 2017).

The Laws of Burgos 1512. Retrieved from://faculty.smu.edu/bakewell/bakewell/texts/burgoslaws.html (Accessed on 6 June 2017).

Todorov, T. 1982. *The Conquest of America: The Question of the Other.* New York: Harper & Rosw Publishers.

Torres-Cuevas, E. & Loyola Vega, O. 2002. *Historia de Cuba 1492-1898. Formación y Liberación de la Nación.* Habana: Pueblo y Educación.

Tricando, M. 1997. El aborigen y la Caridad del Cobre. *El Caribe Arqueológico, 2* (1), 14-120.

Trouillot, M. R. 1995. *Silencing the Past: Power and the Production of History.* Boston: Beacon Press.

Tuhiway Smith, L. 1999. *Decolonizing Methodologies: Research and Indigenous Peoples.* London & New York: Zed Books Ltd.

Turner, H.W. & MacKenzie, P. R. 1977. *Rudolf Otto: The idea of the Holy: Commentary on a shortened version: A guide for students.* Aberdeen: Aberdeen Peoples Press.

Ulloa Hung J. 2014. *Arqueología en la Línea Noroeste de La Española. Paisajes, cerámicas e interacciones.* Santo Domingo: Instituto Tecnológico de Santo Domingo.

Ulloa Hung, J. & Herrera Malatesta, E. 2015. Investigaciones arqueológicas en el norte de La Española. Entre viejos esquemas y nuevos datos, *Boletín del Museo del Hombre Dominicano XLII (46)*, 75-107.

Ulloa Hung, J. 2015. Cultura material, patrimonio arqueológico y diáspora africana en la República Dominicana. Un enfoque crítico-epistemológico. *Ciencia y Sociedad 40*(1), 77-107.

Ulloa Hung, J. 2015. Española, entre viejos esquemas y nuevos datos. *Boletín del Museo del Hombre Dominicano, 46,* 75-107.

Ulloa Hung, J. 2016. Colonialismo, Indigenismo, y Arquelogía en República Dominicana: silencios confusos y encubrimiento diversos. In J. Ulloa Hung & Valcárcel Rojas, R. (eds), *Los Indígenas más allá de Colón. Indígenas e indios en el Caribe Presencia, legado y estudio.*

Ulloa Hung, J. & Valcárel Rojas, R. (eds) 2016. *Los Indígenas más allá de Colón. Indígenas e indios en el Caribe Presencia, legado y estudio.* Santo Domingo: Búho.

Urbani, B. & Urbani, F. 2010-2011. Relaciones sobre cuevas en el continente americano durante los siglos XV y XVI, parte I, Suramérica y el Caribe. Bol. Soc. *Venezolana Espeleol.,* 44, 2-34.

Valcárcel Rojas, R. & Pérez Concepción, H. 2014. *Indios de Holguín.* Holguín: La Mezquita.

Valcárcel Rojas, R. 1997. Introducción a la arqueología del contacto indohispánico en la Provincia de Holguín, Cuba. *El Caribe Arqueológico, 2*, 64-77.

Valcárcel Rojas, R. 2012. Interacción colonial en un pueblo de indios encomendados: el Chorro de Maíta, Cuba. Ph.D. dissertation, Faculty Archaeology, Leiden University.

Valcárcel Rojas, R. 2016. *Archaeology of early colonial interaction at El Chorro de Maíta, Cuba.* Gainesville: University Press of Florida.

Valcárcel Rojas, R. 2016. Cuba. Indios después de Colón. In J. Ulloa Hung & Valcárel Rojas, R. (eds), *Los Indígenas más allá de Colón. Indígenas e indios en el Caribe Presencia, legado y estudio*. Santo Domingo: Búho.

Valcárcel Rojas, R. Samson, A. V. M & Hoogland, M. L. P. 2013. Indo-Hispanic Dynamics: From Contact to Colonial Interaction in the Greater Antilles. *International Journal of Historical Archeology.* Springer.

Valdés Bernal, S. 1991. *Las lenguas indígenas de América y el español de Cuba.* La Habana: Editorial Academia.

Vansina, J. 1987. *Oral Tradition as History.* Wisconsin: The University of Wisconsin Press.

Vargas, T. 2002. *Ciencias Sociales 4. Educación básica.* Santo Domingo: Editorial Edisa.

Vega Suñol, J. 2014. Los aborígenes de Cuba en la etnohistoria de Holguín: un acercamiento a los libros bautismales de los siglos XVIII y XIX. In Valcárcel Rojas, R. & H. Pérez Concepción, *Indios de Holguín.* Holguín: La Mezquita.

Vega, B. 1981. *Herencía Indigena en la Cultura Dominicana.* Santo Domingo: Ediciones del Museo Del Hombre Dominicano.

Vega, B. 1988. *Ensayos sobre cultura dominicana* (2a. ed.). Santo Domingo: Fundación Cultural Dominicana: Museo del Hombre Dominicano.

Verschuuren, B., Wild, R., McNeely, J. & Oviedo, G. 2010. *Sacred Natural Sites Conserving Nature and Culture.* London/Washington: Earthscan.

Vespucci, A. (1509). *Diss büchlin saget wie die zwē durchlüchtigstē herrē her Fernandus K. zů Castilien und herr Emanuel K. zů Portugal haben das weyte mör ersůchet unnd funden vil Insulen, und ein Nüwe welt von wilden nackenden Leüten, vormals unbekant.* Gedruckt zů Strassburg: Durch Johānē Grüniger. Retrieved from online catalogue of the British Library.

Vidal, S. M. 2000. Kuwe Duwakalumi: The Arawak Sacred Routes of Migration, Trade, and Resistance. *Ethnohistory, 47*(3), 635-667.

Vidal, S. M. 2011. The Arawak-Speaking Groups of Northwestern Amazonia: Amerindian Cartography as a Way of Preserving and Interpreting the Past. In N. L. Whitehead, *Of Cannibals and Kings. Primal Anthropology in Americas.* Pennsylvania State University: University Press.

Villalón, M. E. & Corradini, H. 2011. Predeterminaciones fatales: la construcción discursiva de la menlancolía entre los E´ñepa de Venezuela. In G. V. Freire (ed.), *Perspectivas en salud indígena. Cosmovisión, enfermedad y políticas públicas.* Ecuador: Abya-Yala.

Viveiros De Castro, E. 1998. *Cosmological Deixsis and Amerindian Perspectivism.* Cambridge: King's College Cambridge.

Voeks, R. & Rashford, J. 2013. *African ethnobotany in the Americas.* New York, London: Springer.

Vonk, J. & Shackelford, T. K. (eds) 2012. *The Oxford handbook of comparative evolutionary psychology.* New York: Oxford University Press.

Vossen T., Towns A., Ruysschaert S., Quiroz D. & van Andel T. 2014. Consequences of the Trans-Atlantic Slave Trade on Medicinal Plant Selection: Plant Use for Cultural Bound Syndromes Affecting Children in Suriname and Western Africa. *PLoS ONE 9*(11).

Walton, G. M. & Cohen, G. L. 2011. A brief social-belonging intervention improves academic and health outcomes of minority students. *Science, 331(6023), 1447-51.*

Watts, D. 1990. *The West Indies: Patterns of development culture and environmental change since 1492.* Cambridge [etc.]: Camnbridge University Press.

Wheat, D. 2016. *Atlantic Africa and the Spanish Caribbean, 1570-1640.* Chapel Hill: University of North Carolina Press.

Whitehead, N. L. 2002. Arawak Linguistic and Cultural Identity through Time: Contact, Colonialism, and Creolization. In J. D. Hill & F. Santos-Granero (eds), *Comparative Arawakan Histories. Rethinking Language Family and Culture Area in Amazonia.* Urbana and Chicago: University of Illinoius.

Whitehead, N. L. 2003. *Histories and historicities in Amazonia.* University of Nebraska Press.

Whitehead, N. L. 2011. *Of Cannibals and Kings. Primal Anthropology in Americas.* Pennsylvania State University: University Press.

Whitehead, N. L. (ed.) 1995. *Wolves from the sea: readings in the anthropology of the native Caribbean.* Leiden: KITLV Press.

Wilbert, W. & Ayala Lefée-Wilbert, C. 2011. Fitoterapia warao: fundamentos teóricos. In G. V. Freire (eds), *Perspectivas en salud indígena. Cosmovisión, enfermedad y políticas públicas.* Ecuador: Abya-Yala.

Wiley, J. 2007. *Landscape.* Oxon: Routledge.

Williams, A. 1998. Therapeutic landscapes in holistic medicine. *Soc. Sci. Med., 46*(9), 1193-1203.

Willow, A. 2010. Images of American Indians in Environmental Education: Anthropological Reflections on the Politics and History of Cultural Representation. *American Indian Culture and Research Journal, 34*(1), 67-88.

Wilson, K. 2003. Therapeutic Landscapes and First Nations peoples: an exploration of culture, health and place. *Health & Place. 9*(2): 83-93.

Wilson, S. 2007. *The archaeology of the Caribbean.* New York: Cambridge University Press.

Wylie, J. 2007. *Landscape.* London etc.: Routledge.

Yaremko, J. 2016. *Indigenous passages to Cuba, 1515-1900.* Gainesville: University Press of Florida.

Yero Masdeu, J. 2016. *El aporte de los aborígenes a la conformación de la sociedad criolla en los de la actual provincia de Granma.* Retrieved from://www.crisol.cult.cu/index.php/actualidad/articulos/926-el-aporte-de-los-aborigenes-a-la-conformacion-de-la-sociedad-criolla-en-los-territorios-de-la-actual-provincia-de-granma.html.

Zambrano, H. 2009. *Historia de Boyá.* Monte Plata: Impresos de Monte Plata.

Zent, E. L & Zent, S. 2011. Ser y volverse jodi: la construcción del yo, el cuerpo y la persona a través de las prácticas curativas indígena. In G. V. Freire (eds), *Perspectivas en salud indígena. Cosmovisión, enfermedad y políticas públicas.* Ecuador: Abya-Yala.

Attachment

Photos from Various Locations

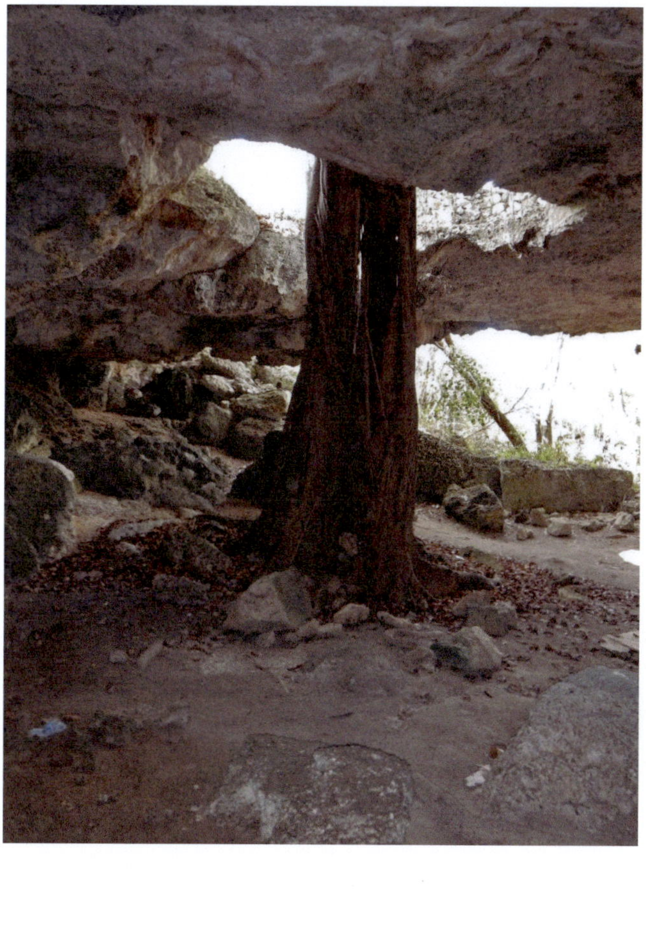

Figure 80 A cavern in Boca de Yuma used by followers of Evangelism, Dominican Repulic.

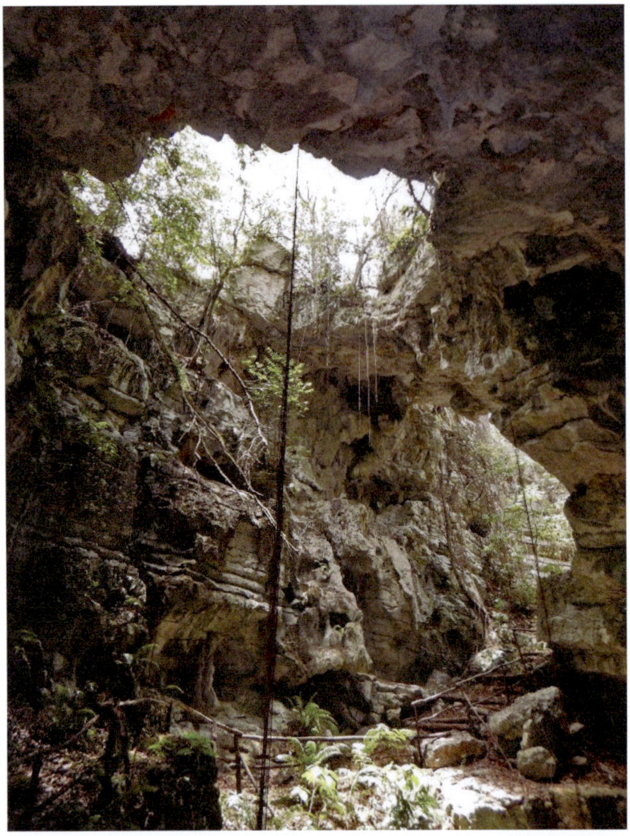

Figure 81 One of caves in Pommier where flower offerings are brought, Dominican Republic.

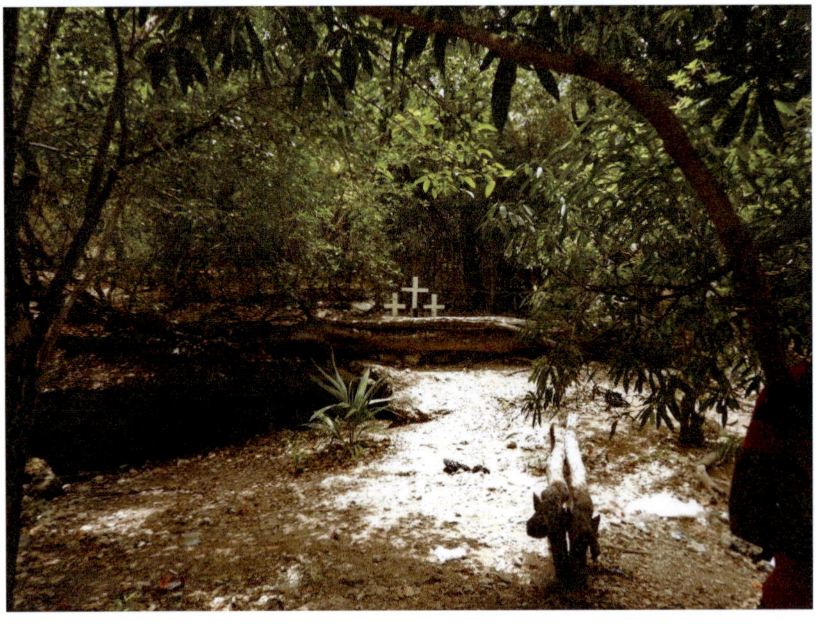

Figure 82 A location at Cepi Cepi where the celebrations of Holy Cross take place, Dominican Republic.

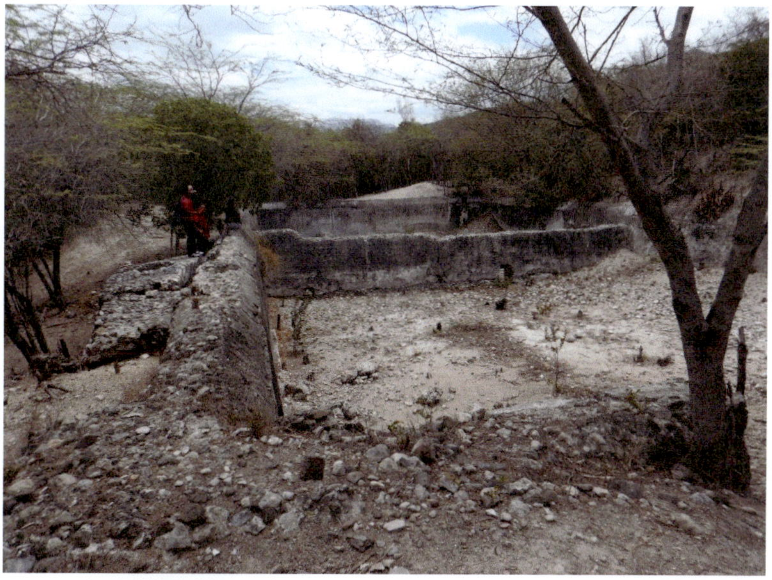

Figure 83 Part of archeological site Cepi Cepi.

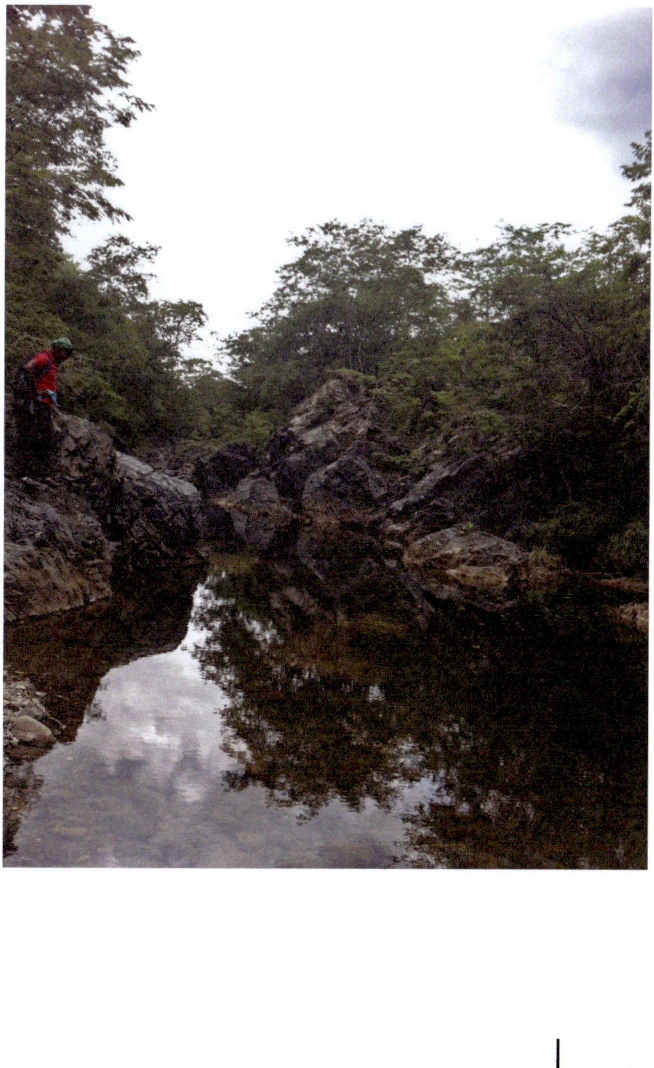

Figure 84 Chacuey river, the Pool of Indigenous Misterios, Dominican Republic.

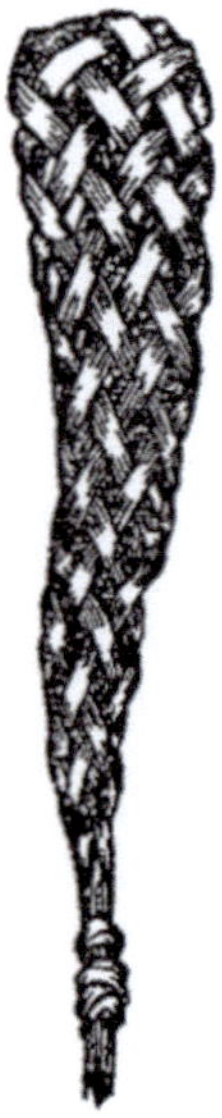

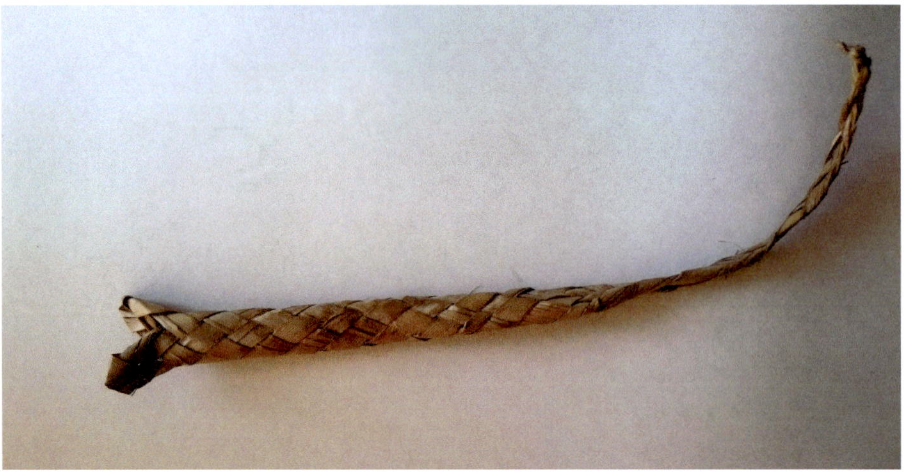

Figure 85 Left: "Attrappe-la-main" or "wife leader" in Taylor (1938), above: atrapa dedo from Pedro Santana, Dominican Republic.

Plant use overview

Abre camino	*Vitex trifolia* L *Koanophyllon villosum* (Sw.)	Baths	Old World (native: Africa, Asia, Pacific).the second native to Americas
Anica	*Critonia aromatisans*	Baths good luck, boneache	New World (West Indies)
Ajonjolí	*Sesamum radiatum* *Sesamum orientale L.*	Against witchcraft	Old World (West Africa)
Álamo	*Ficus religiosa L.* *Alamo blanco*= Thespesia populnea *(L.)*	To lose weight, for cleaning livers, dries out sores, baths for good luck	Old World Thespesia Old and New World
Albahaca morada	*Ocimum campechianum* *Albehaca blanca* Ocimum basilicum *L.*	Sweet baths against withcraft	New World Old World
Algarroba	*Hymenaea courbaril* L.	Immune system	New World
Amapola	*Erythrina poeppigiana*	Pneumonia	New World (CA)
Anacaüita	*Sterculia foetida L.*	Headache	New World
Anamú	*Petiveria alliacea* L.	Cold	New World
Apazote	*Chenopodium ambrosioides* L.	Parasites	Central America, South America,
Arroz		Roots Poisonous	Old World
Broquelejo	*Piper peltatum* L.	Cleansing after giving birth, for women trying to get pregnant	New World
Bayahonda	*Prosopis juliflora* (Sw.)	For the Cross	New World
Bejuco Indio	*Gouania polygama* (Jacq.)	Baths for child for skin, mabí	New World
Bejuco lombri	*Vanilla spp.* *Philodendron consanguineu*	Parasites	Both New World

Table 6 Medicinal Plant Use in Boyá.

Bejuco caro	*Cissus spp.*	Kidneys	New World
Bruca hembra	*Senna obtusifolia*	Bronchytis	New World
Cadillo de tres pies	*Pavonia spinifex* (L.)	Kidneys infection	New World
Café Leaf		(leaf) Parasitos	Old World
Capa puertoriqueño		Indigestión, cleansing of body, baths for good luck	New World
Caña brava	*Gynerium sagittatum* (Aubl.) *Bambusa bambos* (L.)	Misterio	New World Old World
Cardo Santo	*Argemone mexicana L.*	Infections	New World
Ceiba	*Ceiba petandra L.*	Misterio, Baths, Tootache (cotton)	New World
Cereza	*Malpighiaceae* *Malpighia glabra L. Malpighia glabra L.*	Flu	New World New World
Coco	*Cocos nucifera* L.	Coconut Nacidos, Skin infection (aceite)	Old World
Cola de caballo	*Chloris ciliata* Sw.	Kidneys	New World
Cuaba	*Pinus occidentalis* Sw.	Rheumatism, Diabetis,	New World
Cundeamor	*Momordica charantia* L.	Cold, Baths, Smallpox	Old World from West Africa with the slave trade.
Escoba amarga	*Parthenium hysterophorus* L.	Clean from inside	New World
Flor de libertad	*Moringa oleifera* Lam.	Cough	Old World (native: India)
Guacima		Infections, Ahogo/ pressure in the chest that does not allow to breath properly	New World
Guahabo	*Senna alata* (L.)	Parasites, purgative	New World
Guanábana		Flu	New World
Guayaba	*Psidium guajava* L.	Diarrhea, Flu,	New World
Higo	*Ficus carica* L., Ficus umbrifera, Urostigma laurifolium	Has misterio	Old World, New World
Higüero	*Crescenia cujete*	Clean from inside, vaginal infections	New World
Jagua	*Genipa americana* L.	Refreshment of blood	New World
Juan prieto	*Varronia curassavica* Jacq.	Chiqunguya	New World
Juana La Blanca	*Spermacoce spp.*	Cholesterol	New World
Lechoza	*Carica papaya* L.	Parasites	New World
Magüey	*Agave spp.*	Clean from inside, Vaginal Infections, Headache	New World
Magueyito	*Tetramicra canaliculata* (Aubl.)	Headache	New World
Mala madre			Unidentified
Mamón	*Annona reticulata* L.	Diarrhea	New World
Maravelí	*Securidaca virgata* Sw.	Clean from inside	New World
Marcasá	*Mecardonia dianthera*	Infection of uterus	New World New World,
Mate negro	*Sapindus saponaria L.*	Amulets for protection of children	New World
Miona	*Unidentified*	Kidneys	Unidentified

Table 6 (continued) Medicinal Plant Use in Boyá.

Mora	*Solanum nigrum L. var. Americanum*	Nerves, kidneys,rheumatism	Unidentified
Marilopez	*Turnera ulmifolia* L.	Vaginales inf.	New World
Guano		Viernes santos	New World
Naranja agria (l.)	*Citrus x aurantium* L.	Flue, Hepatitis (+cinnamon) for Anemia	Old World
Oregano		Diarrhea	Old World
Osua	*Myrcianthes fragrans* (Sw.) *Pimenta racemosa* (Mill.)	Flu, fever	New World New World
Periquito	*Ruellia tuberosa* L.	Infections	New World
Piñón	*Erythrina berteroana* Urb. *Jatropha curcas* L.	Together with Bruca for smallpox Misterio	Both New World
Quibey	*Hippobroma longiflora* (L.)	Poisonous	New World
Quina	*Unidentified*	Blood	
Ruda	*Ruta chalenpensis*	Protection against evil, baths	Old World
Sábila	*Aloe vera* (L.)	Against witchcraft, baths	Old World (SW. Arabian Pen.)
Sen	*Cassia acutifolia* *Senna bicapsularis (L.) Roxb. var. bicapsularis (Fl. Ind., ed. 1832, 2: 342. 1832.)*	Parasites	Old World New World
Tamarindo	*Tamarindus indica* L.	Hepatitis	Old World (native: Africa, Asia),
Tautau	*Jatropha gossypiifolia L.*	Stomache, Parasites	C, CA, SA
Timacle	*Chiococca alba* (L.)	Kidneys	New World
Tobacco	*Nicotiana tabacum*	Wounds, Stomach pain, headache, calling lwas	New World
Tuna de España	*Nopalea cochenillifera* (L.)	For clothes ,Infections	New World (CA, SA)
Uayama	*Cucurbita pepo* L.	Parasites, Hearth diseases	New World
Verbena	*Glandularia hybrida* *Bouchea prismatica* (L.) *Stachytarpheta jamaicensis* *Verbena officinalis*	Indigestion, baths	New Wolrd West Indies West Indies Old World
Verdolaga	*Trianthema portulacastrum* L.	Stomachache, Flatulence	Old and New World Pantropical
Verón		Baths for good luck	
Yucca	*Manihot esculenta* Crantz	(leaf) Kidneys, (almidón de) =>skin rush	New World
Yerba de calentura/	*Cymbopogon citratus* (DC.)	Tea served during nine days wake, together with jengibre, clavo dulce, osua.	Old World

Table 6 (continued) Medicinal Plant Use in Boyá.

This overview was based on the information provided by Mrs. Dorotea Mejía.The scientific name of plants was based on the publication of Roig (1974). For the origin of the plants was used publication of Acevedo-Rodríguez & Strong (2012), based on the scientific names indicated by Roig. As it is often difficult to distinguish between precolonial and colonial migration of plants from Mesoamerica, South America and Caribbean, the category New World was used to distinguish from plants brought in the colonial time from regions known to Europeans previously to 1492, so-called Old World. The abbreviation of the regions are as follow: C stands for Caribbean, can indicate several, but not all every time all Caribbean islands. A stands for Americas, CA refers to Central America, SA to South America , NA to North America, TA to Tropical America, and similarly also the plant can live in one, or several lands of this region.

Common Name	*Latin Name*	Use	Origin
Abre Camino	*Vitex trifolia* L.	Spiritual purification, matrimonial problems	Old World (native: Africa, Asia, Pacific)
Achiote	*Bixa orellana*	Alimentation, to defend against enemies	New World
Agrimonia	*Teucrium cubense* Jacq.	Diabetis	New World
Aguate	*Persea americana*	Infection, Parasites, Diabetis	New World
Ají	*Capsicum frutescens var. Baccatum*	Diabetis	New World (but also Tropics of Old World)
Ajo	*Allivium sativum*	Cancer, Boneache, Parasites	Old World
Albahaca	*Ocimum spp.*	Gives the hope Against headache	
Albahaca morada	*Ociumum sanctum (Roig)*	Pain, Diabetes, High blood pressure, Stress, Gastritis, to Ward off spirts and evil spells	Old World (Tropics of Old World)
Algodón morado	*Gossypium spp.*	Flu, Baths for removing harmful spirits and spells	Tropics, Subtropics
Almendro de India	*Terminalio catappa*	Parasites	Asia
Amansaguapo	*Gymnanthes albicans*	Spiritual purification	New World
Anacagüita	*Sterculia apetala*	Love, inhabited by potentially dangerous spirits	New World (Colombia)
Anamú, also called espante de muerto	*Petiveria alliacea*	Catarrh, Colon Cancer, blood circulation, Toothache Spiritual, purification, to remote malevolant spirits	New World (A)
Anis	*Decarinium latifolium, Pimpinella anisum*	Digestion, Catarrh, to calm down	Caribbean, NA,SA, Mediterrean
Anon	*Annona squamosa L.*	Stomach, Indigestion	CA, SA
Apasote	*Chenopodium ambrosioides L.*	Parasites, Evil eye, draw away the bad luck	New World (Chenopodium spathu-latum also New and Old World)
Ármica	*Jatropha multifida L.*	Blood Circulation	C, CA, SA
Ateje	*Cordia rariflora A.*	Sore throat	New World (C)
Auyá	*Zanthoxylum martinicense*	Evil eye, for good and harmful spells	New World (C, SA)
Behuco Indio	*Gouania polygama* *Gouania lupuloides* (L.)	Prú	Both New World (C, CA, SA)
Behuco ubí	*Cissus sicyoides L.*	Necklace for horses	New World (C, TA)
Bijagua	*Colubrina obtusata*	Eczema	New World (CA, NA)
Bora	*Unidentified*	Disrupt the evil spells	Unidentified
Cabalongo	*Thevetia peruviana*	Evil eye	C, TA, native to Mexico
Cactus	*Opuntia spp.* *Nopalea spp.*	To protect the home	New World
Caimito de Cimarón	*Hirtela spp.* *Chrysophyllum cainito L.*	Spiritual purification	All New World
Calabaza	*Curcubita maxima* *Cucurbita pepo L.*	Good luck, prosperity	Old World (India) Roig New World (CA, NA)
Caña mejicana	*Cheilocostus speciosus*	Kidneys	Asia
Caña santa	*Cheilocostus speciosus*	Fever	Old World (Tropical Asia and Malesia)

Table 7 Medicinal plants Jiguaní.

Common Name	*Latin Name*	Use	Origin
Canafistola	*Cathartocarpus fistula*	Diabetis, infections of blood	Old World (Tropical Asia)
Caoba	*Swietenia mahagoni L.*	Atleets fotos, Spiritual protection, cross	C
Ceiba	*Ceiba pentandra (L.)*	to Ward off malecious spell, all saints, offers, vows to Virgen	C, CA, SA
Coco	*Cocos nucifera L.*	Kidneys´ infection, Prosperity, Cleansing, purifying	Native to Malesia and Pacific Region coastal regions.
Contraguao	*Guettarda calyptrata Ouratea agrophylla Urban.*	To diminish the reaction to guao tree	Both endemic to Cuba
Cuabá	*Amyris balsamifera L.*	Baths	C, SA
Cuayahabo	*Unidentified*	Evil eye	Unidentified
Cundiamor	*Momordica charantia* L.	Stomach, Against Parasites, Abortive	Old World (Pantropical)
Damajagua	*Pariti tiliaceum*	Hair	C, CA, SA
Escoba amarga	*Parthenium hysterophorus L.*	Fever	New World (C, CA, SA, NA)
Frijol carita		Cleansing	
Garañon/maya	*Bromelia karatas L.*	Prostata, infection of prostate, stones	C, CA, SA
Guacima	*Guazuma ulmifolia*	Kidneys	C, CA, SA
Guaguací	*Zuelania guidonia*	Diarrhea, Kidneys, Rheumatism, Hair loss	C
Guajaca	*Tillandsia usneoides L.*	Blood pressure	C, AT
Guama	*Lonchocarpus domingensis*	Colon pain	C
Guanabana	*Annona muricata L*	Indigestion, Flu, Blood pressure, Cancer, Attracting good, economic prosperity	New World (CA, SA)
Guayaba	*Psidium guajava L.*	Diarrhea, Pain, Stomache	New World (C)
Güira	*Crescentia cujete* L.	Flu, Vaginal infections, constipations	New World
Guizazo de baracoa	*Xanthium strumarium L.*	Kidneys	NA
Gupito	*Unidentified*	During childbirth, Ward off evil spirits, To avoid problems	Unidentified
Guyacán	*Guaiacum officinale L.*	Desinfection during epidemics with the smoke, Before pulling tooth to loosen it up, Amulets for protection	New World (C, CA, SA)
Hierba Buena	*Mentha spicata L.*	Indigestion, the stomachpain dolor de Stomach, Gastric problems	Old World
Hierba de Aura	*Hyptis spicata*	Spiritual purification	C, CA, SA
Hoja de Aire	*Kalanchoe pinnata*	Inflammation of the ears, To ward off evil	Madagascar
Jaboncillo	*Sapindus saponaria L.*	Prú, Amulets for protection of children	New World (Caribbean)
Jagüey	*Ficuss spp.*	Hunting the birds	C, Americas
Jíba	*Erythroxylon havanense*	cross amulets for children, wood	Cuba
Jiquí	*Pera bumeliaefolia*	Toothache	Cuba, DR
Jiribía	*Dichanthium caricosum L.*	Add to clay called cocoa for construction of houses and burénes	Distribution: Exotic in Cuba and Lesser Antilles (Barbados), native to Asia and Malesia
Jobaban	*Trichilia hirta L.*	Leukemia, prostate, inflamaciones, cancer de prostata	Cuba, C, CA, SA
Jobo	*Spondias mombin L.*	Baths, cleansing	New and Old World
Maguey	*Agave legrelliana also Agave Americana*	Soap, rope	1st Cuba, 2nd A

Table 7 (continued) Medicinal plants Jiguaní.

Common Name	*Latin Name*	Use	Origin
Magüiro	*Enallagma latifolia*	Stomach	C
Majagua	*Hibiscus elatus*	Bath for children	C
Manahú	*Unidentified*	Astma	U Unidentified
Mango	*Mangifera indica*	Flu	Old World
Mano poderosa	*Syngonium podophyllum*		Native to Asia and Malesia.
Manzanilla	*Matricaria chamomilla*	Stomache, Skin, diabetis	Old World (Europe, Africa, Asia)
Manzanillo	*Hippomane mancinella L.*	Diabetis	New World (C, CA, AT)
Masqüiro	*Unidentified*	Vaginal infections	Unidentified
Mata Negro	*Rourea sympetala*	Poisonous	C, CA, SA
Matuerzo	*Lepidium viriginicum L.,*	Flatulence, kidneys, To disturp the life of others, ward off negative	Caribbean, NA
Maya	*Bromelia pinguin L.*	Parasites	Caribbean, CA, SA
Mejorana	*Origanum majorana* L.	Diarrhea, parasites, digestion, stomach, ear infections, hemeroids, To avoid the bad luck	Old World
Melon	*Citrullus vulgaris*	Fever	Africa Tropical
Mora	*Solanum nigrum L. var. Americanum*	Poisonous, Stomach, Vaginal infections, inflamations	Euroasia
Moringa	*Moringa oleifera Lam*	Osteoarthritis, Nerves, Nutritive, Cancer	Tropical Asia
Nomeolvide	*Unidentified*	Love	Unidentified
Oregano	*Origanum vulgare*	Catarrh	Europe Asia
Palo Brazil	*Caesalpinia bahamensis* Lam. subsp. *bahamensis*	Kidneys, To lower the level of blood sugar, To cause the fights	Native Antillas, CA,
Palo de Caja	*Allophylus cominia L.*	Diabetis	Caribbean, CA, SA,
Paraíso	*Melia azedarach L.*	For spritual development	Asia
Peonia	*Abrus Precatorius L.*	To cause fights	Caribbean, American and Old World Tropics
Pimpinilla	*Poterium sanguisorba*	Skin diseases, Parasites, Vaginal Infections, Abortive	Old World
Piñon	*Jatropha curcas L.*	Evil eye	Caribbean, Americas
Pirulí	*Codiaeum variegatum (L.)*	To cause disruption, fights	Asia
Pulcillana	*Unidentified*	Matrimonial problems	Unidentified
Quebracho	*Ehretia tinifolia L.*	Spiritual purification	Caribbean, CA,
Queremernucho	*Unidentified*		Unidentified
Romerillo	*Bidens pilosa L.*	Catarrh	C, A, and Old World Tropics
Romero	*Rosmarinus officinalis*	Hair, Love	Mediterranean
Rompezaraüey	*Eupatorium odoratum L.*	Stomache, To avoid bad luck, to disrupt the evil spells, matrimonial problems	C, AT
Ruda	*Ruta chalenpensis*	Stomach, Digestion, Good luck	Old World
Sábila	*Aloe vera* (L.)	Parasites, accelerate healing of scars, desifects, anticancerigeno, skin, infections of uterus, Sore throat	Old World (SW. Arabian Pen.)
Salvadera	*Hura Crepitans L.*	Cough	C, SA, CA
Salvía	*Salvia oficinalis*	Catarrh, Sore throat, To rescue the souls	Old World

Table 7 (continued) Medicinal plants Jiguaní.

Common Name	*Latin Name*	Use	Origin
Sasafrán	*Bursera graveolens*	Stomach, everything	New World (CA, SA)
Sen	*Cassia acutifolia* *Senna bicapsularis (L.) Roxb. var. bicapsularis (Fl. Ind., ed. 1832, 2: 342. 1832.)*	Poisonous, abortive	Old World New World
Siguaraya	*Trichilia glabra L.*	Communication with the family members, baths for ward off the negative (spirits, spells)	C, CA
Tabacco	*Nicotiana tabacum*	Headache	New World
Tamarindo	*Tamarindus Indica*	Gallbladder, Stomach	Old World India
Toronjil	*Mentha citrata*		Exotic to Caribbean
Tuatua	*Jatropha gossypiifolia L.*	Blood purification, diarhea, Parasites, vomitive, Stomach, Diarea, vomitar depende como uno de la manera de arranas	C, CA, SA
Vencebatalla	*Unidentified*	Matrimonial problems	Unidentified
Vencedor	*Vitex agnus-castus L.*	Cough, Spiritual purification, to combat evil spirits	Exotic to Caribbean
Vervena	*Verbena domingensis* *Verbena officinalis*	Stomach, gastritis, constipation, antiinflamatory, baths for kids to protect the skin, digestion, kidneys, Baths de purification, to attrack good luck, matrimonial problems	Old and New World
Yaba	*Andira inermis*	To separate someone from own life path, protection of home	New World (CA, SA)
Yagruma	*Cecropia peltata L.*	Lungs, Uterus infections, catarrh, It has two faces, asking permit, spiritual cleansing, ward off the evil, to be placed behind the main door	C, SA, CA
Yamagua	*Guarea trichiloides L.*	Menstruation	
Yaya	*Oxandra lanceolata*	Wounds	Endemic to Greater Antilles
Yaya/salva hombre	*Oxandra lanceolata*	Prostate, Wounds, To reinforce something *e.g.* relation	C
Yerba de criollo	*Unidentified*	Parasites	Unidentified
Yerbaluisa	*Aloysia triphylla*	Stomach	SA
Yopuedomásquetu	*Unidentified*	Spiritual purification	Unidentified
Yucca	*Manihot esculenta*	Tea from leaves alleviates the pain caused by stone (not specified if kidneys, bladder etc.), sores	Caribbean, native to SA

Table 7 (continued) Medicinal plants Jiguaní.

This overview of medicinal properties on plants from Jiguaní was based on the information provided by following contributors: Manuela de Oro Dieüz, Lino Castillo Cubillo, Juana Figuerero Capote, Orestes Iganacio Zalazar Gonzáles. The interview with Harvin Ramírez Reyes was not included because even if he grow up as espiritista, he was trained in Regla de Ocha. As this religion has not so much tradition in this location we have focused only on the information provided by the previous contributors.

Common name	Latin name	Use	Origin
Alamo		Good luck	
Anamú	*Petiveria alliacea* L.	To ward off malecious spirit	New World
Ajonjoli	*Sesamum orientale* L.		Old World
Anica	*Critonia aromatisans check*		New World
Albehaca morada	*Ocimum tenuiflorum* L.	Good luck, to Ward of negative energy	Old World (native: Asia to N. Australia)
Albehaca	*Albehaca cimarona Ocimum campechianum Mill.* *Albehaca blanca Ocimum basilicum L.*		Cimarona New World Blanca Old World
Apasote	*Chenopodium ambrosioides* L.	Parasites	South America and Old World
Azahar	*la flor de limon y naranja*	wellbeing, baths for good luck	Old World
Artemisa	*Ambrosia paniculata* *Cimarona= A. domingensis Urb.* *Artemisia abs.= Altamisa blanca* *Gnaphalium domingense Lam.*	To Ward off the malicious spirit	Cimarona New World Absinthum North America native
Bruca hembra	*Senna obtusifolia*		New World
Bayahonda	*Prosopis juliflora* *Vachellia farnesiana (L.)* *b. blanca* *Parkinsonia aculeata*	For the Cross	New World Old World + New World New World
Cañafistola	*Cassia fistula L.*	Stomache, Refreshment of body	Old World
Flor de Jericó -	*Anastatica hierochuntica*	Protection, Good luck	Old World
Cundiamor	*Momordica charantia* L.	Abortive	Old World
Guandule	*Cajanus cajan*		Old World Africa
Guano	*Coccothrinax barbadensis* *Coccothrinax boschiana* *Coccothrinax argentea*	Against malicious spirits	New World Boschiana endemic Native West Indies
Limón		Baths for good luck	
Maíz		Offerings	New World
Maní	*Arachis hypogaea L.*	Offerings	New World
Mamey	*Mammea Americana L.*	A spell against other peoples, for bath curing eczema	New World
Mejorana	*Origanum majorana* [A]		Old World
Mostaza	*Brassica juncea* (L.)	Against witches	Old World
Moringa, flor de libertad	*Moringa oleifera* Lam.	To attract good luck	Old World
Naranja	*Cistrus sp.*	Wellbeing, baths for good luck	
Pachulí	*Vetiveria zizanioides* (L.)	Baths for good luck, economic prosperity	Old World
Palode pejo, Palode pez	*Picramnia pentandra* Sw.,	For spiritual protection	New World

Table 8 A brief overview of ritual plants used in various Dominican locations.
[A] *In Cuba could be also Croton bispinosus C.*

Common name	Latin name	Use	Origin
Valeriana	*Valeriana sp.*	Roots used for dreaming, for insomnia	Old World/diff. variant New World
Romero	*Rosmarinus officinalis*	Good luck, purification	Old World
Rompezaraüey	*Eupatorium odoratum L*	To remove bad luck from home and business, boiled in water and mixed with lime Stone, and salt is used to wipe out the house	
Ruda	*Ruta graveolens*	Against courses, evil eye, against black magic	Old World
Verbena	*Glandularia hybrida* *Bouchea prismatica* (L.) *Stachytarpheta jamaicensis* *Verbena officinalis*		
Vencedor	*Vitex agnus-castus L.*		
Toronjín		Good luck	
Tobacco		To call lwas, offering	New World
Verbena	*Glandularia hybrida* *Bouchea prismatica* (L.) *Stachytarpheta jamaicensis* *Verbena officinalis*		New World West Indies West Indies Old World
Sábila	*Aloe vera* (L.)	Protect the house from malecious spirits	Old World
Yerba luisa	*Aloysia citriodora*		New World
Sangre de Cristo	*Columnea sanguinea* *Verbesina alata* *Hibiscus rosa-sinensis*		New World New World Old World
Zanten		Estomago	

Table 8 (continued) A brief overview of ritual plants used in various Dominican locations.

Scientific name	Vernacular names and uses in Jiguaní and Boyá	Dominica
Annona spp.	*A. reticulata*: Mamón Agaist diarrhea *A.muricata: Guanabana* Fruits edible, As medicine for Indigestion, Flu, Blood pressure *A. Squamosa:* Stomach, Stomach, Indigestion	*A. reticulata*: Custard Apple, Bullock's Heart, Cachima, Cachima Coeur de Boeuf, alakáliua (m), kasíma (w). In a tea against fever. *A.muricata:* Soursop, Corossol, ualápana Beverages, a tea for gonorrhea, ritual tea, against diarrhea, fever, colds, or women in labor, leaves also used for bathes *A.squamosa:* Sweetsop, Sugar Apple, Pomme Canelle, kalíkiri: For a painful spleen
Bixa orellana L.	Bija, achiote Seasoning for dishes, as a charm to defend against enemies	Bíset Favoring meat or sauces, ritual bath
Capsicum frutescens	Ají Foodways. Medicinal for diabetis	Red Pepper, Piment, buémuē, ualéiri (m), áti (w) Alimentation as a relish and for seasoning sauces. For wounds and sores.
Cecropia peltata L.	Yagruma Lungs, Uterus infections, catarrh Spiritual cleansing, ward off the evil, to be placed behind the main door	Trumpet-Tree, Trumpet-Woo – Bois Canon. The leaves as a poultice to wounds and sores. The wood for light catamarans, known as «piperie».
Ceiba pentandra (L.)	Ceiba Misterio, Baths, Tootache (cotton), to Ward off malecious spell, all saints, offerings, vows to Virgen	Kapok, Silk Cotton Tree, Fromager, kumáka Canoes, boats, tubs, home of spirits, who would be angry if their house was disturbed. In period from March to May at which time it is believed the tree spirits are absent can be felled.
Chenopodium ambrosioides	Apazote Against parasites, collect, to ward off the evil energies, against evil eye	Wormseed, Semen Contra As a beverage, to deworm children. Leaves one of constituents of a ritual bath given to the mother after childbirth
Chiococca alba	Timacle Kidneys	Flowers for a tea as abortive
Crescenia cujete	Various kitchen utensils	Calebasse, matálu (m), uíra (w). As utensils Shamans' rattles, called sísira (w) or maláka (m), were also made from the calabash.
Ficus spp.	*Ficus carica* L. (Higo) Alamo Ficus religiosa L., Jagüey: medicinal Higo has misterio Alamo: To lose weight, for cleaning livers, dries out sores, baths for good luck	The larger spreading species of figuier are considered by Kalinagos to be the homes of the "tree-spirit"– and as with Ceiba pentandra and Mammea americana L. – these trees are never felled or otherwise disturbed for fear of making the spirit angry. Leaves of figuier are one of many ingredients (see Ipomoea pes-caprae) in a ritual bath given for any sickness caused by pyjai.
Genipa americana	Jagua Refreshment of blood	Edible fruits. Formerly the dark fruit stain for face decoration. Against yaws and skin disease
Gossypium spp.	Algodon morado, Flu, baths removing harmful spirits and spells	Cotton. – ikálotopue, māulu (m) (cf. Tupi amandiyu-b). For hammocks, head and leg bands, for mending clothes. Stuffing pillows and mattresses. A ritual bath, given to the mother after childbirth.
Gynerium sagittatum	Caña brava Has a misterio	Arrow, Wild Cane. – Roseau. – buléua (m) («arrow», «pierce»), mabúlu, mabúru
Jatropha spp.	Piñon One of components for treatment of smallpox To deworm, Against Stomache. This trees is believed to have misterio.	(J. gossypifolia: medecinier noir, J. curcas: medecinier) Seeds as purgative or as an emetic. A tea given as a cure for general sickness. A special purgative tea after child birth. This tea is brewed from: medecinier noir, leaves of balie doux (Scoparia dulcis), leaves of momben (Spondias mombin), sprigs of verveine (Stachytarpheta spp.), and ricinus oil (Ricinus communis).

Table 8 A brief comparison of plant use in Dominica and Jiguaní and Boyá.

Scientific name	Vernacular names and uses in Jiguaní and Boyá	Dominica
Manihot esculenta	Yucca Cassava bread, Leaves for kidneys, the porridge from its starch for skin rush Tea from leaves alleviates the pain caused by stone (not specified if kidneys, bladder etc.) and sores.	Cassava. – Manioc (Amer), Manioc Doux, Camanioc. – kiére (m), kāī (w) Bitter Manioc. iúbue (m), kamániā, kumánana – Sweet Manioc. For cassava bread and for a beer (uéku).
Momordica charantia L. (Old World)	Cundiamor, Cundeamor Cold, Baths, Smallpox, Stomach, parasites	Wild Balsam Apple. – Pomme Coolie, Pavecka. As a brew for childrens' colds.
Nicotiana tabacum	Tabaco Wounds, Stomach pain, headache, calling lwas	Tobacco, Tabac Pays. – iúli, iúri (w), itámāle (m). The smoke is blown on ailing infants for their wellbeing and streghts. Its juice is used as an emetic. Powdered tobacco was burnt as an offering to the «Maitre Tête-Chien» and other spirits. Its powder also consumed for leisure.
Ocimum spp.	Albahaca (vaca, morada) Headache, Pain, Diabetes, High blood pressure, Stress, Gastritis, Sweet baths against witchcraft	O. micranthum Various ritual baths, after childbirth, for unlucky canoes, for colds
Oxandra laurifolia (Sw.) Rich.	Yaya, Salva hombre Wounds, prostate	Bois Pian For the treatment of yaws («pians»).
Petiveria alliacea L	Anamú, Espante Muerto Catarrh, Colon Cancer, blood circulation, Toothache, To ward off malicious spirit	Kudjuruk. – émeruáiuma, lemúru. In a ritual bath taken at the time of the new moon. It is rubbed on the body as a protection against evil spells. Prepared as «tea» it is considered an antidote to poisoning, as well as an aid to women in childbirth.
Pimenta racemosa *(Mill.)*	Osua Flu, fever, tea in wake	Bay Tree, Bay Rum Tree. – Bois d'Inde, Black Cinnamon. – asúru, hasuru Its wood for «boucans» (barbecues), pestles for wooden mortars, crude singlepost presses for sugarcane, house-piles, forked posts for mwìna (primitive type native dwelling), and formerly also for war clubs. Its leaves and fruits for a tea drunk as a cure for colic and stomach ache, or in a shampoo for washing the hair or body.
Psidium guava	Guayaba Against diarrhea, stomach pain, and flu. The fruit is edible	Guava. – Gouyave, Goyave. – balíkasi, kuiábu (white variety), balúbui (m), ualíapa (w) (red variety). Against diarrhea or intestinal chill.
Sapindus saponaria L.	Mate negro Amulets for protection of children, as soap and beverage called prú	Soapberry, Soap Tree. – Bois Savonette. – túlisi (m), lúluru (w) Washing purposes. Its bark for soap and to stop dysentery
Stachytarpheta spp.	*S. jamaicensis: Verbena* Indigestion, baths	S. cayennensis and S. jamaicensis Verveine. – kuiékuiéti («slippery, slimy»), kuríbīū ákuani («birdbath» or «twist-bath»). A tea from verveine in ritual bathing (for undoing spells, etc.), for colds, and in fact for «any illness». A purgative tea that is given after childbirth.

Table 8 (continued) A brief comparison of plant use in Dominica and Jiguaní and Boyá.

The information on the plant use on Dominica has been retrieved from Hodge and Taylor (1957).

Abstract

Indigenous Ancestors and Healing Landscapes: Cultural Memory and Intercultural Communication in the Dominican Republic and Cuba

The research and its objectives

Until recently, only a few studies have investigated in depth the impact of the European colonization on the indigenous populations of the Caribbean. The aim of the Nexus 1492 project is to bring new insights into the histories and legacies of the indigenous Caribbean across the historical divide created by European colonization and the ensuing complex intercultural dynamics over the past five centuries. Within Nexus 1492, the subproject Landscape Transformations, this study focuses on current healing practices in relation to European colonization and the profound demographic changes that have taken place. More specifically, this research examines current Dominican and Cuban healing landscapes from a cultural memory perspective.

The main problem that informs this research is: how do healing landscapes encapsulate cultural memories of the indigenous past? In order to gather a better understanding of the contemporary healing landscapes, this study offers insights into how contemporary medicinal cultures have been historically constructed. Fieldwork was carried out in order to explore how community members relate some landscape features to the indigenous past and how these associations play a role in traditional healing practices. A further analysis of the historical and ethnographic data allows us to situate the concept of healing landscapes within current landscape theories.

By presenting data on current, non-institutional healing practices, this study highlights their continuous importance and recognizes their significant value as a part of Caribbean heritage. This research draw attention to the need to include contemporary local epistemologies as an important departure point for inclusive medicinal histories.

In combination with other projects within Nexus 1492, this investigation provides glimpses into results of landscape transformations in the Caribbean after the European conquest, and by this means it hopes to contribute to the deconstruction of colonial discourse about the past. More specifically, the collected data on healing landscapes offer a contrast to the prevalent representations of present-day Caribbean societies in terms of uprooted hybridity or impurity, and as being too fragmented (among others by colonization) to have any spiritual relation with local landscapes.

Theoretical and methodological perspective

By combining data from ethnographic fieldwork and critical historical analysis, this thesis explores the contemporary character of the healing landscapes and their historical background. Concretely, it follows the recommendations of previous studies to examine the relation of medicinal practices with indigenous ancestors. Before discussing the medicinal history as well as the ideas, narratives and cultural practices that are presented in the second part of this dissertation, it was necessary to reflect upon the origins of the historical genesis of representation of the indigenous peoples of the Dominican Republic and Cuba through the lenses of colonial authors.

A review of the primary and secondary historical sources focused on cultural and religious transformations and their role in the medicinal histories of the region. This concerned documents relating to colonial history of the indigenous peoples on both islands after the encomienda period. This review was further situated within the broader demographic history of the region and local histories of sites where the fieldwork was conducted.

The main corpus of knowledge originates from ethnographic fieldwork, interactions with local experts and mentors in the field. This data collection in the field focused on healing landscapes that were defined as agents that were said to promote physical, mental, and spiritual health. Following this definition this study has collected many examples of the human interaction with divine and ancestral beings residing or manifested in places, vegetation, and natural features. The concept healing landscape integrates insights from previous botanical and anthropological studies with landscape theories and fieldwork data on present-day healing practices.

The memory approach was motivated by the popular ideas about contemporary healing practices as being indigenous heritage. These ideas seemed to contradict the widely accepted narratives about the national history wherein indigenous ancestors did not survive the European conquest and colonization. The concept of 'cultural memory' helped this study reflect upon how people engage with the past through healing practices, and how these practices in turn are continuations and/or reinterpretations of past beliefs, knowledge and customs. Previous memory studies offered us broader insights into the power dynamics, particularly their influence on people's perception and engagement with the past. This approach allowed us to consider the emic vision of the past as an integral part of the context and mechanism of transmitting medicinal cultures. The combination of landscape and memory studies allowed us to contextualize the ideas about spacialization of memory as an integral part of people becoming reflexive of their own past within the Caribbean context.

Main results

The history of healing landscapes has developed within a profound landscape transformation, including material and conceptual aspects. The colonization of the landscape implied large scale expropriation of lands and natural resources, spiritual conquest, and profound loss of ancestral medicinal cultures and knowledge. The colonization of Hispaniola and Cuba triggered also introduction of new religions and cultural synergy of medicinal cultures, while part of indigenous botanical knowledge was circulated through the world. Various authors (Pané, Fernandez de Oviedo, Monardes, Mendéz Nieto, Breton, Sloane, Górdon y de Acosta) provide information about the indigenous co-authorship of the biography of healing landscapes. The indigenous healer and carriers of the knowledge were longer active then previously argued. Simultenously, the circulation of medicinal knowledge was marked by high intra and interregional mobility of the carriers of this knowledge. The healers from across the Atlantic Ocean and even from the American mainland equally contributed to the rich current medicinal practices.

The overview of the demographic and medicinal histories of Hispaniola and Cuba suggest that Ortiz' hypothesis of the failed indigenous transculturation needs to be revised. Some registers kept brief references about the long-continued presence and social integration of the indigenous descendants in several urban and rural settlements in both study regions during the colonial period. Without doubts, the ancestors of originally non-Caribbean background numerically outweighed the numbers of indigenous descendants. The question about the indigenous contribution to the transculturation process of medicinal cultures remains open. The colonial emphasis on race should not blind us to the multiple ways in which indigenous descendants were able to maintain distinct ethnic identities, continue medicinal cultures and transfer their knowledge and culture to the next generations.

Part II, which comprises chapters 6 through 9, presents some facets of the present-day healing landscapes, including landscape symbolism that emerges from the significance of natural resources in daily life, agricultural, ritual time and the liminal life period of diseases.

Landscapes hold great importance in individual health and wellbeing as well as for communal quality of life. The realm of ecological knowledge in the domain of foodways, crafts, and agriculture also reflects cultural and linguistic continuities and changes in the use of flora from the time of the ancestors. The collective prayers, the use of the lunar calendar and other customs securing the harvest or invoking rain were among the discussed examples.

Among the most important actors that promote physical, mental and spiritual health are healers, ritual specialist and spiritual mediums that act as mediators between the visible and invisible worlds. Healers, ritual specialists and devotees interact with various landscape features in order to improve their health and wellbeing. Various examples from 21 Division, Roman Catholicism, Regla de Ocha and Spiritism of Cord show how Dominican and Cuban landscapes are charged with rich symbolism and values which are often activated during healing practices. The diagnosis and remedies are sought through careful application of plants, interactions with divine, spiritual, and ancestral beings that are invoked at home altars, but also at natural shrines, or manifested in different natural elements.

The religious life and healing practices at various caverns and bodies of water tell about the more or less conscious ways of remembering the indigenous ancestors. The invocation of the indigenous ancestors within the present-day Cuban and Dominican religions shows how contemporary communities in their own terms reconnect to the surrounding landscapes and locate themselves within their past. The selection of these places and their symbolism offer a contrast with historical descriptions; others suggest continuities and discontinuities of ancestral practices of different origins. The multiple meaning of certain trees such as the silk-cotton tree, places like the Waterfall in Barajagua or the patronal celebration of Saint Francis in cave in Bánica are testimonies about the richness of the cultural heritage of these communities. Also, many other examples show us how new meanings of places and flora were created in conjunction with the memory of the indigenous predecessors.

The journey seeking information on healing practices in the context of the Greater Antilles in terms of continuities of particular ancestral worldviews is highly complex and without definitive conclusions. This discussion offers us points of reflection about the importance of recognition of subaltern ancestral voices in medicinal histories. Following Ortiz's metaphor of the counterpoint this study concludes that cultural memory can serve as one of two sides of the counterpoint by creating a contrast to the bias inherent in colonial archives. Needless to say, this memory is, to a certain degree, carries imprints of the five hundred yeards of cultural hegemony. The fragmentation of the memory by conquest, colonization, and forced assimilation together with the profound demographic and cultural changes have created obstacles to reconstruct the histories of those ancestors that have been historically marginalized.

Cuban and Dominican medicinal histories tell about devastation, diseases, deaths and appropriation of the natural resources and knowledge. At the same time, together with the information retrieved from present-day healing landscapes, these are also testimonies of survival, creativity, resilience and capacity to heal, and find unity in dehumanizing and alienating atmospheres of violence and exploitation. The contemporary healing landscapes are also testimonies of multidirectional exchanges of peoples, their worldviews, illnesses and remedies. The current medicinal practices show how Cuban and Dominican ancestors improvised and learned in new unknown environments, passed on ecological insights often articulated in a set of cultural practices and teachings to the next generations.

Future directions

Healing traditions still constitute an important part of medicinal cultures (even those in the Diaspora) and are combined/integrated with institutional medicine. More systematic and interdisciplinary studies combining phytochemical, pharmacological evaluation of herbal medicine, the dispensing practices, dosage in combination with other herbs and medicine are necessary to secure the wellbeing of the population. The existing medicinal cultures, which are complex and manifest in various ways, deserve more attention from an emic perspective, which often benefits from long term observations and learning.

Future studies on medicinal histories will be able to create inclusive histories, including the history of healing traditions of historically marginalized peoples. Despite their biased nature, the colonial sources are often the only references to the medicinal practices of enslaved population and indigenous descendants. Likewise an analysis of components of the organic residues of the pharmaceutical containers as encountered at sites such as the convent in La Vega Vieja are likely to create valuable data for medicinal histories. In combination with historical inventories about the medicines these are likely to inform us also about the incorporation of the native and exotic remedies within these settings.

The rich oral traditions presented here provide valuable historical information and invite further studies to consider their value in the historiographies. The spatial character of remembering, combined with various cognitions of time, are important starting points for studies and policies aiming at understanding and securing the preservation of tangible and intangible heritage.

The quality of any future systematic study of religiously important sites and ancestral places such as caverns relies upon the respectful inclusion of the spiritual leaders and local mentors in the field. The future research including archeological excavations of spiritual important ancestral sites needs to respect the rights of the communities to co-design and co-direct investigations as a part of their Free, Prior and Informed Consent.

Resumen

Ancestros indígenas y paisajes curativos: Memoria cultural y comunicación intercultural en la República Dominicana y Cuba

La investigación y sus objetivos

Hasta poco, sólo unos cuantos estudios han investigado en profundidad el impacto de la colonización europea sobre las poblaciones indígenas en el Caribe. El objetivo del proyecto Nexus 1492 es aportar nuevos conocimientos sobre las historias y los legados del Caribe indígena a través de la división histórica creada por la colonización europea y las complejas dinámicas interculturales de los últimos cinco siglos. Dentro de Nexus 1492, el subproyecto Transformaciones del Paisaje se centra en las prácticas actuales de sanación en relación con la colonización europea y los profundos cambios demográficos que han tenido lugar. Más específicamente, esta investigación examina los paisajes curativos dominicanos y cubanos actuales desde la perspectiva de la memoria cultural.

El principal problema que informa esta investigación es: ¿cómo encapsulan los paisajes curativos las memorias culturales del pasado indígena? Con el fin de obtener una mejor comprensión de los paisajes curativos contemporáneos, este estudio ofrece una visión de cómo se han construido históricamente las culturas medicinales contemporáneas. Se llevó a cabo un trabajo de campo para explorar cómo los miembros de la comunidad relacionan algunas características del paisaje con el pasado indígena y cómo estas asociaciones juegan un papel en las prácticas curativas tradicionales. Un análisis más profundo de los datos históricos y etnográficos nos permite situar el concepto de paisajes curativos dentro de las teorías actuales del paisaje.

Al presentar datos sobre las prácticas actuales de sanación no institucionales, este estudio destaca su importancia continua y reconoce su valor significativo como parte del patrimonio caribeño. Esta investigación llama la atención sobre la necesidad de incluir las epistemologías locales contemporáneas como un punto de partida importante para las historias medicinales inclusivas.

En combinación con otros proyectos dentro de Nexus 1492, esta investigación proporciona vislumbres de los resultados de las transformaciones del paisaje en el Caribe después de la conquista europea, y por este medio espera contribuir a la deconstrucción del discurso colonial sobre el pasado. Más específicamente, los datos recopilados sobre paisajes de curación ofrecen un contraste con las representaciones predominantes de las sociedades caribeñas actuales en términos de hibridez o impureza desarraigadas, y por estar demasiado fragmentadas (entre otras cosas por la colonización) para tener alguna relación espiritual con los paisajes locales.

Perspectiva teórica y metodológica

Combinando datos del trabajo de campo etnográfico y del análisis histórico crítico, esta tesis explora el carácter contemporáneo de los paisajes de curación y sus antecedentes históricos. Concretamente, sigue las recomendaciones de estudios anteriores para examinar la relación de las prácticas medicinales con los antepasados indígenas. Antes de discutir la historia de la medicina, así como las ideas, narraciones y prácticas culturales que se presentan en la segunda parte de esta disertación, era necesario reflexionar sobre los orígenes de la génesis histórica de la representación de los pueblos indígenas de la República Dominicana y Cuba a través de los lentes de los autores coloniales.

Una revisión de las fuentes históricas primarias y secundarias se centró en las transformaciones culturales y religiosas y su papel en las historias medicinales de la región. Se trataba de documentos relativos a la historia colonial de los pueblos indígenas de ambas islas tras el período de la encomienda. Esta revisión se situó además dentro de la historia demográfica más amplia de la región y de las historias locales de los sitios donde se llevó a cabo el trabajo de campo.

El principal corpus de conocimiento se origina del trabajo etnográfico de campo, las interacciones con expertos locales y los mentores en el campo. Esta recolección de datos en el campo se centró en paisajes curativos que fueron definidos como agentes que promueven la salud física, mental y espiritual. Siguiendo esta definición, este estudio ha recopilado muchos ejemplos de la interacción humana con seres divinos y ancestrales que residen o se manifiestan en lugares, en la vegetación y rasgos naturales. El concepto de paisaje curativo integra los conocimientos de estudios botánicos y antropológicos anteriores con teorías del paisaje y datos de trabajo de campo sobre las prácticas de curación actuales.

El enfoque de la memoria fue motivado por las ideas populares sobre que las prácticas curativas contemporáneas son patrimonio indígena. Estas ideas parecían contradecir las narrativas ampliamente aceptadas sobre la historia nacional, en la que los antepasados indígenas no sobrevivieron a la conquista y colonización europea. El concepto de "memoria cultural" ayudó a este estudio a reflexionar sobre cómo las personas se relacionan con el pasado a través de las prácticas de sanación, y cómo estas prácticas son a su vez continuaciones y/o reinterpretaciones de creencias, conocimientos y costumbres del pasado. Estudios anteriores sobre la memoria nos ofrecieron una visión más amplia de la dinámica del poder, en particular su influencia en la percepción de las personas y su compromiso con el pasado. Este enfoque nos permitió considerar la visión emic del pasado como parte integral del contexto y mecanismo de transmisión de las culturas medicinales. La combinación de estudios sobre el paisaje y la memoria nos permitió contextualizar las ideas sobre la espacialización de la memoria como parte integral de las personas, convirtiéndose en un reflejo de su propio pasado dentro del contexto caribeño.

Resultados principales

La historia de los paisajes curativos se ha desarrollado dentro de una profunda transformación del paisaje, incluyendo aspectos materiales y conceptuales. La colonización del paisaje implicó la expropiación a gran escala de tierras y recursos naturales, la conquista espiritual y la pérdida profunda de culturas y conocimientos medicinales ancestrales. La colonización de la Española y Cuba desencadenó también la introducción de nuevas religiones y la sinergia cultural de las culturas medicinales, mientras que parte del conocimiento botánico indígena circuló por el mundo. Varios autores (Pané, Fernández de Oviedo, Monardes, Mendéz Nieto, Bretón, Sloane, Górdon y de Acosta) ofrecen información sobre la coautoría indígena de la biografía de paisajes curativos. El curandero indígena y los portadores del conocimiento estuvieron más tiempo activos que anteriormente argumentado. Simultáneamente, la circulación de los conocimientos médicos se caracterizó por una elevada movilidad intra e interregional de los portadores de estos conocimientos. Los curanderos del otro lado del océano Atlántico e incluso del continente americano contribuyeron igualmente a las ricas prácticas medicinales actuales.

La visión general de las historias demográficas y medicinales de La Española y Cuba sugiere que la hipótesis de Ortiz sobre la transculturación indígena fallida necesita ser revisada. Algunos registros guardaban breves referencias sobre la presencia y la integración social de los descendientes indígenas en varios asentamientos urbanos y rurales de ambas regiones de estudio durante el período colonial. Sin duda, los antepasados de origen no caribeño superaban numéricamente el número de descendientes indígenas. La cuestión de la contribución indígena al proceso de transculturación de las culturas medicinales sigue abierta. El énfasis colonial en la raza no debe hacernos perder de vista las múltiples formas en que los descendientes de los indígenas fueron capaces de mantener las distintas identidades étnicas, continuar con las culturas medicinales y transferir sus conocimientos y cultura a las próximas generaciones.

La Parte II, que comprende los capítulos 6 al 9, presenta algunas facetas de los paisajes curativos actuales, incluyendo el simbolismo del paisaje que surge de la importancia de los recursos naturales en la vida diaria, la agricultura, el tiempo de los rituales y el período de la vida liminal de las enfermedades.

Los paisajes tienen una gran importancia para la salud y el bienestar individual, así como para la calidad de vida comunitaria. El ámbito del conocimiento ecológico en el ámbito de la alimentación, la artesanía y la agricultura también refleja las continuidades culturales y lingüísticas, y los cambios en el uso de la flora desde la época de los antepasados. Las oraciones colectivas, el uso del calendario lunar y otras costumbres que aseguran la cosecha o la invocación de la lluvia, fueron algunos de los ejemplos discutidos.

Entre los actores más importantes que promueven la salud física, mental y espiritual se encuentran los curanderos, los especialistas rituales y los médiums que actúan como mediadores entre el mundo visible y el invisible. Los curanderos, especialistas rituales y devotos interactúan con diversos elementos del paisaje para mejorar su salud y bienestar. Varios ejemplos de la División 21, el Catolicismo Romano, la Regla de Ocha y el Espiritismo de Cordón muestran cómo los paisajes dominicanos y cubanos están cargados de un rico simbolismo y valores que a menudo se activan durante las prácticas de sanación. El diagnóstico y los remedios se buscan a través de la aplicación cuidadosa de plantas, interacciones con seres divinos, espirituales y ancestrales que se invocan en los altares del hogar, pero también en los santuarios naturales, o que se manifiestan en diferentes elementos naturales.

La vida religiosa y las prácticas curativas en varias cavernas y cuerpos de agua hablan de las formas más o menos conscientes de recordar a los ancestros indígenas. La invocación de los antepasados indígenas dentro de las religiones cubanas y dominicanas actuales muestra cómo las comunidades contemporáneas, en sus propios términos, se reconectan con los paisajes circundantes y se sitúan dentro de su pasado. La selección de estos lugares y su simbolismo ofrecen un contraste con las descripciones históricas; otros sugieren continuidades y discontinuidades de prácticas ancestrales de diferentes orígenes. El significado múltiple de algunos árboles como la ceiba, lugares como la El Saltadero de Barajagua o la fiesta patronal de San Francisco en la cueva de Bánica son testimonios de la riqueza del patrimonio cultural de estas comunidades. Además, muchos otros ejemplos nos muestran cómo se crearon nuevos significados de lugares y flora en conjunción con la memoria de los predecesores indígenas.

El viaje de búsqueda de información sobre las prácticas curativas en el contexto de las Antillas Mayores en términos de continuidad de visiones particulares del mundo ancestral es altamente complejo y sin conclusiones definitivas. Esta discusión nos ofrece puntos de reflexión sobre la importancia del reconocimiento de las voces ancestrales subalternas en las historias medicinales. Siguiendo la metáfora de Ortiz del contrapunto, este estudio concluye que la memoria cultural puede servir como uno de los dos lados del contrapunto al crear un contraste con el sesgo inherente a los archivos coloniales. No hace falta decir que esta memoria es, hasta cierto punto, portadora de huellas de los quinientos años de hegemonía cultural. La fragmentación de la memoria por conquista, colonización y asimilación forzada, junto con los profundos cambios demográficos y culturales, han creado obstáculos para reconstruir las historias de aquellos antepasados que han sido históricamente marginados.

Las historias de la medicina cubana y dominicana hablan de devastación, enfermedades, muertes y apropiación de los recursos naturales y el conocimiento. Al mismo tiempo, junto con la información recuperada de los paisajes curativos actuales, también son testimonios de supervivencia, creatividad, resistencia y capacidad de curar, y de encontrar unidad en atmósferas deshumanizadoras y alienantes de violencia y explotación. Los paisajes curativos contemporáneos son también testimonios de intercambios multidireccionales de pueblos, sus cosmovisiones, enfermedades y remedios. Las prácticas medicinales actuales muestran cómo los antepasados cubanos y dominicanos improvisaban y aprendían en nuevos entornos desconocidos, transmitiendo conocimientos ecológicos que a menudo se articulan en un conjunto de prácticas culturales y enseñanzas a las siguientes generaciones.

Orientaciones futuras

Las tradiciones curativas siguen siendo una parte importante de las culturas medicinales (incluso las de la diáspora) y se combinan/integran con la medicina institucional. Se necesitan estudios más sistemáticos e interdisciplinarios que combinen la evaluación fitoquímica y farmacológica de la medicina herbal, las prácticas de dispensación, la dosificación en combinación con otras hierbas y la medicina para asegurar el bienestar de la población. Las culturas medicinales existentes son complejas y se manifiestan de diversas maneras, merecen más atención desde una perspectiva emic, que a menudo se beneficia de las observaciones y el aprendizaje a largo plazo.

Los estudios futuros sobre las historias de los medicamentos podrán crear historias inclusivas, incluyendo la historia de las tradiciones curativas de los pueblos históricamente marginados. A pesar de su naturaleza sesgada, las fuentes coloniales son a menudo las únicas referencias a las prácticas medicinales de la población esclavizada y de los descendientes de indígenas. Asimismo, un análisis de los componentes de los residuos orgánicos de los envases farmacéuticos que se encuentran en sitios como el convento de La Vega Vieja y otros sitios, es probable que generen datos valiosos para las historias medicinales. En combinación con los inventarios históricos sobre los medicamentos, es probable que nos informen también sobre la incorporación de los remedios autóctonos y exóticos en estos entornos.

Las ricas tradiciones orales que se presentan aquí proporcionan valiosa información histórica e invitan a realizar estudios adicionales para considerar su valor en las historiografías. El carácter espacial de la memoria, combinado con las diversas cogniciones del tiempo, son puntos de partida importantes para los estudios y las políticas destinadas a comprender y garantizar la preservación del patrimonio material e inmaterial.

La calidad de cualquier estudio sistemático futuro de sitios de importancia religiosa y lugares ancestrales como las cavernas depende de la inclusión respetuosa de los líderes espirituales y mentores locales en el campo. La investigación futura, incluidas las excavaciones arqueológicas de sitios ancestrales de importancia espiritual, debe respetar el derecho de las comunidades a codiseñar y codirigir las investigaciones como parte de su consentimiento libre, previo e informado.

Samenvatting

Inheemse voorouders en helende landschappen. Cultureel geheugen en interculturele communicatie op de Dominicaanse Republiek en Cuba

Het onderzoek en zijn doelstellingen

Tot voor kort bestonden er slechts enkele studies waarin de impact van de Europese kolonisatie op de inheemse bevolking van het Caribisch gebied grondig is onderzocht. Het doel van het Nexus 1492 project is om nieuwe inzichten te brengen in de geschiedenissen en erfenissen van de inheems-Caribische bevolkingen van voor en tijdens de Europese kolonisatie en de daaruit voortvloeiende complexe interculturele dynamiek van de afgelopen vijf eeuwen. Als onderdeel van het subproject '*Veranderingen van Landschappen*' van het Nexus 1492 project, wordt er in deze studie geconcentreerd op bestaande genezingspraktijken in relatie tot de Europese kolonisatie en de gerelateerde demografische veranderingen. De huidige Dominicaanse en Cubaanse genezende landschappen zijn de meer specifieke onderwerpen van studie en worden bezien vanuit een perspectief van een cultureel geheugen.

De voornaamste probleemstelling die aan dit onderzoek ten grondslag ligt, luidt: hoe incorporeren genezende landschappen culturele herinneringen aan het inheemse verleden? Om een beter begrip van helende/genezende landschappen te kunnen bewerkstelligen, verschaft deze studie inzicht in de wijze waarop huidige medische culturen historisch geconstrueerd zijn. Er is etnografisch veldwerk uitgevoerd om te onderzoeken hoe leden van de gemeenschap kenmerken van het landschap in verband brengen met het inheemse verleden en op welke wijze deze culturele associaties een rol spelen in de traditionele genezingspraktijken. Een verdere analyse van de historische en etnografische gegevens stelt ons in staat het concept van genezende landschappen binnen huidige landschapstheorieën te situeren.

De gepresenteerde gegevens betreffende huidige non-institutionele genezingspraktijken benadrukken hun voortdurende belang en waarde als onderdeel van het Caribische erfgoed. In dit onderzoek wordt de aandacht gevestigd op de noodzaak hedendaagse lokale epistemologieën op te nemen als een belangrijk vertrekpunt voor meer inclusieve medicinale geschiedenissen.

Tezamen met andere projecten binnen Nexus 1492 verschaft dit onderzoek een blik op de resulterende landschapstransformaties in het Caribisch gebied na de Europese verovering, en hoopt zo bij te kunnen dragen aan de deconstructie van het koloniale discours over het verleden. Meer specifiek zijn het de verzamelde gegevens over genezende landschappen die een contrast vormen met de heersende beeldvorming over de huidige Caribische bevolkingen in termen van ontwortelde hybriditeit of onzuiverheid, en als te gefragmenteerd (onder andere door kolonisatie) om enig spirituele verband met lokale landschappen te kunnen hebben.

Theoretisch en methodologisch perspectief

Door het combineren van de data van het etnografische veldwerk en die van de kritische historische analyse, wordt in deze dissertatie het hedendaagse karakter van de helende landschappen en hun historische achtergrond verkend. Hiermee worden concrete aanbevelingen van eerdere studies opgevolgd om de relatie tussen medicinale praktijken en inheemse voorouders te onderzoeken. Voorafgaand aan het bespreken van de medicinale geschiedenis en de ideeën, verhalen en culturele praktijken in het tweede deel van dit proefschrift, werd het noodzakelijk geacht eerst de oorsprong van de historische beeldvorming aangaande de inheemse volkeren van de Dominicaanse Republiek en Cuba te bespreken.

Er volgt een overzicht van de primaire en secundaire historische bronnen over culturele en religieuze transformaties en hun rol in de medicinale geschiedenis van de regio. Het betreft hier documenten met betrekking tot de koloniale geschiedenis van de inheemse volkeren op beide eilanden na de encomienda-periode. Dit overzicht wordt vervolgens verder gesitueerd in het kader van de bredere demografische geschiedenis van de regio en in relatie tot de lokale geschiedenissen van de plaatsen waar het veldwerk is uitgevoerd.

De belangrijkste kennis is afkomstig van het etnografisch veldwerk, uitwisselingen met lokale experts en mentoren in het veld. Het verzamelen van gegevens uit het veld concentreerde zich op genezende landschappen die werden gedefinieerd als actoren die de fysieke, mentale en spirituele gezondheid zouden bevorderen. Aan de hand van deze definitie zijn er in deze studie vele voorbeelden verzameld van menselijke interactie met goddelijke en voorouderlijke wezens die verblijven ofwel zich manifesteren in plaatsen, vegetatie en natuurlijke landschapskenmerken. Het concept genezend landschap integreert inzichten uit eerdere botanische en antropologische studies met landschapstheorieën en veldwerkgegevens over hedendaagse genezingspraktijken.

De benadering vanuit het concept cultureel geheugen werd gemotiveerd door de populaire theorieën over hedendaagse genezingspraktijken als inheems erfgoed. Deze theorieën leken in tegenspraak met de algemeen aanvaarde verhalen vanuit de nationale geschiedenis, waarin inheemse voorouders de Europese verovering en kolonisatie niet zouden hebben overleefd. Het concept van het 'cultureel geheugen' heeft in deze studie geholpen te reflecteren op de manier waarop mensen met het verleden omgaan door middel van genezingspraktijken, en hoe deze praktijken op hun beurt voortzettingen en/of herinterpretaties zijn van vroegere overtuigingen, kennis en gewoonten. Eerdere cultuurgeheugen studies boden ons bredere inzichten in de machtsdynamiek, en in het bijzonder de invloed daarvan op de perceptie van mensen en hun betrokkenheid met het verleden. Deze benadering stelt ons in staat om de *emic* visie op het verleden te beschouwen als een integraal onderdeel van de context en het mechanisme van de overdracht van medicinale culturen. De combinatie van landschap en cultureelgeheugen studies stelt ons in staat om de ideeën over het belang van ruimtelijke aspecten van het geheugen te contextualiseren als een integraal onderdeel van het reflectief worden van mensen over hun eigen verleden in de Caribische context.

Belangrijkste resultaten

De geschiedenis van helende landschappen heeft zich ontwikkeld binnen een radicale transformatie van landschappen, zowel in materieel als conceptueel aspect. De kolonisatie van het landschap impliceerde grootschalige onteigening van land en natuurlijke bronnen, spirituele verovering en diepgaand verlies van voorouderlijke medicinale culturen en kennis. De kolonisatie van Hispaniola en Cuba leidde ook tot de introductie van nieuwe religies en culturele synergie van medicinale culturen, terwijl een deel van de inheemse botanische kennis over de hele wereld werd verspreid. Verschillende auteurs (Pané, Fernandez de Oviedo, Monardes, Mendéz Nieto, Breton, Sloane, Górdon y de Acosta) geven informatie over de inheemse co-auteurschap van de biografie van helende landschappen. De inheemse genezers en dragers van de kennis waren langer actief dan voorheen werd beredebeerd. Bovendien werd de circulatie van medicinale kennis gekenmerkt door een hoge intra- en interregionale mobiliteit van de dragers van deze kennis. De genezers van de andere kant van de Atlantische Oceaan en zelfs van het Amerikaanse vasteland droegen in gelijke mate bij aan de rijke huidige medicinale praktijken.

Het overzicht van de demografische en medicinale geschiedenis van Hispaniola en Cuba suggereert dat Ortiz's hypothese van de mislukte inheemse transculturatie moet worden herzien. Sommige registers bevatten korte referenties aan een langdurige aanwezigheid en sociale integratie van de inheemse nakomelingen tijdens de koloniale periode in verschillende stedelijke en landelijke nederzettingen in beide studiegebieden. De voorouders met de oorspronkelijk niet-Caribische achtergrond wogen numeriek ongetwijfeld zwaarder dan het aantal inheemse nazaten. De vraag naar de bijdrage van de inheemse bevolking aan het transculturatieproces van medicinale culturen blijft open. De koloniale nadruk op ras mag ons niet blind maken voor de vele manieren waarop inheemse afstammelingen in staat waren om verschillende etnische identiteiten te behouden, medicinale culturen voort te zetten en hun kennis en cultuur over te dragen aan de volgende generaties.

In Deel II, bestaand uit hoofdstukken 6 tot en met 9, worden enkele facetten van de huidige genezende landschappen gepresenteerd, waaronder landschapssymboliek welke voortkomt uit de betekenis van natuurlijke hulpbronnen in het dagelijks leven, de landbouw, rituele tijd en de liminale levensperiode van ziektes.

Landschappen zijn van groot belang voor de gezondheid en het welzijn van het individu alsook voor de gemeenschappelijke kwaliteit van leven. Het geheel van ecologische kennis op het gebied van praktijken omtrent voedsel, ambachten en landbouw weerspiegelt ook de culturele en taalkundige continuïteit en veranderingen in het gebruik van flora uit de tijd van de voorouders. De collectieve gebeden, het gebruik van de maankalender, het aanroepen van regen, zijn andere voorbeelden om de oogst veilig te stellen zijn enkele van de besproken voorbeelden.

Tot de belangrijkste actoren die de fysieke, mentale en spirituele gezondheid bevorderen behoren genezers, rituele specialisten en spirituele mediums die optreden als bemiddelaars tussen de zichtbare en onzichtbare werelden. Genezers, rituele specialisten en toegewijden interacteren met verschillende landschapselementen om gezondheid en welzijn te verbeteren. Verschillende voorbeelden uit de geloofsrichtigen van 21 Divisies, Rooms-katholicisme, Regla de Ocha en Espiritismo de Cordón laten zien hoe Dominicaanse en Cubaanse landschappen geladen zijn met rijke symboliek en waarden die vaak geactiveerd worden tijdens genezingspraktijken. De diagnoses en remedies worden gezocht door zorgvuldige toepassing van planten, interacties met goddelijke, spirituele en voorouderlijke wezens die aan huisaltaars worden aangeroepen, maar ook bij natuurlijke heiligdommen, of zich manifesteren in verschillende natuurlijke elementen.

Religieuze rituelen en genezingspraktijken die plaatsvinden in verschillende grotten en bij waterlichamen vertellen over de min of meer bewuste manieren waarop inheemse voorouders worden herinnerd. De aanroeping van de inheemse voorouders binnen de huidige Cubaanse en Dominicaanse religies laat zien hoe hedendaagse gemeenschappen zich op hun eigen termen opnieuw verbinden met de omringende landschappen en zich in hun verleden situeren. De selectie van deze plaatsen en hun symboliek bieden een contrast met historische beschrijvingen; anderen suggereren continuïteiten en discontinuïteiten met voorouderlijke praktijken van verschillende oorsprong. De veelzijdige betekenissen van bepaalde bomen zoals de kapokboom, plaatsen zoals de waterval in Barajagua of de patroonsfeesten van Sint Franciscus in de grot in Bánica, zijn de getuigenissen van de rijkdom van het cultureel erfgoed van deze gemeenschappen. Tevens laten vele andere voorbeelden zien hoe nieuwe betekenissen van plaatsen en flora werden gecreëerd in samenhang met de herinnering aan de inheemse voorgangers.

De zoektocht naar informatie over genezingspraktijken in de context van de Grote Antillen in termen van voortzettingen van bepaalde voorouderlijke wereldbeelden is zeer complex en zonder definitieve conclusies. De discussie erover biedt ons echter de gelegenheid om na te denken over het belang van de erkenning van subalterne voorouders in de medicinale geschiedenis. In navolging van Ortiz's metafoor van de '*contrapunto*' wordt er in deze studie geconcludeerd dat het culturele geheugen dient als een van de beide zijden van het contrapunt, contrast creërend met de vooringenomenheid die inherent is aan koloniale archieven. Het spreekt voor zich dat dit geheugen tot op zekere hoogte de sporen draagt van vijfhonderd jaar culturele hegemonie. De fragmentatie van het geheugen door verovering, kolonisatie en gedwongen assimilatie, samen met ingrijpende demografische en culturele veranderingen, hebben obstakels gecreëerd voor de herconstructie van de geschiedenis van die voorouders die historisch gemarginaliseerd zijn.

Cubaanse en Dominicaanse medicinale geschiedenissen vertellen over verwoesting, ziekten, sterfgevallen en toe-eigening van de natuurlijke bronnen en kennis. Samen met de informatie voorkomend uit de hedendaagse genezende landschappen zijn dat echter ook getuigenissen van overleving, creativiteit, veerkracht en het vermogen om te genezen en eenheid te vinden in mensonterende en vervreemdende atmosferen van geweld en uitbuiting. De hedendaagse genezende landschappen zijn ook getuigenissen van multi-directionele uitwisselingen van volkeren, hun wereldbeelden, ziekten en geneesmiddelen. De huidige medicinale praktijken laten zien hoe Cubaanse en Dominicaanse voorouders improviseerden en leerden in nieuwe onbekende omgevingen, en hoe zij ecologische inzichten, vaak verwoord in een set van culturele praktijken en leerstellingen, doorgaven aan de volgende generaties.

Toekomstige studies

Genezingstradities vormen nog steeds een belangrijk onderdeel van medicinale culturen (zelfs die in de diaspora) en worden gecombineerd met en/of geïntegreerd in de institutionele geneeskunde. Meer systematische en interdisciplinaire studies die de fytochemische en farmacologische evaluatie van de kruidengeneeskunde (de dosering in combinatie met andere kruiden en de geneeskunde) combineren, zijn noodzakelijk om het welzijn van de bevolking te waarborgen. De bestaande medicinale culturen die vaak complex zijn en zich op verschillende manieren manifesteren, verdienen meer aandacht vanuit een emic perspectief, welke vaak gebaat zijn bij lange periodes van observaties en leren.

Toekomstige studies over medicinale geschiedenissen zullen in staat zijn om inclusieve geschiedenissen te creëren, waarin ook de geschiedenis van genezingstradities van historisch gemarginaliseerde volkeren is inbegrepen. Ondanks hun bevooroordeelde aard zijn de koloniale bronnen vaak de enige verwijzingen naar de medicinale praktijken van de tot slaaf gemaakte bevolkingen en inheemse afstammelingen. Ook bijvoorbeeld een analyse van de bestanddelen van de organische resten van de farmaceutische containers, aangetroffen op vindplaatsen zoals het klooster in La Vega Vieja, heeft potentieel om een waardevolle contributie te leveren aan de medicinale geschiedenis. In combinatie met historische inventarissen over de geneesmiddelen zullen deze ons waarschijnlijk ook informeren over de integratie van de inheemse en exotische geneesmiddelen in deze omgevingen.

De rijke orale tradities die in deze studie worden gepresenteerd, bieden waardevolle historische informatie en nodigen uit tot verdere studies om hun waarde in de historiografieën te overwegen. Het ruimtelijke karakter van het herinneren, in combinatie met de verschillende concepten van de tijd, zijn belangrijke uitgangspunten voor studies en beleid gericht op het begrijpen en veiligstellen van het behoud van materieel en immaterieel erfgoed.

De kwaliteit van elke toekomstige systematische studie van belangrijke religieuze vindplaatsen, en voorouderlijke plaatsen zoals grotten, is afhankelijk van de respectvolle betrokkenheid van de spirituele leiders en lokale mentoren in het veld. Het toekomstige onderzoek, met inbegrip van archeologische opgravingen van spiritueel belangrijke voorouderlijke vindplaatsen, moet de rechten van de gemeenschappen om onderzoek mee vorm te geven en mee uit te voeren, respecteren als onderdeel van hun Vrije, Voorafgaande en Geïnformeerde Toestemming (FPIC).

Acknowledgments

Many people have influenced the journey that resulted in this manuscript. I am grateful to my supervisor Prof. Corinne Hofman for having given me the opportunity to participate in a project full of inspiring colleagues, teaching me about histories and cultures of the Caribbean and facilitating me the contact with the Caribbean scholars. Since the beginning of this project Dr. Jorge Ulloa Hung and Dr. Roberto Valcárcel took time to orient me in the great amount of the historical and existing archeological studies, and offered me crucial support in the preparation of and conduct of fieldworks. They not only provided me with feedback on this work but inspired me as a person. I am also grateful to have received the support of my colleague Dr. Jimmy Mans who especially in the first half of the trajectory offered me his guidance, and shaped my approach by providing me recommendations of seminal works. I owe a great debt of gratitude to Prof. Maarten Jansen for his patience, vital guidance, recommending me literature and including me in discussions and meetings of the department of the Heritage and rights of indigenous peoples. The work presented here would not be also possible without the caring support and inspiration of Aurora Jiménez Peréz, a scholar and defender of indigenous rights, who made me aware of persisting social struggles of the indigenous peoples throughout the world.

Special thanks and gratitude deserve those who accompanied me on my journeys in the Dominican Republic: Adrian Rivera, Roberto Torres, Richard Peña, and Abelito Gonzáles. This whole dissertation would never be possible without the kindness, patience and knowledge that many Cuban and Dominican contributors have shared with me. I opted for the term contributors as it better reflected the importance of their collaboration and participation. Various local mentors and specialists have trusted me, shared with me their wisdom about medicinal plants, their worldviews and traditions. The list of those to whom I am grateful is very long but to mention just a few, I would like to thank again my Dominican contributors: Giovanni Guzmán from Haina, J. A. (Toño) Arías Peláez, Glenys Tavarez, Arlene Alvarez, the family Torres especially Lucilo Torres Valdéz from La Luperona, José Sadí and Estela Pérez from Loma de Guayacanes, family Gonzáles from Loma Atravesada. Likewise I am grateful for the time and information provided by Mrs. Esperanza from Guananico, brothers Morillo Martínez from Caño Miguel, Mrs. Felicia Ulloa from la Trinchera, Eloi Cruz, Cundo, Bonilla, Mrs. Mayra Dominques from Villa Isabela, families Álvarez, González, and Mr. Álvarez from Chacuey. From the Valverde region conversations also with the following were very helpful: Clementio Olivo, Maria Tati, José Fermín Ramón, Ramón Nevera, Mamita

Rojas, Francisco Muñoz Fermiz, Antonio Almonte Cruz, Margarita Martínez, Juan Julio Castillo, Papito Polanco, Domingo Antonio Batista Costa, Ramón Díaz, Solillo Acosta, Cirillo Acerado Hernández, Francisco Basilillo, Ramon Díaz and Ciprín Cruz, Martin Nuesis, Maria Nomencía Flora, and Domingo Antonio Batista Costa. Various consults with healers such as Boby, Benito, Bololo, Dany, Dora, Dulce, Estela, Evita, Florinda, Flor, Juancito, Librado, Kukita, Mayra, Maribel, and Simona from Valverde region were important.

Similarly, many inhabitants of Bánica contributed in various way to this study. Among them were H. Gómez, L. De La Rosa Alcántara, Benjamin Alcántara, León Alcántara, Filomeno M. Alcántara, Hermania Alcántara, María García Alcántara, Carmela Alcántara, De La Rosa de Oro, Javier De Los Santos, Manuel M. Moreta De Los Santos, and Arturo Valenzuela from Pedro Santana. Among the inhabitants of Boyá my gratitude and best whishes go to: Dorotea Mejía, María Mejía, Juan Peña Valera, Héctor Zambrano, Felipe Ortiz from Naranjo, Ramona González Moreno. Several inhabitants of Boca de Mana shared with me their knowledge about fascinating local traditions; among these were: Julián De La Rosa, Juan Pablo Rosario Araujo, José Isabel Jiménez de Los Santos, Candelaria Bautista De La Rosa, Estefanía De La Rosa, and Mirella from Boca de Mana.

Throughout my fieldwork in Cuba I was accompanied by Julio Corbea Calzado, Hugo Armas, María Palmares, J. Yero Masdeu, Lourdes Perez Iglesias, Juan J. Guarch Rodriguez, Benedicto Paz, David Lester and Marcos Rodríguez Matamoros (R.I.P). The knowledge of Cuban contributors has also enriched the construction of this work. I would like to thank again my co-supervisors´ families and especially their spouses Idalmis Hernández and Jypsis Matos Mora for creating for me a stable temporal home. Various Jiguaniceros have contributed, particularly Celida Hernández Reyes, Harvin Ramírez Reyes, Santos Anayas Castillo, Jínez Sánchez, Alberto Pérez. I owe also gratitude to Caridad Rodríguez Cullel (R.I.P.), M. Sánchez González, L.R. Fout Cruz, D. M. Rodríguez Sánchez, T. Rodríguez González, J. M. Gutiérrez Parrón, F. Zaldívar Rojas, D. Rodríguez Morales from Fray Benito, J. Gutiérrez from Chorro de Maíta, R. Segura Hidalgo, C. Portelles, E. Avila Rojas, M. Alvárez Hernández from Barajagua, O. I. Zalazar Gonzáles, A. D. Campo Tarrago from Managuaco, Escalona Galán and his grandfather from Barajagua, family Los Zaldívar from Fray Benito, Jerónimo Santana,Torre Anguilera, José Corella Varona and Tomás Rodríguez Gonzáles from Gíbara. This dissertation was also not posible without the support of Cristian Martínez (Museo Del Hombre Dominicano) and Elena Guarch Rodríguez (CITMA). In short, I am very grateful to all people that I have met during my fieldwork have facilitated me important information or shaped the content of this study.

Many thanks also to Andy Ciofalo and Angus Martin who with great patience have edited the grammar of this manuscript. To Daniel Antonio Guarch Pérez, Jypsis Matos Mora, for helping me with the transcription of some interviews and to Simone Cassale for creating the maps displayed in this dissertation. I am also very grateful to my colleagues who provided me with constructive feedback during our review sessions and team support and in particular to Adrian Gomes and Sony Jean who commented on some of these chapters. I am thankful to my family, friends and Tashunka for their support and patience throughout my PhD trajectory.

Agradecimientos

Muchas personas han influido en el viaje que resultó en este manuscrito. Agradezco a mi supervisora, la profesora Corinne Hofman, por haberme dado la oportunidad de participar en un proyecto lleno de colegas inspiradores, enseñándome sobre las historias y culturas del Caribe y facilitándome el contacto con los estudiosos del Caribe. Desde el inicio de este proyecto el Dr. Jorge Ulloa Hung y el Dr. Roberto Valcárcel se tomaron el tiempo de orientarme en la gran cantidad de estudios históricos y arqueológicos existentes, y me ofrecieron un apoyo crucial en la preparación y realización de trabajos de campo. No sólo me dieron su opinión sobre este trabajo, sino que me inspiraron como persona. También estoy agradecido por haber recibido el apoyo de mi colega el Dr. Jimmy Mans, quien especialmente en la primera mitad de la trayectoria me ofreció su guía, y dio forma a mi enfoque proporcionándome recomendaciones de trabajos fundamentales. Tengo una gran deuda de gratitud con el Prof. Maarten Jansen por su paciencia, su guía vital, recomendándome literatura e incluyéndome en las discusiones y reuniones del departamento de Patrimonio y Derechos de los Pueblos Indígenas. El trabajo que aquí se presenta no sería posible sin el apoyo y la inspiración de Aurora Jiménez Pérez, estudiosa y defensora de los derechos de los indígenas, quien me hizo tomar conciencia de las persistentes luchas sociales de los pueblos indígenas en todo el mundo.

Especial agradecimiento y gratitud merecen quienes me acompañaron en mis viajes por la República Dominicana: Adrián Rivera, Roberto Torres, Richard Peña y Abelito Gonzáles. Toda esta disertación no sería posible sin la amabilidad, paciencia y conocimiento que muchos colaboradores cubanos y dominicanos han compartido conmigo. Opté por el término colaboradores porque reflejaba mejor la importancia de su colaboración y participación. Varios mentores y especialistas locales han confiado en mí, compartiendo conmigo su sabiduría sobre las plantas medicinales, sus cosmovisiones y tradiciones. La lista de aquellos a quienes estoy agradecido es muy larga, pero por mencionar sólo unos pocos, me gustaría agradecer nuevamente a mis colaboradores dominicanos: Giovanni Guzmán de Haina, J. A. (Toño) Arías Peláez, Glenys Tavarez, Arlene Alvarez, la familia Torres especialmente Lucilo Torres Valdéz de La Luperona, José Sadí y Estela Pérez de Loma de Guayacanes, familia Gonzáles de Loma Atravesada. Igualmente agradezco el tiempo y la información que me han brindado la Sra. Esperanza de Guananico, los hermanos Morillo Martínez de Caño Miguel, la Sra. Felicia Ulloa de la Trinchera, Eloi Cruz, Cundo, Bonilla, la Sra. Mayra Dominques de Villa Isabela, las familias Álvarez, González, y el Sr. Álvarez de Chacuey. Desde la región de Valverde las conversaciones también con los siguientes fueron de gran ayuda: Clementio Olivo, Maria Tati, José Fermín Ramón, Ramón Nevera, Mamita Rojas, Francisco Muñoz Fermiz, Antonio Almonte Cruz, Margarita Martínez, Juan Julio Castillo, Papito Polanco, Domingo Antonio Batista Costa, Ramón Díaz, Solillo Acosta, Cirillo Acerado Hernández, Francisco Basilillo, Ramón Díaz y Ciprín Cruz, Martín Nuesis, María Nomencía Flora y Domingo Antonio Batista Costa. Varias consultas con curanderos como Boby, Benito, Bololo, Dany, Dora, Dulce, Estela, Evita, Florinda, Florcito, Librado, Kukita, Mayra, Maribel y Simona de la región de Valverde fueron importantes.

De manera similar, muchos habitantes de Bánica contribuyeron de diversas maneras a este estudio. Entre ellos se encontraban H. Gómez, L. De La Rosa Alcántara,

Benjamín Alcántara, León Alcántara, Filomeno M. Alcántara, Hermania Alcántara, María García Alcántara, Carmela Alcántara, De La Rosa de Oro, Javier De Los Santos, Manuel M. Moreta De Los Santos, y Arturo Valenzuela de Pedro Santana. Entre los habitantes de Boyá mi gratitud y mis mejores deseos: Dorotea Mejía, María Mejía, Juan Peña Valera, Héctor Zambrano, Felipe Ortiz de Naranjo, Ramona González Moreno. Varios habitantes de Boca de Mana compartieron conmigo sus conocimientos sobre fascinantes tradiciones locales, entre ellas: Julián De La Rosa, Juan Pablo Rosario Araujo, José Isabel Jiménez de Los Santos, Candelaria Bautista De La Rosa, Estefanía De La Rosa, y Mirella de Boca de Mana.

A lo largo de mi trabajo de campo en Cuba me acompañaron Julio Corbea Calzado, Hugo Armas, María Palmares, J. Yero Masdeu, Lourdes Pérez Iglesias, Idalmiz Hernández, Juan J. Guarch Rodríguez, Benedicto Paz, David Lester y Marcos Rodríguez Matamoros (R.I.P). El conocimiento de los colaboradores cubanos también ha enriquecido la construcción de esta obra. Me gustaría agradecer de nuevo a mis familias co-supervisores y especialmente a sus cónyuges Idalmis Hernández y Jypsis Matos Mora por crear para mí un hogar temporalmente estable. Varios jiguaniceros han contribuido, en particular Celida Hernández Reyes, Harvin Ramírez Reyes, Santos Anayas Castillo, Jínez Sánchez, Alberto Pérez. También debo agradecer a Caridad Rodríguez Cullel (R.I.P.), M. Sánchez González, L.R. Fout Cruz, D. M. Rodríguez Sánchez, T. Rodríguez González, J. M. Gutiérrez Parrón, F. Zaldívar Rojas, D. Rodríguez Morales de Fray Benito, J. Gutiérrez de Chorro de Maíta, R. Segura Hidalgo, C. Portelles, E. Ávila Rojas, M. Alvárez Hernández de Barajagua, O. I. Zalazar Gonzáles, A. D. Campo Tarrago de Managuaco, Escalona Galán y su abuelo de Barajagua, familia Los Zaldívar de Fray Benito, Jerónimo Santana, Torre Anguilera, José Corella Varona y Tomás Rodríguez Gonzáles de Gíbara. Esta tesis tampoco fue posible sin el apoyo de Cristian Martínez (Museo del Hombre Dominicano) y Elena Guarch Rodríguez (CITMA). En resumen, estoy muy agradecida a todas las personas que he conocido durante mi trabajo de campo que me han facilitado información importante o han dado forma al contenido de este estudio.

Muchas gracias también a Andy Ciofalo y Angus Martin que con gran paciencia han editado la gramática de este manuscrito. A Daniel Antonio Guarch Pérez, Jypsis Matos Mora, por ayudarme con la transcripción de algunas entrevistas, a Simone Casale por crear los mapas que se muestran en esta disertación y a Giselle Schrils por traducir este resumen. También estoy muy agradecida a mis colegas que me proporcionaron comentarios constructivos durante nuestras sesiones de revisión y apoyo del equipo y, en particular, a Adrian Gomes y Sony Jean que comentaron algunos de estos capítulos. Agradezco a mi familia, amigos y Tashunka por su apoyo y paciencia a lo largo de mi trayectoria de doctorado.

Curriculum vitae

Jana Pešoutová was born in Český Brod, Czech Republic in 1987. After obtaining her bachelor's degree in applied linguistics at Palacký University in Olomouc in 2010, she moved to the Netherlands where she completed her Master in the Management of Cultural Diversity. Drawing on theories from social psychology, her master's thesis focused on the impact of the social exclusion and its relationship with extremism among the youth. From 2013 she carried out her doctoral research as a part of the 1492 Nexus project at Faculty of Archeology, Leiden University, The Netherlands.